Human and Organizational Dynamics in e-Health

Edited by

David C Bangert

Associate Professor
Department of Management
University of Hawaii

and

Robert Doktor

Chair and Professor
Department of Management
University of Hawaii

Assistant Editor

Michael Valdez

Research Assistant
Department of Management
University of Hawaii

Radcliffe Publishing
Oxford • Seattle

Radcliffe Publishing Ltd
18 Marcham Road
Abingdon
Oxon OX14 1AA
United Kingdom

www.radcliffe-oxford.com
Electronic catalogue and worldwide online ordering facility.

British Library Cataloguing in Publication Data

A catalogue record for this book is available from the British Library.

ISBN 1 85775 666 5

Typeset by Anne Joshua & Associates, Oxford
Printed and bound by TJ International Ltd, Padstow, Cornwall

26014157

Contents

The CD

- Human factors and the acceptance of telemedicine
  Marilyn J Field © 1996

  Based on a background paper drafted by John C Scott and Neal I Neuberger. This was located in Chapter 4: The policy context of telemedicine, in Field MJ (1996) *Telemedicine: a guide to assessing telecommunications in health care*. National Academy Press.

- Cultural constraints in management theories
  Geert Hofstede © 1993

- Will disruptive innovations cure health care?
  Clayton M Christensen, Richard Bohmer and John Kenagy © 2002

- Organizational innovation: the influence of individual, organizational, and contextual factors on hospital adoption of technological and administrative innovations
  John R Kimberly and Michael J Evanisko © 2001

- Quasi firms: strategic interorganizational forms in the health care industry
  Roice D Luke, James W Begun and Dennis D Pointer © 2001

- Examining the technology acceptance model using physician acceptance of telemedicine technology
  Paul J Hu, Patrick YK Chau, Olivia R Liu Sheng and Kar Yan Tam © 1999

- Organizational learning, diffusion of innovation and international collaboration in telemedicine
  David F Robinson, Grant T Savage and Kim Sydow Campbell © 2003

List of contributors

IH Monrad Aas PhD
Project Director
The Work Research Institute
Oslo
Norway
mon-a@online.no

Lynne P Baldwin PhD
Assistant Head (Teaching and Learning)
Centre for Health Informatics and Computing
Department of Information Systems and Computing
Brunel University
Uxbridge, Middlesex
United Kingdom
lynne.baldwin@brunel.ac.uk

David C Bangert
Associate Professor
Department of Management
University of Hawaii
Honolulu, HI
dbangert@hawaii.edu

Bobbye Berg RN, MSN, PNP
The University of Texas Medical Branch
Department of Pediatrics
Center for Restorative Care
Galveston, TX

David Bomba PhD
Lecturer
Centre for Health Service Development
University of Wollongong
Wollongong, NSW
Australia
bomba@uow.edu.au

Robert J Bulik PhD
Associate Professor
Director, Telemedicine Research; Center for Telehealth & Distance Education
Associate Director, Office of Educational Development

The University of Texas Medical Branch
Galveston, TX
rjbulik@utmb.edu

Kathleen K Bultman RN, MS
School of Nursing
Alverno College
Milwaukee, WI
kathleen.bultman@alverno.edu

Barbara R Chrispin PhD
Professor & Chairperson – Management
School of Business and Public Administration
California State University, Dominguez Hills
Carson, CA
bchrispin@soma.csudh.edu

Malcolm Clarke PhD
Lecturer and Director, MSc Telemedicine and eHealth
Centre for Health Informatics and Computing
Department of Information Systems and Computing
Brunel University
Uxbridge, Middlesex
United Kingdom
malcolm.clarke@brunel.ac.uk

Mikael Collan MSc
Turku Centre for Computer Science
IAMSR
Abo Akademi University
Finland
mikael.collan@abo.fi

Charles R Doarn MBA
Assistant Professor
Executive Director, MedITAC
Virginia Commonwealth University
Richmond, VA
crdoarn@hsc.vcu.edu

Robert Doktor
Director, PhD Program in International Management
Professor, Department of Management
University of Hawaii
Honolulu, HI
doktor@cba.hawaii.edu

Patty Ellison MSN, RN, CFNP
Assistant Professor
Stephen F Austin State University
Division of Nursing
Nacogdoches, TX

Christina Esperat RN, PhD, CSFNP
Professor and Associate Dean for Practice & Research
Texas Tech University Health Services Center
School of Nursing
Lubbock, TX
christina.esperat@ttuhsc.edu

Arthur D Fisk PhD
Professor
School of Psychology
Georgia Institute of Technology
Atlanta, GA
af7@prism.gatech.edu

Pamela G Forducey PhD
Director, Clinical Development
INTEGRIS Jim Thorpe Rehabilitation Hospital
Oklahoma City, OK
pam.forducey@integris-health.com

John Fulcher PhD
Professor
School of Information Technology and Computer Science
University of Wollongong
Wollongong, NSW
Australia
john@uow.edu.au

Alexia Green RN, PhD
Dean and Professor
Texas Tech University Health Services Center
School of Nursing
Lubbock, TX
alexia.green@ttuhsc.edu

Ville Harkke MSc
Turku Centre for Computer Science
IAMSR
Abo Akademi University
Finland
ville.harkke@abo.fi

Rosanne Harrigan EdD, APRN-Rx, FAAN
Associate Dean
University of Hawaii
John Burns School of Medicine
Honolulu, HI
harrigan@hawaii.edu

Peter Hu MS, CNE
Instructor and Director
Information Services and Integration
The Charles McC Mathias Jr National Study Center for Trauma and EMS
University of Maryland School of Medicine
Baltimore, MD
peter@anesthlab.ummc.umaryland.edu

Nancy Johnson MSN, APRN
Associate Professor
Chair, Nursing Division
UH Maui Community College
Kahului, HI
nancyjoh@hawaii.edu

Deborah K Justis RN, MSHA
Clinical Coordinator, Telemedicine
Virginia Commonwealth University Health System
Richmond, VA
sebastiandb@vcu.edu

James Katzenstein PhD
Professor of Management
School of Business and Public Administration
California State University, Dominguez Hills
Mission Viejo, CA
jimkatzenstein@compuserve.com

Kawaljeet Kaur PhD
Medical College of Wisconsin
Department of Internal Medicine
Milwaukee, WI
kawal@sbcglobal.net

David Lam MD
Adjunct Associate Professor and Faculty
The Charles McC Mathias Jr National Study Center for Trauma and EMS
University of Maryland School of Medicine
Baltimore, MD
lam@tatrc.org

Colin F Mackenzie MB, ChB, FRCA, FCCM
Professor and Director
The Charles McC Mathias Jr National Study Center for Trauma and EMS
Human Factors Research Group
Baltimore, MD
cmack003@umaryland.edu

Ronald C Merrell MD, FACS
Stuart McGuire Professor & Chairman
VCU Department of Surgery
Director – MedITAC
Richmond, VA
ronald.merrell@vcu.edu

Margreet B Michel-Verkerke PhD
Professor
Department of Technology and Management
University of Twente
Faculty BBT
Enschede
The Netherlands
m.b.michel@sms.utwente.nl

Steve Moser MD
Medical Director
Maui Memorial Medical Center
Wailuku, Maui, HI
smoser@hhsc.org

Timothy A Nichols MS
PhD Candidate
School of Psychology
Georgia Institute of Technology
Atlanta, GA
gte966q@mail.gatech.edu

Claudia Oglivie RN, MS
Program Director
The Charles McC Mathias Jr National Study Center for Trauma and EMS
University of Maryland School of Medicine
Baltimore, MD
oglivie@tatrc.org

Jean A Pezzoli PhD
UH Maui Community College
Kahului, Maui, HI
pezzoli@hawaii.edu

Thomas J Pfeil MD
Assistant Professor
Family Medicine – Galveston
University of Texas Medical Branch
Galveston, TX
tpfeil@utmb.edu

Jeanette D Rasche MSMI
Center for Total Access/US Army
Fort Gordon, GA
jeanette.rasche@se.amedd.army.mil

Sally S Robinson MD
QT Box Distinguished Professor, Pediatrics
Director, Division of Pediatric Inpatient Services and Children's Restorative Care
  Unit
Medical Director, Children's Hospital
The University of Texas Medical Branch
Department of Pediatrics
Center for Restorative Care
Galveston, TX
ssrobins@utmb.edu

Wendy A Rogers PhD
Professor
School of Psychology
Georgia Institute of Technology
Atlanta, GA
wr43@prism.gatech.edu

Cynthia Scheideman-Miller
MHA Director, Rural Telemedicine Project
INTEGRIS Health
Oklahoma City, OK
cynthia.scheideman-miller@integris-health.com

Roel W Schuring PhD
Professor
Department of Technology and Management
University of Twente
Faculty BBT
Enschede
The Netherlands
r.w.schuring@sms.utwente.nl

Deborah E Seale MA
Assistant Professor
Information and Communication Sciences
Southern Illinois University

School of Medicine
Springfield, IL
dseale@siumed.edu

Rufus G Sessions PhD
Chief Scientific Officer
Clinical Applications Division
Telemedicine and Advance Technology Research Center (TATRC)
Frederick, Maryland
Fort Derick, MD
sessions@tatrc.org

Lori Smith MSci
Clinical Development Manager
INTEGRIS Jim Thorpe Rehabilitation Hospital
Oklahoma City, OK
lori.smith@integris-health.com

Ton AM Spil PhD
Assistant Professor
Department of Technology and Management
University of Twente
Faculty BBT
Enschede
The Netherlands
a.a.m.spil@utwente.nl

CB Sridhar MD
Professor and Head Department of Medicine, Diabetes, Endocrinology
MVJ Medical College and Research Hospital
Bangalore
India
sridharcb@vsnl.net

Aideen J Stronge MS
PhD Candidate
School of Psychology
Georgia Institute of Technology
Atlanta, GA
gte968q@prism.gatech.edu

Deena Suresh MSc
Manager, Medical Services
Recon Healthcare Ltd
Basavanagudi, Bangalore
India
duttashri@vsnl.net

Glenda Walker RN, DSN
Director
Stephen F Austin State University
Division of Nursing
Nacogdoches, TX
glenda.walker@tamut.edu

Rita Webb MSN, APRN
Nurse Practitioner
Veterans Administration Clinic
Kahului, Maui, HI
rita.webb@med.va.gov

Sherry Wulff MA
Associate Professor
Professional Communication Department
Alverno College
Milwaukee, WI
sherry.wulff@alverno.edu

Yan Xiao PhD
Associate Professor and Director
Human Factors and Technology
Department of Anesthesiology
University of Maryland School of Medicine
Baltimore, MD
yxiao@umaryland.edu

Acknowledgement

Whenever we talk about 'our' book – this tome, which was seeded in a primary research effort examining telemedicine at Tripler Hospital in Hawaii eight years ago – the ownership inherent in 'our' extends to many. From conceptualization to realization, the process has been sustained by generous resources of all kinds: vision, experience, ideas, collaboration, partnership, time, language, friendship and support. Such resources cascaded abundantly in the development of this book to the editors, as well as to our valued contributors. To acknowledge a few:

Our abiding appreciation goes first to those who wrote the many thoughtful, focused, fluent articles in this text. It is only through their willingness, collegiality, time commitment and efforts to enhance state-of-the-art development of e-health that this book could emerge. They all worked very hard, indeed. All of the contributors to this book went through a two-stage review process. First drafts were reviewed by the editors, and revisions suggested. Second drafts were all subject to internal reviews, during which the contributors made suggestions to each of all the other authors in their section of the book. External reviews by subject-matter experts were organized by the editors when appropriate and feasible.

Resources also abounded from our academic colleagues at the University of Hawaii's College of Business Administration (CBA) and Medical School; thanks to CBA Interim Dean Jim Wills and his predecessor, Dean David McClain, for encouraging and supporting our research of management issues in e-health; thanks to Dean Edwin Cadman and his staff at the Medical School for supporting and facilitating our interdisciplinary studies.

With great respect, we also thank our colleagues at the US Army Medical Command, and TATRC in particular, for their willing collaboration, stalwart encouragement and their financial commitment to providing this valuable resource to the e-health community of practice. For going the extra mile, we appreciate the support efforts of Dr Rufus Sessions, Col Harrison Hassell, Col Ronald Poropatish, Cheryl Merritt and Jessica Kenyon, to name a few.

Last and not least we give thanks to our families for their understanding, comfort and allegiance during the four years from gestation to publication of this book. Special thanks to Leilani, Kristie and Sa'ili for understanding when Bob wasn't there; to Marianna for her encouragement and support of Michael; and to Linda for her life and career partnership with David and making his words understandable.

David C Bangert
Robert Doktor
Michael Valdez
Honolulu, HI
November 2004

We dedicate this work to Dr Rufus Sessions.

As an agent of change, he gave birth to the idea of this book and championed it with vigor and grace.

Dr Sessions' work and life made a difference to all of ours!

Introduction

Many Americans, now over 60 years of age, may think back nostalgically to the medical care we received as youths. Perhaps the memories are similar to Bob's: he recalls lying on the living room couch, bundled in soft blankets, in his lower-middle class home in the suburbs. When reporting a sore throat in the evening, his mother would say: 'No school for you tomorrow; I'm calling Dr Siegel!' In the morning, Mother would call the school principal's office at 7.30am, 'Bob is sick and will be absent from school today.' She'd call Dr Siegel at 8.30am, during his morning call hour. The doctor would answer the phone himself. Mother would explain the situation: temperature 103°, sore throat, can't swallow. Dr Siegel would say: 'I'll be there at 2.'

At 2.30pm Dr Siegel's Jaguar sedan would appear in Bob's driveway. With black bag in hand, Dr Siegel would walk up the steps, ring the doorbell and find Mother there to greet him at the front door. He looked for the patient while standing on tiptoes – for Dr Siegel was but 5'3". This same doctor had delivered Bob 11 years before at Memorial Hospital.

Mother would lead Dr Siegel to the sick bed. Out of the black bag came a thermometer and a stethoscope: 'Open wide,' he'd say, and in would go the thermometer. 'Take a deep breath and hold it' would be the warning as the cold steel of the stethoscope touched skin. He would feel Bob's neck for swelling. 'Open wider' echoed as that terrible wooden tongue depressor thrust toward the sore throat. A look at the thermometer: 'Looks like it might be strep so I'm going to give him a shot. Have him gargle with warm water and salt, and here is a prescription to get at the pharmacy,' he'd say while scribbling a prescription on a pad. 'Take one teaspoon every eight hours for seven days; Bobby should be better in 48 hours. If he still has a fever above 99 on Wednesday morning, please call me between 8 and 9am. If you want to, he can have up to two aspirins a day; one in the morning and one before bedtime.'

Dr Siegel would then collect his gear as Mother would scurry to the bedroom returning with cash in hand. She would give Dr Siegel $25. There was no insurance, no paperwork and no government red tape. He would put the money in his wallet and Mother would see him out.

As Bob watched the good doctor leave, pining for a ride in that baby blue Jaguar with the white leather seats, Mother would telephone Schmidt's Pharmacy, three blocks away. Mr Schmidt would send Ray, the delivery boy, on his bike, to the house with the prescription before 4pm. Ray would pick up the prescription paper and the $4.95 for the liquid. Mother gave Ray $5.25 – inclusive of a 30 cent tip!

All in all, the medical treatment cost $30.25 – not cheap! That two-bedroom, one-bath home, two years earlier, was purchased for $11 000. Money was tight. All in all, from the awareness of the illness to the medical advice spanned 19 hours, the initial set of likely needed medication came 21 hours after awareness. Bob was well and back to a normal routine 60 hours after initial awareness of illness.

That healthcare of 50 years ago was good! We were satisfied consumers! Dr Siegel was financially comfortable and Pharmacist Schmidt drove a Cadillac Eldorado. Ray thought $0.30 a good tip. Mr Schmidt was paying him $1.00 per hour. Ray already planned on becoming a doctor when he grew up. Life was good.

Things are different now. Consider a typical scenario in Hawaii 2004. Both of Leilani's parents are financially comfortable college teachers. Their house is big; it's on a golf course and only 200 meters from a beautiful beach.

Leilani reports a sore throat at 7pm. Mother says: 'I'll call Dr Sia in the morning.' His office is 13 miles away, downtown at Kapiolani Medical Center. As a participating doctor in the family's Blue Cross/Blue Shield medical plan, costs can be kept down. Lei's parents pay (with their employer) $575 per month for health insurance for the family of three. There are some non-participating pediatricians nearer the family home, but to go to them might add $200–300 to the bill. Dr Sia is considered one of the best around and Leilani's parents are happy he has room in his practice for her.

At 7.30am, Mother calls the school to say Leilani will be absent; she calls Dr Sia's office at 8.30. The recording states: 'Please leave your name and telephone number and a short message as to your problem. We will call you back as soon as we can.' At 9.45 the phone rings. Mother explains that Leilani complained of a sore throat and had a fever of 103° last evening. The lady calling says you cannot bring Leilani in right away because mornings are reserved for well-baby check-ups. She can try to fit Leilani in that afternoon – around 3pm.

Mother packs up 11-year-old Leilani at 2pm; the drive takes 45 minutes – traffic is normal. Arriving at the parking garage at 2.45, Mother takes a parking ticket from an automated machine and carefully puts it in her purse to avoid penalties of $15 to $20 for losing a ticket or not having it stamped. All the spaces on the first and second floor of the garage are reserved for doctors and staff and they all seem to be full of Mercedes. Between cars backing out, cars taking many moves to get into tight spaces and full parking spaces on all floors, it takes Mother 20 minutes to land a space on the ninth floor of the garage. It is now 3.05pm, so Mother rushes Leilani out of the car. They hurry to the garage elevator, for they are now late for their 3pm emergency appointment. The elevator is slow and stops many times on its way down. Getting on at floor 5 is a women carrying a baby and dragging a sick young boy (coughing and coughing and coughing). Mother and Leilani finally get out and rush down the hallway at 3.15. In all the waiting rooms along the way, patients are coughing and sneezing – it must be flu season.

Mother and Leilani finally reach the elevator to the medical offices! Pediatricians are all on the ninth floor. There is a large crowd at the elevator door area and lots more coughing! When the elevator finally arrives, Mother and child pile into a full elevator and a loud buzzing begins. Knowing that someone has to get out, an older gentleman with a cane smiles and departs. The elevator is again on the move, but stops at floors 2, 3, 4, 5, 6, 7 and finally 9. Out they go, down the hall, left and into Dr Sia's waiting room. It is now 3.25pm. The nurse looks at mother and child, looks at the clock, raises her eyes and clicks a note of disdain. Mother explains that they arrived at the medical center at 2.45 but parking was a problem. The nurse responds: 'Tell me about it. I have to park at a lot four blocks away. And they charge me $250 a year for that!'

The nurse tells Mother and child to take a seat. Mother takes a seat by the nurse's desk and directs Leilani to take the only other empty one across the room. One boy, the cougher from the garage elevator, is about her age. Mother took off work today, so she calls the office to be sure that her class 'Intro to Geography' will be 'covered' by a colleague. Her secretary says all is well, 'But stop by the university before 5pm to sign some papers for next year's book orders that are due today.' Because it is now only 3.35, Mother says 'Of course'; the university is only a 10-minute drive from the medical center.

Four o'clock comes and goes. At 4.45 the nurse finally calls Leilani's name and escorts them to a small room for the examination. A nurse takes Lei's temperature, blood pressure and asks questions of the problem. She makes notes on a form, and says: 'Dr is running a little late, make yourselves comfortable.'

At 5.15 Dr Sia appears – cheery as ever. 'Hi Leilani, what's up?' Lei tells of her sore throat. Dr Sia feels her throat and uses a wooden tongue depressor to press her tongue down. With a cotton swab, he takes a sample from the reddened area. 'OK Leilani, we will have to check this out – see if it is strep or a virus' he counsels. 'Lots of viruses going around. We should get the results back in two days. See the nurse and schedule a follow-up on Wednesday afternoon' the good Dr orders.

When Mother explains that Leilani had a high temperature the night before, Dr Sia suggests Tylenol for the fever. He explains that viruses are not affected by antibiotics – lab results are needed before prescriptions can be made. Giving antibiotics inappropriately could lead to resistant strains of bacteria. And that is a problem for all of us.

Mother reschedules for 4pm Wednesday. The lab will be ready by noon on Wednesday. Mother and Lei leave at 5.30 to find the exit to the parking garage backed up. Mother forgot to get the parking ticket stamped, so at 5.45, the parking attendant says: '$15 please'. With traffic in rush hour mode, an exhausted Mother and child get home at 7pm. Mother calls on an old family ritual and gives Leilani a cool bath to bring the fever down. One child's Tylenol, a bowl of soup and Lei is off to bed. Mother forgot the 5pm deadline to sign papers at her work. As a consequence, books for her class next semester will arrive 10 days after the class begins, causing all kinds of complaints from her students and from her department chair.

Leilani's condition seems worse on Tuesday morning, but after another cool bath, some soup and Tylenol, she is OK with a temperature of 102°. She was miserable on Tuesday night as were Mother and Father. Their little girl was sick and all they could do was provide love, a cool bath, soup and Tylenol. Mother now starts to cough as well. Thinking that she picked something up at the medical center, Mother cancels her class to stay with Leilani. Tuesday night Leilani wakes the family three times with coughing and pain from her throat. Father suggests the emergency room at 3am but Mother argues that it is better to wait. Getting some sleep and seeing Dr Sia on Wednesday seems like a wiser course of action. Mother attends to her emails at 2am: students are looking for clarification on their assignments due to the cancelled class. By 7am, now sick with 102° temperature herself, Mother goes to bed. Father calls to cancel his scheduled class and makes soup for Mother and child. They both get Tylenol as well. At 1pm on Wednesday afternoon Father and Leilani leave for Dr Sia's office. They arrive at the parking structure at 1.45. By 2pm they are in the waiting room. The nurse says they are early. At 2.30 Dr Sia returns from a late lunch. Leilani is called at 3pm – an hour before her 4pm appointment. Dr Sia's nurse takes her temperature and blood pressure before Dr Sia arrives at 3.15. 'You have strep, young lady' he says. 'Lab tests are positive. Do you have any allergies or bad reactions to any antibiotics?' Father says 'No' as Dr Sia writes a prescription. Father and child leave the office for the pharmacy on the first floor at 3.30. Behind a line of five at the pharmacy, their prescription is taken at 3.45. The clerk says the wait will be about 45 minutes. Father and child wait with a room full of coughing, nose-blowing, eye-rubbing people. Three babies are crying in their mother's arms. At 4pm Leilani's name is called. The payment required is $52, inclusive of the co-pay. Parking only cost $3 because the pharmacy stamped the ticket. At 4.30 Father and child set out in early rush hour to make the one hour drive home. Leilani takes the first dose of her medication at 5.31pm. It had been 70.5 hours from first awareness of illness to the initial medication. It would be another 48 hours until Leilani is feeling alright – a total of 118.5 hours of feeling ill. Of course, inappropriate distribution of antibiotics had been avoided. The family spent 9.5 hours of travel and waiting time at the doctor's office. Parking cost $18, in addition to the cost of $575 per month for health insurance, a $52 payment for pharmaceuticals, and Dr Sia's bill of $73 for two visits and lab tests. The family used gasoline and clogged the road at rush hours. Mother became ill and missed her classes for two days. Father was fine, but he too cancelled one of his classes. Healthcare was effective, but no consideration of time lost or the cascading effect of that lost time of patients and patient helpers was calculated into the systems efficiency model. All was modeled around the efficient use of the healthcare provider, staff and facility. This kind of care results in families who are unhappy consumers. Dr Sia knew the parents were upset and appeared to wish that this family would find another doctor. Mother would most likely follow the same path, the next day, which Leilani had traversed. Students of Mother and Father were inconvenienced. That night, father had a sore tickle in his throat. How would this medical scenario ever change?

Let's jump ahead to 2034 when Leilani's 11-year-old son comes down with a sore throat. It is 7pm when Colin's temperature is registered at 103°. Leilani and Dave live in a middle-class neighborhood, with a modest home purchased two years earlier. The home has a standard model Arrowsmith Telehealth Center located in an alcove in the eat-in kitchen. Leilani turns on the system. The Arrowsmith interactive software immediately springs to life. Arrowsmith is an online interactive telehealth system functioning in millions of homes. It uses the latest artificial intelligence technologies and is capable of learning. All interactions between Arrowsmith modules and patients are, after appropriate security and privacy routine, stored in central memory; the database is continually analyzed allowing it to contribute to Arrowsmith's learning from experience of results of diagnosis and treatments. It asks Leilani what is wrong. When she tells Arrowsmith that Colin seems ill, Arrowsmith focuses the camera in Colin's room on him and activates the measurement component in Colin's mattress, checking temperature, blood pressure and pulse probe. Arrowsmith says Colin has a 102° fever, high pulse rate and normal blood pressure. Arrowsmith asks where Colin has pain. When Colin says his throat hurts, Arrowsmith requests a swab be taken by Leilani and placed within his digital and spectral analyzer. Thirty seconds later Arrowsmith confirms 'Strep!' After checking Colin's stored medical records for allergies and other medications being taken, Arrowsmith automatically registers a prescription for antibiotics with the telepharmacy. The antibiotics will arrive three hours later by FedEx delivery. Arrowsmith explains to Leilani that the new antibiotic capsule should arrive before 10pm and she should give one to Colin tonight and one in the morning. They are so effective that Colin goes to school the following morning feeling fine. Arrowsmith asks Leilani if she wants to be connected to a human health counselor for their further guidance. She declines and Arrowsmith signs off. At 9.45 the home delivery service arrives with the two pills for Colin. He sleeps well. From awareness of illness to guidance takes five minutes. From awareness of illness to medication takes two hours and 45 minutes. Colin is well within 11 hours of the initial awareness of the illness. Mother and Father are unaffected.

No physicians were visited personally; no long waits at pharmacies, nor long trips to medical centers. This tells the story of an advanced application of a subset of e-health called 'telemedicine' at work, and this is no fish story, it's the truth to be. It is a system which looks at efficiency, not just from the perspective of healthcare providers and facilities, but from a whole system point of view, avoiding many of the dysfunctional cascading effects to the lives of patients and their helpers which today's healthcare system does not take into consideration.

This book is about the pioneering of a revolution in healthcare that is stemming from the advent of information technology combined with healthcare technology . . . what we call e-health.

In the pages that follow, experts from diverse fields and different parts of the globe will share their research and opinions about problems and solutions of putting e-health, such as telemedicine, to work for society's benefit.

Telemedicine is at the forefront of clinical e-health systems. Globally, both in government and private sectors, professionals agree that telemedicine is a good idea and here to stay; most agree it is central to the future delivery of healthcare services. Yet, many stakeholders report that telemedicine seems more like a failure than a success. In case after case, soon after the implementation of telemedicine, the utilization and interest curves skate downhill – sometimes to the point where the system becomes unused. While there are notable exceptions to this trend, the reported failures of telemedicine foster a reputation that distinctly challenges leaders who seek to adopt this promising technology. Further, the same dynamics relevant to the adoption of telemedicine may foreshadow adoptions of different and/or more advanced clinical e-health technology to come.

Across cultures around the world, failures are disheartening, especially for advocates of the efficacy of telemedicine and other clinical e-health solutions. To them, telemedicine clearly presents a constellation of opportunities, some of which are:

- to increase access to healthcare of the highest quality
- to improve the quality of healthcare by providing earlier, more effective interventions
- to improve the quality of healthcare by providing a mechanism for continuing clinical learning and rapid, widespread knowledge dissemination.

And, intuitively, despite a recent study in *British Medical Journal* that concludes 'there is no good evidence that telemedicine is a cost effective means of delivering healthcare', healthcare professionals and government policy planners believe that telemedicine holds the promise of decreasing the cost of healthcare services.

Why do so many telemedicine systems fail? What are the dynamics underlying the failure to thrive; how can we preclude such failure? Why is success so rare? What enables the successes and what can we learn from them? Research, especially the examination of the impact of organizational and individual dynamics on telemedicine, may hold the answers to these questions, not only for telemedicine but also for clinical e-health systems in general.

Normally, the root of telemedicine failure (relative to cost-effectiveness) is not the technology, but rather the human system in which the technology is implanted. When the technology is not utilized to its potential, a low number of interactions is expensed to the initial investment; the program is thus deemed too costly. Insufficient utilization is central to the failure of telemedicine: the source is neither consumer acceptance nor inadequate technology. The utilization problem is a human dynamic expressing an interesting ambiguity: healthcare providers accept the new delivery system as a good development and yet resist using it. The organizational and individual resistance may come from human–machine interface, change in organizational processes and culture, individual behavior, clinical conditions and user preconceptions of telemedicine. Any of these dynamics within the field of human factors may stem the drop in the utilization rates to the point where cost is excessive.

This book is dedicated to understanding and resolving organizational and individual resistance to telemedicine, and prescribes specific solutions that are inordinately relevant to current challenges – as well as to more complex clinical e-health technology of the future. The book's international comparative perspective fuels the discovery and transfer of the wisdom of diverse cultures to all others.

Facilitating utilization is a key to unlocking the potential of e-health technology. Understanding and managing people within an organization during a change of technology such as telemedicine is a complex, interactive and systemic challenge, particularly since the reality of being able to isolate and control one aspect of an issue without impacting other aspects is highly unlikely. High rates of utilization of telemedicine significantly reduce the cost per consult and result in telemedicine being viewed as a success by healthcare leaders, which then allows continuation, innovation, increased access, improved quality and reduction of the overall cost of healthcare. Understanding, mediating and managing complex human factors in the adoption of clinical e-health solutions is thus essential to the evolution of global healthcare.

In this book we identify human and organizational factor issues in clinical e-health utilization. And, we acknowledge that such artificial, analytic decomposition and disintegration belies the true interconnectedness and interactivity of the healthcare social system.

Having made this disclaimer, we proceed to deconstruct the real world, international phenomena of acceptance/resistance to telemedicine and construct culturally competent strategies to overcome individual and organizational resistance to such e-health technology.

We conceptualize the challenge of managing successful telemedicine and e-health adoptions as peeling an onion. Revealing (understanding) each layer contributes to achieving success at the core. In this book, we peel off each layer successively, examining each before proceeding, always recognizing that these layers are constructions of our own minds; they are helpful in our understanding of nature, but are not the reality of nature. (The map is not the territory.) The reality lies in the natural symbiosis of all these aspects as coherent whole. Thus, we view the issue as depicted in Figure 1.

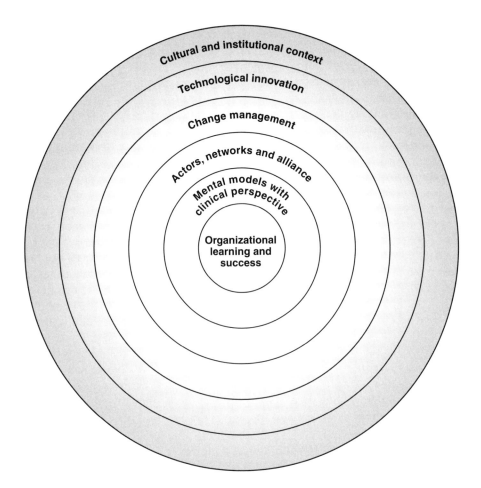

Figure 1 The Study of Human Factors model.

The design of our book seeks to present the best expert analysis of each layer of the onion in Figure 1, and to explore each layer in consideration of concurrence, sequence and integration with each and all other layers. That is, while each expert may emphasise one layer of the onion, they have been encouraged to make note of its interactivity with all others. They may discuss it within any or all of the subfields of management and organization. Contributions from the experts may be the result of rigorous investigation, thought pieces, reviews of literature or case studies. In addition to these expert contributions, included in discussion of each layer are 'classic' articles (found in the supplemental CD to this volume) from the broader literature on the adoption of technology and the impact of the resulting changes on the organization. Expert referrals to the 'classics' are tied to the current state of e-health and overarching principles of management and organization.

In Section 1 of the volume, Stronge, Nichols, Rasche, Sessions, Fisk and Rogers discuss the human factors' issues (training, workload, communication, usability testing) most relevant to the challenge of facilitating the effective utilization of e-health systems. Human factor methods (task analysis, decision–action diagrams and questionnaires) are used to demonstrate how helpful this line of research can be in providing recommendations to improve 'usability' of e-health systems. In the next section, the viewpoint is widened.

In Section 2, Katzenstein and Chrispin, and Sridhar and Suresh investigate what role culture (national, organizational and/or professional) plays in the use of e-health, and how implementation strategies may need to be 'custom-designed' for different cultural environments. Here, the work of culture researchers and sociotechnical systems experts are combined to help in the understanding of the necessary institutional design parameters for successful use of e-health. Examples of 'design innovation' in both African and Indian cultures enliven this section with real-world experiences in implementing an e-health innovation.

In existing institutions, problems arise as new technologies often fit poorly with old design parameters. This is the subject of the third section of the book: putting to use new technologies, which may be disruptive to the way things have been done. Harkke and Collan, Fulcher, and Baldwin and Clarke give examples of new e-health technologies adopted in Finland, the UK and Australia. E-health techno-logies of EHRs (Electronic Health Records), AIDMAN (two-way, real-time gen-eralists/specialist teleconsults) and IT (information technology) in general are slow to be accepted. Understanding the causes of poor acceptance and utilization of e-health technological innovations is thus the primary theme of Section 3.

Section 4 focuses on application of change management techniques to aid in the problems identified in Section 3. Herein, we examine change management techniques applied to using new e-health technologies. Unfreezing old attitudes and habits, changing, and then refreezing new behavior and attitudes are key ideas presented. Spil, Schuring and Michel-Verkerke and Forducey, Smith, Kaur and Scheideman-Miller explore implementation approaches in the Netherlands and in Oklahoma. In both studies, early involvement of users with IT designers was seen to greatly enhance the perceived professional advantages and job relevance (unfreezing) of future e-health users. Only after effective unfreezing of important stakeholders do we find change successfully accomplished and implementation a reality. To better understand the ability to unfreeze, one needs better knowledge of the characteristics of the actors, networks and alliances of the stakeholders, and so these are the topics of the next section.

In Section 5, Justis, Doarn and Merrell, Bomba, and Seale, Robinson, Green, Walker, Esperat, Berg and Ellison investigate actors, networks and alliances in e-health. All these factors are necessarily considered in the design of change techniques. In this section, experiences in Sweden, Australia and the US point out the need to go beyond a stated positive attitude towards implementation of e-health, and provide both institutional and societal support for both initial and sustained usage. Networks and alliances are key ingredients in the design of such social usage support systems. Actors, too, must be supportive.

Towards this end, Section 6 explores the mental models of key actors in the utilization paradigm of e-health. Mackenzie, Xiao, Lam, Hu and Oglivie, Johnson,

Webb, Moser, Harrigan and Pezzoli, and Bulik, Wulff, Butman and Pfeil share their thoughts on the role mental models and the clinical perspective have upon implementation success and failure. It is the mental model held not just by the primary care provider, but also the mental model of the specialist and the mental model of the patient, all of which interact and result in a greater or lesser likelihood of e-health implementation success. This section makes it apparent that e-health implementation success depends greatly upon the attitudes and cognition held by all involved. If primary and/or specialist providers come to the table with clinical perspectives that denigrate the utility of alternative technological communication channels, and believe only face-to-face communication can be the gold standard, then implementation failure is almost always assured. If patients can achieve enhanced education and guidance so as to 'upgrade' their mental models of their illness, and most importantly, understand the reasons for their treatment regimes, then the likelihood of implementation success can be enhanced. In the next section, we return to the macro-picture as we explore the mental models not of individuals, but of organizations.

Section 7 is all about the shared mental models of collectivities, often called organizational culture, and how these collective models are learned and modified. Aas and Bangert and Doktor look at examples in Norway, France, the UK, US, Italy and South Korea in an effort to understand the role organization culture and learning have upon implementation of e-health. Users of an e-health system generally agree that they learn while using the system. Most of the learning of which they speak is, of course, context related to healthcare treatments. Nonetheless, there is also, no doubt, a substantial amount of learning related to modification of their mental models of e-health, and therefore to the shared collective mental model of e-health and its usability. As form follows function, it is possible that use of e-health has the potential to cause modifications in form (organizational structures and procedures) such that the newer organizational forms will be more conducive to e-health utilization: 'Use it and you likely will not lose it'. It's a circle; more conducive structures and procedures lead to even more enhanced organizational utilization of e-health. Primary in these redesigns is the necessity to match the organization to the expectations about the organization held by key stakeholders. These expectations change with social trends. Thus, the advent of e-health may make today a justified time to question current organizational designs in healthcare from the bottom up.

The brave new world of e-health presents immense challenges to the healthcare field. To date, we have only seen the tip of the iceberg. So much more is to come; and to come quickly as the healthcare profession is at the dawn of a turbulent day, but a day filled with promise as well as challenge. It is to this promise that this book is directed.

Section 1

Overview of human factors in healthcare technology utilization

Chapter 1

An application of human factors methods to teledermatology

Aideen J Stronge, Timothy A Nichols, Jeanette D Rasche, Rufus G Sessions, Arthur D Fisk and Wendy A Rogers

The United States Department of Defense (DoD) manages the world's largest healthcare system[1] and has been instrumental in the development of healthcare innovations. During the Civil War, the first Ambulance Corps was formed to transport wounded soldiers rather than postpone treatment until a medic arrived.[2] The Civil War also marked one of the first instances when military personnel used telecommunications technology to transmit healthcare information; the telegraph was used to send messages about casualties and to request medical supplies.[3] Since then, various telecommunications technologies have been used in the military with the same overall goal as the first Ambulance Corps, to increase access and decrease the waiting time to healthcare treatment.

Telemedicine is the natural progression of telecommunications technology. It may be defined as the communication of health information across space and/or time through the use of technology. The DoD has launched numerous telemedicine programs ranging from teleoncology[4] to telemental health[5] as a way to practice 'good medicine in bad places'.[6] DoD interest in telemedicine stems from two practical reasons: to reduce disruptions in healthcare due to frequent changes in location, and to provide cost-effective, easily accessible healthcare to military personnel deployed internationally in small units.[2] Reductions in military healthcare costs have been well documented and can be quite substantial.[5,7–9] These reduced costs include a reduction in lost work hours and travel for specialist care[5,7,8] as well as reduced treatment time, with personnel returning to work earlier.[8] However, there are costs associated with implementing and using a telemedicine system such as hardware, software, support personnel and so on.[10] If a telemedicine system is not adopted and widely used, the financial benefits to the organization will not be realized.[11]

Unfortunately, many military telemedicine systems fail to be included in the standard healthcare process. A common misconception within many organizations is that telemedicine technologies, once provided, will automatically be accepted and used.[12] The field of 'human factors' (also known as ergonomics or engineering psychology) is a scientific discipline that strives to optimize the relationship between technology and the human user.[13] Human factors practitioners focus on increasing efficiency and minimizing error in the design, implementation and use of a human–machine system. Bangert and Doktor's onion model (see Figure 1, Introduction) illustrated critical human factors issues in the implementation and evaluation of a telemedicine system. We have extended this model by adding specific human factors issues within each level or 'layer' (*see* Figure 1.1). For the purposes of this chapter, the levels or 'layers' of this model will be discussed as they relate to macroergonomic issues, user characteristics and technology issues. These categories are not meant to be mutually exclusive; however, they are useful for grouping related issues.

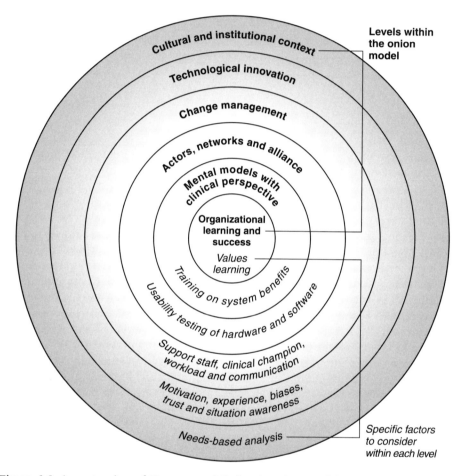

Figure 1.1 An extension of Bangert and Doktor's onion model to incorporate human factors issues.

Factors contributing to system success

Macroergonomic issues

Macroergonomic issues concern organizational issues and the design of work-place systems (*see* reference 14 for a review). One macroergomic issue to consider is the cultural or institutional context in which the telemedicine technology is implemented (the first layer within the onion model). This issue is particularly salient when evaluating a telemedicine system within the US military, as each military branch has its own distinctive organizational culture. Moreover, some branches may be more receptive to telemedicine technologies based on their population's needs. For example, US Navy personnel may be more likely to adopt a telemedicine system than other military branches due to the population's distance from specialist care. As a result of these distinct organizational climates, an evaluation of any telemedicine system must include a needs analysis. A needs analysis is conducted to define the needs of the user population and their expectations of the system.[15] A telemedicine system will not be easily adopted if the user population does not perceive a need for telemedicine regardless of whether such a system could benefit the organization.

When evaluating the cultural climate within an organization, one also should consider whether the organization values learning (the sixth layer within the onion model). A telemedicine system is more likely to succeed within an organization that incorporates educational opportunities for the development of new skills.[7] An organization needs to be supportive of the telemedicine technologies and willing to devote the resources necessary to train users on the system's components.

The development of effective training programs is an essential macroergonomic issue as it leads to clinician acceptance.[11,12,16] In a survey of a store-and-forward ophthalmic telemedicine system used by the US Army, users reported difficulty viewing images because they did not know how to use the software.[16] However, a training program should not be limited to training on the technology and/or software used within the system. Bangert et al.[11] assessed the training needs of military healthcare providers by distributing surveys to users and non-users of telemedicine programs. Participants were asked to rank the importance of different learning objectives. Their responses were grouped according to four categories and it was found that the clinical aspects of telemedicine were considered most important for a training program (e.g. specifics about conducting a consultation), followed by the training of telemedicine technologies, organizational/management issues (e.g. funding) and the fundamentals of telemedicine (e.g. history of telemedicine).

Training also should be viewed as an opportunity to explain the organizational benefits to using telemedicine systems. Physicians within a telemedicine system may have limited mental models concerning how telemedicine can benefit them (layer five within the onion model – mental models with clinical perspective). In fact, telemedicine technologies offer benefits to both physicians and patients within the military environment. Telemedicine can increase the opportunities for physicians to interact professionally with specialists, provide educational opportunities and reduce the number of unnecessary patient referrals.[4] For example, one telemedicine system offered physicians the opportunity to earn continuing medical education credits through online courses and hosted online conferences where physicians could meet to share information about consultations.[17]

Physicians will be more receptive to a telemedicine technology if their peers endorse it.[10] In particular, physicians have knowledge of the clinical issues related to telemedicine and can explain to other physicians how the system can benefit their practice.[9] However, the initial acceptance of physicians must lead to continued acceptance for the success of the telemedicine system. To achieve success, the telemedicine system needs the support of a physician at each site (i.e. a clinical champion) to ensure its continued use.

This clinical champion also can serve as a leader or manager to facilitate the organizational changes that need to occur as a result of the telemedicine system (layer three within the onion model – change management). For example, the clinical champion can manage how workload is distributed among the different team members. The use of a telemedicine system may increase the overall workload for physicians and their clinical staff,[6] and there should be assistants in place to handle the administrative aspects of the system to reduce workload.[9] Workload is also an issue at the organizational level. It is important that specialists receive recognition for the consults that they answer.[7] Currently, a DoD working group has been tasked with the responsibility to complete the workload credit for a teleconsultation (Dingbaum, personal communication). Though not complete, it provides guidance on how to obtain workload credit for a teleconsultation. However, at this time, a teleconsultation is not considered equal to a face-to-face consultation. Thus, the inclusion of an organizational support staff would be essential in managing overall workload in a military environment. The support staff should manage the number of consultations that a specialist receives to avoid overburdening them and losing their participation within the system.

The support staff also could be responsible for managing communication between team members located at different sites. Within a telemedicine system, information is transferred between users and there can be multiple streams of information (i.e. patients). The support staff need to maintain an overall awareness of the status of information within the system. Users also need to be aware of the information within the system, such as where the information originated, who should receive the information and who to contact if they have further questions. As a result, user roles should be well defined within a telemedicine system to optimize communication between users. In addition, the telemedicine system should provide users with feedback about their communications. In particular, users should receive feedback about which consults have been answered, which consults need to be answered and whether there are any additional requests for information.

User characteristics

The implementation of telemedicine technologies should be driven by the needs of its users rather than by the latest technologies.[10] A telemedicine system can be designed using the latest technology, but unless there is an understanding of the user's capabilities, limitations, needs and preferences there is no assurance of a successful human–machine system. User characteristics relevant to telemedicine center on the concept of embracing technological innovations (layer two within the onion model). To understand the acceptance (or lack thereof) of telemedicine technologies, it is critical to consider the factors that motivate a user to begin and continue using a telemedicine system:

- experience and knowledge about the system and its components
- any preconceived biases about telemedicine technologies
- perceived trust in the telemedicine system.

Perhaps the most important user characteristic is perceived trust in the system. Any automated system relies on user trust to ensure its use.[18] In a study of a teledermatology system, the referring physicians requested face-to-face consultations because they did not feel comfortable evaluating a patient solely on the information provided via the telemedicine system (i.e. clinical history and images).[6] Thus, the quality of the digital images and the clinical history play a key role in physician trust and, in turn, physician acceptance. A thorough understanding of factors that lead to trust in the system should increase the success of telemedicine technologies.

Technology issues

There are various components within a telemedicine system, including both human actors as well as non-human entities (e.g. software). A goal of telemedicine technologies is to optimize the relationship between these components (layer four within the onion model – actors, networks and alliances). Developing standards for the hardware and software of telemedicine components would be one strategy to improve the relationship between humans and the equipment used.[10] Another way to optimize this relationship would be to make the equipment more user-friendly by increasing its usability.[10] Usability can be defined as how easy an interface is to use, including how this affects learning, error recovery and efficiency.[19] The usability of a software interface in a telemedicine system is critical and it has been asserted 'telemedicine application software is chosen . . . with ease of use a primary consideration equal to clinical effectiveness' (Carlos and Pangelinan, 1999, p. 61). As a result, organizations should include usability testing as part of their evaluation of a telemedicine system (*see* Dix *et al.*, 1988 for a review of these techniques[20]).

Furthermore, when users experience difficulty using the telemedicine system, technical assistance should be available. Technical difficulties influence the use of a telemedicine system[6] and organizations may need to include additional technical assistance to support telemedicine systems.[7] Technical problems can also be related to macroergonomic issues, in particular how the organization views the telemedicine system. In the analysis of one teledermatology system used within the military, it was found that many of the technical problems associated with the system were due to additional programs added to the consult computer.[9] These added programs resulted in about two calls per month in which the user reported difficulty using the telemedicine system. As a consequence of this finding, the organization enforced an agreement with the users that they would not alter the telemedicine workstation.

Human factors and ergonomics methods

Human factors and ergonomics methods can be used to evaluate telemedicine systems and identify the issues that contribute to their success. The field of human factors utilizes various assessment methods to understand the capabilities and limitations of people to design 'systems, organizations, jobs, machines, tools, and consumer products for safe, efficient, and comfortable human use' (Helander, 1997, p. 4).[21] As discussed in the previous section, the human factors issues related to the success of telemedicine systems fall under the general categories of macroergonomic issues, user characteristics and technology issues. However, human factors and ergonomics methods can also identify potential errors and problems, propose suggestions for how to fix those errors and problems (i.e. it can be prescriptive), and provide guidance in the development of new systems and predict where errors and problems may occur.

The human factors and ergonomics techniques used to collect data about macroergonomic issues, user characteristics and technology issues include task analysis, decision–action diagrams and tools to elicit information from system users such as questionnaires, structured interviews and focus groups (*see* Nichols *et al.*, 2004, for a review of these methods[22]). Although it is not required, it is recommended that there should be a progression from the task analysis and decision–action diagrams to the tools targeted at system users, as each method can build off the previous one.

Task analysis is the detailed description about the work activities of the people who are involved with the specific system (*see* Luczak, 1997, for a review[23]). A task analysis consists of a listing of activities and behaviors that are required to complete a given task, including the hardware involved in the task (e.g. telemedicine equipment) and performance requirements (e.g. turn-around time for a consultation). Each task is divided into the subtasks required to carry out the task and each subtask can be analyzed on factors such as the feedback information the user receives from the system and potential sources of error.

To aid in the conceptualization of the system tasks, decision–action diagrams are often developed. Decision-action diagrams are defined as 'a procedure for decomposing or identifying the sequence of functions or actions that must be performed by a system' (Chapanis, 1996, p. 93[24]). Decision-action diagrams represent the flow of information in the system and can be useful in identifying communication issues, how workload is distributed among team members and where problems or errors could cause a breakdown in the flow of information. Although task analyses and decision–action diagrams are useful for understanding individual tasks and how to optimize their performance, they are not a substitute for the knowledge that can be gained through interactions with actual users of the system. However, they can provide guidance in the development of questionnaires, structured interviews and focus groups to assess users' knowledge, beliefs and opinions about the system.

A questionnaire approach facilitates the collection of information from a large number of users in an efficient manner. If the sample is large enough, questionnaires can be useful for collecting quantitative data (e.g. how many times a problem is encountered or how frequently a particular error occurs). However, questionnaires provide only limited data that is qualitative in nature (e.g. what is the nature of the error being made, what is the context under which communication difficulties arise). The goal of structured interviews and focus groups is to gather rich, qualitative information from participants, such as their beliefs, opinions and experiences interacting with a telemedicine system.[25]

A structured interview is a questionnaire administered in person with the opportunity to ask follow-up questions. In general, data collection and data analysis for structured interviews is more time-intensive than for questionnaires because only one person is interviewed at a time and the data are qualitative and must be coded. Focus groups involve the administration of the questionnaire in a group setting; as a result they may be less structured in nature than structured interviews, but they are also useful for collecting qualitative data to assess users' beliefs and opinions about telemedicine. During a focus group, a moderator engages a group of system users about a given topic giving them the opportunity to follow up on various comments. Similar to structured interviews, the analysis of the qualitative data can be time-intensive, although data collection itself is less time-intensive as multiple participants are interviewed at the same time. However, within the group situation it is important to employ an experienced moderator as some participants may be overly influenced by others within the group.[26]

The current system evaluation

Telemedicine systems vary in their clinical applications (e.g. teleoncology, telepsychiatry), the type of information transferred (e.g. video, audio, text) and whether the communication is synchronous (i.e. real time) versus asynchronous (i.e. store-and-forward).[27] Synchronous telemedicine systems typically employ video-conferencing technologies to enable real-time patient–doctor communications that are similar to a face-to-face consultation.[28] However, there are limitations to synchronous communication in that it requires a large amount of bandwidth and all parties must be present at the same time, which can be a challenge when time zones differ at each location.[28]

In store-and-forward telemedicine systems, patients' medical histories and digital photographs of their condition are transmitted to a healthcare provider[29] and reviewed by that healthcare provider at a later time.[28] In contrast to synchronous telemedicine, store-and-forward systems typically require equipment that is less expensive and lower bandwidth, and members of a team do not all need to be available at the same time.[6] The Internet is particularly useful as the medium to relay information between team members because it is cost-effective while still maintaining an ability to transmit sizeable amounts of information.[6] However, there are also limitations to store-and-forward telemedicine systems because if the patient's history is deficient, incorrect or image quality is poor, the specialist cannot ask immediate follow-up questions concerning the patient's condition (unlike real-time video conferencing).[6] Moreover, long download times for digital images may be frustrating to users. Despite these limitations, store-and-forward systems are potentially very useful, especially in areas such as dermatology where the number of specialists is limited and high-quality images can be transmitted via the Internet. For these reasons, the use of store-and-forward technologies will most likely be the future of teledermatology.[29]

The current system evaluation focused on an asynchronous teledermatology system that is currently used by the US military. There is a need for teledermatology systems within the military as dermatologic conditions in the armed forces are a common cause of death and loss of work days.[30] Teledermatology is defined as the 'interpretation of electronically transmitted images and clinical history to reach a diagnosis and provide recommendations for therapy' (Vidmar, 1999, p. 113[6]). Teledermatology is particularly amenable to the goals of telemedicine because a picture of the condition is easily transferred via the Internet and the dermatologist can make a recommendation based on the picture. Much work in the field of teledermatology has been directed towards the development of software that can compress a large digital image file without losing too much of the image's resolution.[29] These efforts appear to have been fruitful as the general finding in the literature is that dermatologists can be as diagnostically accurate and reliable using store-and-forward telemedicine technologies as they are in face-to-face consultations.[29] For example, one study that compared the level of agreement between teledermatologists and dermatologists who met with patients face-to-face found a 77% agreement between the two groups.[31]

There are four user groups in the teledermatology system we evaluated:

1   primary care managers (i.e. general physicians)
2   consult managers who assist the primary care managers in interactions with the teledermatology system (not all sites have a consult manager)
3   dermatologists
4   technical support personnel consisting of a nurse coordinator and a system administrator.

The system was evaluated using the following human factors methods:

- task analysis
- decision–action diagrams
- a questionnaire targeted at subject matter experts.

Task analysis

A task analysis begins with identification of the high-level tasks involved in using the system. We used multiple methods to acquire information for task analysis of the teledermatology, including discussions with the support staff, analysis of the teledermatology website, evaluation of the training materials and review of the internal documentation managed by the nurse coordinator. The overall teledermatology system consists of four high-level tasks:

1   a patient with a dermatological condition visits a primary care manager
2   the primary care manager (and/or consult manager) processes the patient and completes the online consult form on the teledermatology website
3   the dermatologist reviews the consult and provides recommendations for patient care
4   the primary care manager receives the recommendations and applies them to the patient.

Additionally, the support staff ensure that the consult is approved and responded to in a timely fashion, monitor the communication between the primary care manager and dermatologist, and oversee the quality of the consults.

The system may appear relatively simple and straightforward based on the identification of the high-level tasks. However, one of the goals of a task analysis is to identify all of the subtasks (i.e. steps) required to complete a given task. The first high-level task within this system is when the primary care manager and/or consult manager processes the patient. A task analysis revealed that this task involved a total of 91 possible subtasks (*see* Table 1.1 for subsections from the task analysis). Each subtask was listed in order and the following factors were considered:

Table 1.1 Subsections of the task analysis of the high-level step 'primary care manager/consult manager processes the patient'

Step	Description	Feedback	Potential errors	Design issues
4.4.2.4	Enter unit	User is required to respond before proceeding to the next screen	Organization of fields is confusing. Easy to miss unit and rank	For any required fields, designers should use appropriate grouping cues
4.4.2.5	Enter rank	User is required to respond before proceeding to the next screen		
4.4.6.2	Repeat steps 4.4.6.1.1.3 as necessary for up to 5 images	When an image is submitted and the user presses a back button, there is no feedback	Entire consult is lost, as system will not continue to process the consult	Users should receive feedback that the original picture has been submitted
4.4.6.3	Click next button	User is given feedback that images have been uploaded. Each image is given a unique file name by the system. There is insufficient feedback about what pictures have been attached	User may attach the wrong pictures at this point and not realize it	1 Inserting a thumbnail of each picture would help users see what they have attached. It would also help to have a filename next to the pictures. 2 The button on the menu bar should not be called 'Cancel/main menu'. It should be called 'Cancel this consult' – then on the very last page of the consult, it should be called 'Return to main menu'. In particular, on this page it should not be called the 'Cancel/main menu' button because you cannot cancel the consult at this point – it has already been created

- the feedback the user received from the system
- the potential errors that could occur
- how system efficiency could be improved through design.

An example of a feedback issue is when the primary care manager uploads the pictures of the patient's condition onto the teledermatology website (*see* Table 1, step 4.4.6.3). The system provides the user with feedback for which pictures have been uploaded. However, the feedback that the user receives from this subtask is insufficient because the system assigns a unique file name to each picture that is different from the name that the user assigned the file. As a result of this feedback, a user could attach pictures from another patient, resulting in a misdiagnosis of the current patient's condition.

An example of a potential error is when the user submits an image onto the website (*see* Table 1.1, step 4.4.6.2). If the user hits the back button, it appears that the image has disappeared, and if the user tries to resubmit the image, the entire consult may be lost.

An example of how to improve system efficiency through design has to do with filling out the required information on the online consult form (*see* Table 1.1, steps 4.4.2.4–4.4.2.5). On one screen of the consult form, most of the required fields were grouped together, except for two required fields that were off to the side and easy to miss. A design recommendation for this potential problem would be that for any required fields, designers should use appropriate grouping cues so that important information is entered.

These examples illustrate the importance of analyzing each subtask involved in a particular task to understand where users might encounter difficulties and to make recommendations for design improvements and perhaps training as well. We have provided only a small set of the subtasks analyzed in the complete analysis. These factors were considered for every subtask that needed to be completed within the system.[32]

Decision–action diagrams

Based on the task analyses, decision–action diagrams for each person involved in the system were developed including a decision–action diagram for the overall system. Figure 1.2 is an example of a decision–action diagram for one team member, the dermatologist. The dermatologist logs into the teledermatology website, selects the appropriate consult, reviews the consult and provides recommendations for patient care. One potential breakdown in the flow of information due to a communication issue could occur if there is additional information required. At this point, the dermatologist should contact the primary care manager and request more information. If the primary care manager sends the amendments or additional information through email, this could be a potentially confusing situation because the email will not be tied to the original consult and the dermatologist may have difficulty remembering which consult it refers to. The task analysis and decision–action diagrams serve many purposes, one of which is to identify sources of user difficulties at different levels, ranging from the specific design of the interface to inter-individual communication within an organization.

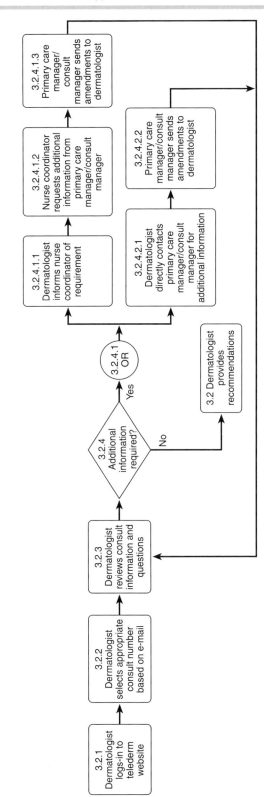

Figure 1.2 Decision–action diagram representing the activities of the dermatologist.

User questionnaires

Task analyses and decision–action diagrams also provide guidance for the development of questionnaires to understand the critical human factors issues that involve macroergonomic issues, user characteristics and technology issues. We designed a questionnaire to assess the human factors issues already identified, as well as questions about issues that could not be identified through the task analysis and decision–action diagrams (e.g. the specific context in which errors might occur or the degree to which training was successful). The questionnaire consisted of multiple-choice, rank-order and open-ended questions (*see* Appendix A for example questions of macroergonomic issues, user characteristics and technology issues).

Five subject matter experts (i.e. experienced users of the system) were queried: two primary care managers, two dermatologists and one consult manager. A questionnaire was used for this sample, as opposed to a structured interview, because we wanted the subject matter experts to critically evaluate the questions we were asking and the form in which we were asking them (this study was a precursor to a structured interview study conducted with a larger sample of participants).[33] A written questionnaire was used to enable the subject matter experts to evaluate the wording of the questions and to provide guidance about the structural organization of the questionnaire. All five subject matter experts were male and reported a range of experience with the system from less than six months to less than five years. Responses to the questionnaire were categorized according to the human factors issues that they referenced and example responses have been included in the following sections to illustrate the type of data that can be gathered through questionnaires.

Macroergonomic issues

We identified four macroergonomic issues:

- workload
- communication
- training
- the involvement of the support staff.

Concerning workload, one dermatologist reported that high workload resulted in his inability to 'complete all consults on a given day'. Another dermatologist reported that it was 'difficult to capture the workload involved with the system because they do not get credit in the military for a patient visit for each consult that is answered'. However, they reported that 'training nursing staff to send the consults to the physicians' would help to reduce this workload.

Communication issues can arise when the primary care manager contacts the consult manager through the system. In the current system, different dermatologists are assigned to work on different days. One primary care manager reported that he sent out a request for more information, the request arrived at a different time and it was not returned to the specific dermatologist. This disrupts communication between the primary care manager and the dermatologist and creates a potentially confusing situation. Primary care managers also reported that they needed to contact the support staff regarding confusion about a dermatologist's recommendations, about errors in the consult, operational issues regarding the website and insufficient information in a consult. These data speak to the need for having support staff accessible to system users to oversee communication within the system.

None of the users reported difficulty in learning to use the system, suggesting that the training for this teledermatology system was sufficient in meeting the needs of its users. This may have been the result of the type of training they received. Most of the users received one-on-one training from the support staff that oversee the system. One subject matter expert reported that potential users should be educated about telemedicine's benefits to 'market service to patients and primary care managers as a useful consultative tool'. Thus, as discussed within the onion model, training programs should not be limited to telemedicine technologies, but should include the benefits of telemedicine technologies.

The support staff responsible for overseeing the entire consult process was reported to be an integral part of this telemedicine system. Users reported that the support staff members were 'very supportive and dedicated', 'wonderful, intelligent and patient', 'easy to get a hold of', and 'eager to help'. The support staff were responsible for facilitating the adoption and continued use of this telemedicine system. However, these comments indicate the potential importance of individual personalities for the overall success of the system.

User characteristics

Motivation to learn and continue using a telemedicine system may contribute to users' willingness to embrace a telemedicine technology. The subject matter experts were asked to rank order the importance of certain factors in motivating them to begin using the system and continue using the system (*see* Appendix A, User characteristics). The majority indicated that they began using the system and continued using the system because it was a useful professional experience. They reported that the telemedicine technologies enhanced their professional experience through 'rewarding exposure to technology/telemedicine with excellent real-world applications', 'helped with feedback, don't usually get feedback from regular consults', and 'one-on-one conversation with specialist talking to them via consult and pictures helps to demonstrate my thinking'.

Technology issues

Technology issues include the usability of the teledermatology website and any technical failures associated with the technology used. One usability issue that emerged was the function of the back button when filling out an online consult form in that 'clicking it will cause loss of comments in the narrative section'. Other technical issues included difficulty accessing the server, trouble filling out the online forms and incorrect email addresses. Although these technical issues are specific to the current system, they can be generalized to provide guidance to designers of future telemedicine systems. For example, telemedicine systems should have online forms that are usable by people with a wide variety of technology experience and they should be designed to guard against loss of information. One strategy would be to give users the option to save information on a page before moving to the next page. Another strategy would be to avoid the need for navigational buttons by designing the online consult form to present the information on a single page that allows the user to scroll down the form. Identifying the technology problems with a system enables designers to improve users' interactions with the system.

Discussion

The US military has established various telemedicine programs. Although the advantages of these programs have been identified, not all telemedicine programs in the military have been adopted and widely used. Human factors methods can be used to evaluate a telemedicine system by emphasizing factors critical to system success. In the present analysis, task analysis, decision–action diagrams and questionnaires operated in conjunction to identify macroergonomic issues, user characteristics and technology issues. Each method provided unique information about how these factors contribute to system success. The task analysis provided detailed information about the tasks involved in using the system, including a focus on the feedback the user received from the system, the potential errors that could occur and how to improve system efficiency through design. The decision–action diagrams were useful in illustrating the flow of information through the system by demonstrating how workload and communication issues might cause a breakdown in the system. Finally, the questionnaire was a valuable method to obtain information from subject matter experts about specific user issues, including the factors that motivated them to begin and continue using this teledermatology system.

Standard techniques of human factors analysis were used to identify overall human factors issues involved in the implementation and adoption of telemedicine technologies. The issues of most relevance could be incorporated as part of Bangert and Doktor's onion model, as illustrated in Figure 1 (*see* Introduction, p. 7). Future research efforts should be directed towards increasing our understanding of the specific issues involved within the different levels of the onion model.

Within the area of telemedicine, one challenge faced by human factors specialists is to develop 'methods and tools for assessing potential users' needs and for matching characteristics of particular telemedicine technologies to these needs' (Institute of Medicine, 1996, p. 79[10]). The methods discussed in the evaluation of the current teledermatology system could serve as a toolkit for evaluations of other telemedicine systems. This toolkit can be used as the basis for the development of an objective assessment tool to aid in the evaluation of human factors issues that can be used with other existing telemedicine systems (i.e. prescriptive) and in the development of future telemedicine systems (i.e. predictive).

Based on our review of telemedicine systems used within the military and our analysis of a teledermatology system, we propose the following recommendations for the successful implementation of a telemedicine system used within the US military. We have grouped these issues into the categories of macroergonomic issues, user characteristics and technology issues.

Macroergonomic issues

- To ensure the successful implementation of a telemedicine system, organizations should value learning and the development of new skills, and emphasize the benefits of using the telemedicine system.
- The development of training programs should include the clinical aspects of telemedicine, training of telemedicine technologies, organizational/management issues, the fundamentals of telemedicine and the organizational benefits of telemedicine systems.
- An enthusiastic support staff and a clinical champion should be recruited to assist with training, oversee communication and monitor the quality of the consults.
- At each referring site, assistants should be included to reduce the administrative workload of physicians.
- Ideally, physicians should receive workload credit for the consults that they answer. However, as this is presently not the case, a support staff should manage workload to ensure that physicians are not overly burdened.
- Communication should be optimized to increase users' awareness of the information transferred within the system.
- Roles within the telemedicine system should be well defined.
- System feedback should be included in the design of any telemedicine system. This feedback information should indicate what consults have been answered, what consults still need to be answered, and so on.
- There must be flexibility within a telemedicine system to support communication between users and a support staff to manage communications within the system.

User characteristics

- An understanding of the users' capabilities, limitations, needs and preferences should drive system design.
- Improving the quality of the digital images and ensuring that the patient's clinical history is complete can increase perceived trust in a telemedicine system.
- Increase users' motivation to begin using and continue using telemedicine technologies by informing them of how this experience will enhance their professional experience.

Technology issues

- Technology used within a telemedicine system should be user friendly; that is, usability analysis should be conducted on all the components of the system to ensure that a variety of users can operate the technology, that the appropriate feedback is provided to the users, that errors are minimized and that error recovery is supported.
- Usability evaluations should be conducted on both the hardware and software applications used within a telemedicine system.

- Technical assistance and support should be available when users experience technical difficulties within the system.
- Online forms should be designed to be usable by people with a range of technical backgrounds and be structured to guard against loss of information.

Conclusion

In sum, the purpose of the present chapter was to demonstrate how human factors methods can be used to identify macroergonomic issues, user character-istics and technology issues that are most relevant to the design and successful use of a telemedicine system. More specifically, these methods are critical in drawing attention to where errors and problems can occur within the system and ultimately lead to the failure of a telemedicine system being successfully adopted and widely used. The results from these methods can be used to provide guidance for the present system as well as in the analysis of other systems and for the development of future systems.

References

1   Chaffee M (1999) A telehealth odyssey. *American Journal of Nursing.* **99**(7): 27–32.
2   Mogel GT (2003) The role of the Department of Defense in PACS and tele-medicine research and development. *Computerized Medical Imaging and Graphics.* **27**(2–3): 129–35.
3   Zundel KM (1996) Telemedicine: history, applications, and impact on librarianship. *Bulletin of the Medical Library Association.* **84**(1): 71–9.
4   Hunter DC, Brustrom JE, Goldsmith BJ *et al.* (1999) Teleoncology in the Department of Defense: a tale of two systems. *Telemedicine Journal.* **5**(3): 273–82.
5   Grady BJ (2002) A comparative cost analysis of an integrated military telemental health-care service. *Telemedicine Journal and e-health.* **8**(3): 293–300.
6   Vidmar DA (1999) The history of teledermatology in Department of Defense. *Dermatologic Clinics.* **17**(1): 113–23.
7   Bangert D and Doktor R (2000) Implementing store-and-forward telemedicine: organizational issues. *Telemedicine Journal and e-health.* **6**(3): 355–60.
8   Brumage MR, Chinn S and Cho K (2001) Teleradiology in a military training area. *Journal of Telemedicine and Telecare.* **7**(6): 348–52.
9   Carlos ME and Pangelinan SI (1999) Teledermatology in Department of Defense Health Services Region 10. *Journal of Healthcare Information Management.* **13**(4): 59–69.
10 Institute of Medicine (1996) The technical and human context of telemedicine. *Telemedicine: a guide to assessing telecommunications for health care.* The National Academies Press, Washington, DC.
11 Bangert D, Doktor R and Johnson E (2001) Designing Web-based telemedicine training for military healthcare providers. *Journal of Continuing Education in the Health Professions.* **21**(3): 162–9.
12 Yellowlees P (1997) Successful development of telemedicine systems – seven core principles. *Journal of Telemedicine and Telecare.* **3**(4): 215–22.
13 Kantowitz BH and Sorkin RD (1983) *Human Factors: understanding people-system relationships.* Wiley, New York.
14 Hendrick H (1997) Organizational design and macroergonomics. In: G Salvendy (ed.) *Handbook of Human Factors and Ergonomics.* Wiley, New York.

15 Beith BH (1999) Human factors and future of telemedicine. *Medical Device and Diagnostic Injury*. Available from: www.devicelink.com/mddi/archive/99/06/009.html. Accessed 5 March 2004.

16 Lattimore MR (1999) A store-and-forward ophthalmic telemedicine case report from deployed US Army forces in Kuwait. *Telemedicine Journal*. **5**(3): 309–13.

17 Mullick FG, Fontelo P and Pemble C (1996) Telemedicine and telepathology at the Armed Forces Institute of Pathology: history and current mission. *Telemedicine Journal*. **2**(3): 187–93.

18 Lee J and Moray N (1992) Trust, control strategies and allocation of function in human–machine systems. *Ergonomics*. **35**(10): 1243–70.

19 Nielsen J (2003) *Usability 101*. Available from: www.useit.com/alertbox/20030825.html. Accessed 5 March 2004.

20 Dix A, Finlay J, Abowd G *et al*. (1998) *Human-Computer Interaction*. Prentice Hall Europe, Essex.

21 Helander MG (1997) The human factors profession. In: G Salvendy (ed.) *The Handbook of Human Factors and Ergonomics*. Wiley, New York.

22 Nichols TA, Stronge AJ, Rogers WA *et al*. (2004) Human factors and ergonomics: bridging psychology and technology in telemedicine applications. *International Journal of Healthcare Technology and Management*. **6**(1): 3–19.

23 Luczak H (1997) Task analysis. In: G Salvendy (ed.) *Handbook of Human Factors and Ergonomics*. Wiley, New York.

24 Chapanis A (1996) *Human Factors in Systems Engineering*. Wiley Inter-Science, Chichester.

25 Kuzel AJ (1999) Sampling in qualitative inquiry. In: BF Crabtree and WL Miller (eds) *Doing qualitative research* (2e). Sage, Thousand Oaks, CA.

26 Krueger RA (1994) *Focus Groups: a practical guide for applied research* (2e). Sage, Thousand Oaks, CA.

27 Hebert M (2001) Telehealth success: evaluation framework development. *Medinformation*. **10**(2): 1145–9.

28 Whited JD (2001) Teledermatology: current status and future directions. *American Journal of Clinical Dermatology*. **2**(2): 59–64.

29 Eedy DJ and Wootton R (2001) Teledermatology: a review. *British Journal of Dermatology*. **144**(4): 696–707.

30 Vidmar DA, Harford RR, Beasley WJ *et al*. (1996) The epidemiology of dermatologic and venereologic disease in a deployed operational setting. *Military Medicine*. **16**(7): 382–6.

31 Taylor P, Goldsmith P, Murray K *et al*. (2001) Evaluating a telemedicine system to assist in the management of dermatology referrals. *British Journal of Dermatology*. **144**(2): 328–33.

32 Stronge AJ, Nichols TA, Rogers WA and Fisk AD (2004) Human factors analysis of a teledermatology system (HFA-TR-0403). Georgia Institute of Technology, School of Psychology, Human Factors and Aging Laboratory, Atlanta, GA.

33 Stronge AJ, Nichols TA, Rogers WA, Fisk AD, Rasche JD and Dingbaum AM (2004) Presented at the 9th Annual American Telemedicine Association Meeting, 2–4 May, Tampa, FL.

34 Nichols TA, Stronge AJ, Rogers WA, Fisk AD, Rasche JD and Sessions GR (2003) *Methodological Considerations in a Human Factors Assessment of a Teledermatology System*. Proceedings of the 47th Annual Meeting of the Human Factors and Ergonomics Society, 13–17 October, Denver, CO.

Appendix A. Questionnaire distributed to experienced users of the teledermatology system (selected questions)

Macro-organizational – Workload

1 For each of the following teledermatology system tasks, indicate on a scale from 'Never' to 'Always', how often you were the person who performed each task (e.g. even if a task occurred once a month, but you were the person who always performed that task, you would check '5').

	← Never performed/ Always performed →				
	1	2	3	4	5
Online (Web) tasks:					
Complete online consult form	☐	☐	☐	☐	☐
Review online consult form for errors	☐	☐	☐	☐	☐
Submit online consult form	☐	☐	☐	☐	☐
Consult-related communication (email) tasks:					
Correspond with dermatologists	☐	☐	☐	☐	☐
Correspond with the CTA: Nik and/or Angela	☐	☐	☐	☐	☐
Correspond with your clinic support staff	☐	☐	☐	☐	☐
Patient interaction tasks:					
Complete a written consult form	☐	☐	☐	☐	☐
Obtain written consent from the patient	☐	☐	☐	☐	☐
Take digital images of the patient	☐	☐	☐	☐	☐
Organizational tasks:					
Communicate with system administrator (i.e. Nik) in the event of technical issues with computer and/or digital camera	☐	☐	☐	☐	☐
Ensure timely progress of online consult and feedback	☐	☐	☐	☐	☐
Keep a record of digital images, forms, etc.	☐	☐	☐	☐	☐
Provide system training/assistance to other staff	☐	☐	☐	☐	☐
Other (please describe):	☐	☐	☐	☐	☐

_____

_____

User characteristics – Motivation to continue using the system

1 What encouraged you to continue to use the teledermatology system? **For those that are relevant, numerically order by importance, with '1' indicating most important.**
   ☐ Encouragement from chain of command/upper management
   ☐ High patient satisfaction
   ☐ High personal satisfaction
   ☐ System provided a faster consultation process
   ☐ System was easy to use (relative to standard referral procedure)
   ☐ Useful professional experience
   ☐ Other (please describe): _____

_____

Technology issues

1   Indicate if you have ever experienced these problems with the system. Check the appropriate box to indicate the frequency with which these problems occurred (check '0' if you have never experienced this problem). Please briefly explain the problem.

	← Less frequent/ More frequent →					
	0	1	2	3	4	5
Hardware problems	☐	☐	☐	☐	☐	☐
Explain: _____						
Losing information entered into online consult	☐	☐	☐	☐	☐	☐
Explain: _____						
Navigation of consult website	☐	☐	☐	☐	☐	☐
Explain: _____						
Online communication with others within the system	☐	☐	☐	☐	☐	☐
Explain: _____						
Other (please describe below)	☐	☐	☐	☐	☐	☐
Describe: _____						

Author note

This research was supported in part by contributions from the Telemedicine and Advanced Technology Research Center, Fort Detrick, MD. We regretfully note that Dr G Rufus Sessions, the Chief Scientific Officer at the Telemedicine and Advanced Technology Research Center and principle investigator of this research project, has passed away.

  Portions of this chapter were presented at the 8th Annual American Telemedicine Association Meeting in Orlando, FL (April 2003) and the Human Factors and Ergonomics Society 47th Annual Meeting in Denver, CO (October 2003) with proceedings.[34] The authors would like to thank David Bangert, Robert Doktor and Anne C McLaughlin for their input on earlier drafts of this chapter.

Section 2

Cultural and institutional context
of e-health

Chapter 2

Designing a telemedicine system in Tanzania: a sociotechnical systems approach

James Katzenstein and Barbara R Chrispin

Introduction

Tanzania contains Africa's highest mountain, Kilimanjaro; its most famous game park, Ngorongoro Crater; its largest game reserve, the Serengeti; and the three largest lakes on the continent lie on its borders. Tanzania embodies the Africa that people envision when they think of Africa. Tanzania is also one of the ten poorest countries in the world, a fact reflected by the woefully substandard state of healthcare in the country. Deaths from communicable and infectious diseases, which represent only 2% of total deaths in Europe, constitute nearly half of all deaths in Africa. There is a chronic shortage of doctors and other healthcare professionals, as well as a lack of national infrastructure to provide transportation and distribution of resources and services. Building healthcare and educational capacity under these conditions is extremely difficult.

Within this void, Dr Hubert C Kairuki, a visionary African physician, and his family started a four-bed clinic in Dar es Salaam, the economic capital of Tanzania. Dr Kairuki and his family made significant strides in delivering healthcare using a unique business model that involved contracting with government-owned enterprises to provide healthcare to their employees on a fee-for-service basis. In ten years, the clinic grew to become a 130-bed general medical center known as Mission Mikocheni Hospital (MMH).

In 1996, the management at MMH invited a group of faculty and students from The Fielding Graduate Institute in Santa Barbara, California, to Tanzania to help assess the viability of their ten-year strategic plan. This nascent, international partnership provided the foundation for developing a plan to link three outlying clinics with a hub site at MMH, mediated by information and communication technology (ICT). This system, used extensively in the US, laid the groundwork for further study into the feasibility of using telemedicine and telemedicine systems to improve healthcare capacity in developing countries such as Tanzania.

Statement of the problem

The 'ah-ha' that surfaced between the authors is that working in Africa 'really' is different from working in the US – each of these two different worlds provides unique historical and cultural perspectives about development, health and wellness, healthcare capacity and the role of technology. The more we talked, the more aware we became of the project's reliance on Western models of technology and telemedicine as the solution to problems of healthcare capacity in Africa. That is to say, while the system configuration took into consideration the appropriateness of the technology for the economic development of Tanzania, it focused on telemedicine primarily as a technological tool that would expand the reach of the current healthcare system. Furthermore, the initial design seemed to imply that telemedicine systems that work in the Western world would work equally well in Africa, and that they would be positively accepted by the Africans themselves.

In healthcare, there is mounting evidence that the introduction of new technologies invariably creates turbulence within an organization, primarily because the new organizational structures associated with the innovation are not assimilated within the existing status quo.[1] The designers of a telemedicine system must be cognizant of existing patterns of social organization and the likely effect the introduction of new technology will have on those patterns. In addition, these new forms of social organization are likely to be different from place to place and country to country. International telemedicine systems exist within a complex set of cultural environments within which these different social systems operate. Telemedicine systems designed in one culture and social system for use in another are unlikely to work. As Hofstede states in the companion article to this section, 'the export of Western – mostly American – management practices and theories to poor countries has contributed little to nothing to their development . . . and should be sufficient argument to doubt their validity in non-Western environments'.[2]

The problem, as we see it, is how to design a telemedicine system so that both the social and the technical systems can function optimally within the cultural environment of Tanzania. In our view, the cross-cultural interface of human beings and information using ICT presents enormous challenges and may be one of the major reasons for the failure of telemedicine in developing countries.

In this chapter, we use sociotechnical systems theory (STS) to explore the relationship between a telemedicine system and its cultural environment. The STS approach lends itself well to the onion metaphor on which this book is based. The analysis and design of a telemedicine system starts with an understanding of the cultural differences between the Western technology and consultants, and the Tanzanian users of the telemedicine system. This macro view of a culture, dealing with the cultural and institutional context, is essentially the outer layer of the onion used to structure this book.

As we develop a cultural profile of Tanzania, the complexity of working in multiple cultures and social systems will become clearer – shedding light on other levels of the onion.

A second issue addressed in this chapter is the complex role of the international design team. Hofstede, in the accompanying article, suggests that outside experts who believe they can develop a country with their so-called modern management techniques and theories are deplorably arrogant. The consulting model that has been used in Tanzania is proposed as a paradigm for working more effectively in developing countries such as Tanzania.

For the purposes of this research, telemedicine is defined as the delivery of healthcare services where distance is a critical factor, by healthcare professionals using ICT for the exchange of valid information for diagnosis, treatment and prevention of disease and injuries, research and evaluation, and for the continuing education of healthcare providers, all in the interest of advancing the health of individuals and their communities.[3]

Sociotechnical systems (STS) theory

One approach that has relevance to the design of telemedicine systems is sociotechnical systems (STS) theory.[4] In the STS approach, any work organization requiring the interaction of people and technology rests on two premises: the first is that the desired output is achieved through the joint operation of a social as well as a technical system; and the second is that every sociotechnical system is embedded in an environment that is influenced by a culture, its values, and the roles and norms of its members.

A key feature of the sociotechnical approach to work design is an emphasis on creating work systems in which the social and the technical aspects of those systems are integrated and as supportive of one another as possible. This involves attempting to 'jointly optimize' the social and the technical systems that operate in work organizations, rather than maximizing the functioning of the technical system at the expense of the social system.

Another important feature of the STS approach is recognition of the fact that all organizations are embedded in, and affected by, an outside environment. To understand how an organization functions and to make constructive changes in an organization one must pay close attention to the environmental forces that operate on it. Especially important are cultural values that specify how organizations should function and the generally accepted roles that individuals, groups or organizations are supposed to play in society. There is constant interchange between what goes on *within* any given work organization and what goes on in its environment – a fact that is dangerous to ignore when work systems are designed or changed.

The cultural environment of Tanzania

As generally understood, the culture of a society comprises the shared values, understandings, assumptions and goals that are learned from earlier generations, imposed by present members of a society and passed on to succeeding generations.[5] Despite differences among social scientists, there are three characteristics on which there is widespread agreement: '. . . it is not innate, but learned; the various facets of culture are inter-related – you touch a culture in one place and everything else is affected; it is shared and in effect defines the boundaries of different groups'.[6] This shared outlook results in a basis for living grounded in shared communication, standards, codes of conduct and expectations.

Just as organizations can be portrayed as sociotechnical systems, cultural environments can best be understood as systems composed of interrelated parts, or subsystems. To achieve understanding of any given culture requires some familiarity with the cultural variables universal to most cultures – language, religion, education, social organizations, the economy, politics and law, technology, and values and attitudes.[7] From these universal variables, one can develop a cultural profile which identifies the specific differences found in each country or people and hence anticipate how the unfamiliar culture will impact the organizational setting.

Using information available from government and university reports, the following sections show how these universal variables can be used to describe the cultural environment in Tanzania.[8]

Overview

The United Republic of Tanzania is one of the world's least developed nations. Situated on the East Coast of Africa, bordering the Indian Ocean between Kenya and Mozambique, it is slightly larger than twice the size of California. The largest city is Dar es Salaam; Dodoma, located in the center of the country, is the newly designated capital. Tanzania's population of 37.2 million is growing at 2.6% annually. About one-third of the population lives in urban areas, and more than half of all Tanzanians are younger than age 20. Ninety-nine percent of the population is African, coming from some 130 ethnic groups. An estimated 70 000 Arabs and 10 000 Europeans reside in Tanzania, with Arabs most numerous on Zanzibar. People of Lebanese, Palestinian and Indian origin dominate the merchant/trader class. Significant refugee populations from neighboring countries live in border areas.

Language

Swahili (Kiswahili), the primary official language in Tanzania, was developed along the coasts of Kenya and Tanzania as a trade language between Africans and Arabs. It is a mixture of various Bantu languages, Arabic and English. English, the second official language, is used in business, government and higher education.

More than 100 languages are spoken in Tanzania. Most people speak the language associated with their ethnic group, but they generally also speak Swahili. Julius Nyerere, the country's first president, made Swahili official at the time of independence from Britain, to foster pride in the people's African identity.

Religion

On the mainland, more than one-third of the population is Christian. Another third is Muslim. On Zanzibar, nearly all inhabitants are Muslim. About one-third of the population follows indigenous beliefs, although many of these people have also accepted some Christian or Islamic tenets. It is not unusual for professed Christians to mix their beliefs with local traditions. Thus, a local priest and a traditional healer might carry equal respect in a 'Christian' village. The two belief systems are not considered contradictory because each has a place in the people's daily lives. The government is neutral in religious matters and has tried to promote religious tolerance throughout the country.

Education

About 70% of all school-aged children begin primary school but fewer than 10% progress past the seventh grade. Boys are more likely than girls to get an education. As a result, there is a wide disparity between the male and female adult literacy rates, being 84% for males and 66% for females. There are several structural problems that cause difficulties in the education system. Primary school instruction is in Swahili, but English is the main language in secondary schools. As a result, students must change languages when they move to secondary school. There is also a chronic shortage of secondary school classrooms and teachers, so that students who would attend can't find room. Also, the government imposes a tax on students who attend secondary schools, which many parents can't afford to pay.

Economic system

Until the mid-1980s the country was committed to a socialist economy that Julius Nyerere optimistically hoped would foster political and economic self-reliance. However, world economic and political issues, together with serious blunders on the part of the Tanzanian government, contributed to a failed effort. The government of Tanzania has since embarked on a program of free-market reforms and has sold off most of its poorly performing parastatal businesses.

Agriculture still dominates the Tanzanian economy, employing 85% of the population and accounting for 85% of all exports. The industrial sector, which accounts for only about 10% of gross domestic product (GDP), is one of the smallest in Africa. Economic liberalization has encouraged private investment and the creation of new export products. Continued democratic reforms are expected to boost economic performance. However, corruption, mismanagement and regional problems still hamper the economy.

Tourism is a growing segment of the Tanzanian economy, accounting for 7.6% of GDP. The segment is growing rapidly, increasing 22% since the early 1990s, and brings in significant foreign exchange, e.g. $392 million in 1997 and $570 million in 1998. The government of Tanzania has established a National Tourism Policy and has set aside 25% of the land for wildlife and botanical sanctuaries, with the goal of attracting one million tourists a year by 2010. The government estimates that this will increase the sector contribution to GDP to 25%. However, significant investment in infrastructure, promotion and service skills must be made in order for this goal to be reached.

Women tend to enjoy equal access with men to income. Overall, however, people have limited availability of resources and opportunities necessary to pursue personal goals and rise above poverty. Half of the population lives in poverty and the real GDP per capita is $501. To generate some cash income, a family will often run an informal shop that sells produce, soda, soap and sundries, or they may find odd jobs to supplement low-paying wages.

Political and legal system

Tanzania is a democratic republic following a political union between Tanganyika and Zanzibar in 1964. It has three branches – an Executive, Legislative and Judicial – and contains 25 regions. The president (Benjamin Mkapa) is chief of state and the prime minister (Frederick Sumaye) is head of government. The National Assembly (Bunge) has 274 seats, 42 of which are reserved for appointees or specific officials. The voting age is 18. A five-level judiciary combines the jurisdictions of tribal, Islamic and British common law. Zanzibar is a semi-autonomous state with a separate parliament and elected president (Amani Karume).

The technology infrastructure

The ICT infrastructure in Tanzania is undergoing rapid modernization, and is no longer the major barrier it has been to the spread of email and full Internet services. The capital city, Dar es Salaam, has seen dramatic improvement of the local infrastructure, with many digital exchanges being installed, the availability of two cellular telephone networks and now, half a dozen Internet service providers.

Nevertheless, network access in areas outside Dar is still very limited. The multi-donor funded Tanzanian Telecommunications Restructuring Programme (TRP), responsible for much of the improvements in Dar, is also upgrading the links to many secondary towns. Fiber cable is being laid in Moshe and Arusha and the Dodoma-Dar-Zanzibar-Tanga-Moshe-Arusha microwave links are being digitized, as are links to Morogoro and Mwanza. Currently, telecommunication links in northern Tanzania (Arusha) are more reliable to Kenya than to the capital in the south.[9]

Value dimensions

Values are a society's ideas about what is good and bad, right or wrong, and will influence people to behave differently under similar circumstances. As a powerful component of a society's culture, values are communicated through the sub-systems described above and are passed from generation to generation. Most of the variations between cultures stem from underlying value systems, which cause people to behave differently under different circumstances. One framework for understanding how basic values underlie organizational behavior was proposed by Geert Hofstede, as the result of his research on over 116 000 people in over 53 countries.[10] Hofstede, who describes culture as the 'collective programming of the mind', identified five independent dimensions of national culture differences. He suggests that these five dimensions of values – each rooted in a basic problem, with which all societies have to cope, but on which their answers vary – can explain the differences among cultures. The dimensions are as follows:

- individualism versus collectivism
- power distance
- uncertainty avoidance
- masculinity versus femininity
- long-term versus short-term orientation.

Individualism refers to the tendency of people to look after themselves and their immediate families, rather than others. *Collectivist* cultures value the overall good of the group. The expectation is that people will subordinate their individual interests and needs for the benefit of the group. Hofstede's findings indicate that most countries scoring high on individualism have both a higher gross national product and a freer political system than those scoring low on individualism. Additionally, all countries scoring low on individualism score high on power distance. Tanzania, which scores low on individualism, predictably is poor and has an unequal distribution of power. In Tanzania, people typically look after each other in exchange for loyalty, emphasize belonging and make group decisions. Because being part of the group is so important it is often very clear how people in the group should behave.

Power distance is the extent to which less powerful members of organizations accept that power is unequally distributed. It ranges from small to large. A small power distance society such as the US is less comfortable with power differences such as social class distinction or organizational ranking. In a large power distance culture, differences among people with different ranks are accepted, and an individual's societal or organizational position influences how he acts and how others treat him. In Tanzania, a person in a high-level position treats those at lower levels with dignity, but the differences in rank are always clear. Delegating decision making implies incompetence because the rank of a high-status person requires him to make decisions himself. Employees in countries that rank high on power distance are more likely to prefer an autocratic leadership style and some paternalism because they are more comfortable with a clear distinction between managers and subordinates rather than with a blurring of decision-making responsibility.

Uncertainty avoidance, which ranges from strong to weak, focuses on the level of tolerance for uncertainty and ambiguity within the society. A low uncertainty avoidance ranking indicates the country has less concern about ambiguity and uncertainty and has more tolerance for a variety of opinions. This is reflected in a society that is less rule-oriented, more readily accepts change, and takes more and greater risks. Strong uncertainty avoidance countries like Tanzania have a low tolerance for uncertainty and ambiguity. This creates a rule-oriented society that institutes laws, rules, regulations and controls in order to reduce the amount of uncertainty. Such countries have a high need for security, concern for doing things correctly and great respect for experts.

Masculinity refers to the degree of typical 'masculine' values, such as assertiveness, materialism and lack of concern for others. *Femininity* in a society emphasizes concerns for others, relationships with others and quality of life. A high masculinity ranking indicates the country experiences a high degree of gender differentiation. In these cultures, males dominate a significant portion of the society and power structure, with females being controlled by male domination. A low masculinity ranking indicates the country has a low level of differentiation and discrimination between genders.

Long-term versus short-term orientation is a new dimension of national cultures that is independent of the four originally identified by Hofstede. Based on a Chinese values survey (CVS) developed by Michael Harris Bond, it appears to be based on items reminiscent of the teachings of Confucius, and refers to a valuing for persistence and thrift. East Asian countries scored highest on long-term orientation while Western countries scored on the low side. Some Third World countries scored the lowest.

In an attempt to explain why Africa, and particularly southern Africa, remains a 'development economist's headache', Hofstede set out to determine if there might be an 'African dimension' that would help to explain why Western recipes for development don't seem to work in Africa.[10] Development of an 'African values survey' failed to produce any new independent dimensions, but one factor opposed the African to the Asian countries on long-term orientation and thus did provide a possible explanation for their differences in development rate. This factor, called 'Wisdom', was comprised of items such as: 'It is important to show hospitality to strangers'; 'Wisdom is more important than knowledge'; 'Wisdom comes from experience and time, not from education'; and 'It is better to discuss a decision than to impose a decision'. Attributed wisdom that is not based on knowledge and education, however, is a dubious foundation for the development of a country. In his book, *Dark Star Safari*, travel journalist Paul Theroux provides a vivid description of the wisdom versus knowledge divide in Tanzania:

> *At one small halt in this great sun-baked emptiness a single tree grew, a mango of modest size but leafy with dense boughs. There was a circle of shade beneath it. Within that circle were thirty people, pressed against one another to keep in the shade, watched by a miserable goat tethered in the sunshine. What looked like a group game was obviously an afternoon routine of survival. As interesting to me as this packed-together mob of villagers around the lone tree trunk was the idea that no one in this hot exposed place had thought to plant more mango trees for the shade they offered. It was simple enough to plant a tree – this mango itself contained a thousand seeds – yet no one had planted one, or if anyone had, the tree had been cut down. The sight of these Africans in this tiny place in central Tanzania struggling to keep within a patch of shade stayed with me as a vivid instance of forward planning, or rather the lack of it.[11]*

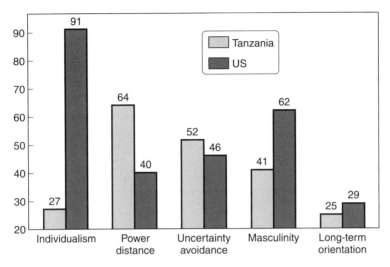

Figure 2.1 Hofstede's cultural dimensions.

Comparing the cultural profile of Tanzania to that of the US on Hofstede's five dimensions, one notes significant differences on several dimensions (*see* Figure 2.1). While the US can be described as very high on individualism and low on power distance, Tanzania is a culture high on collectivism (low individualism). As with most collective cultures, it is a poor country with high power distance. Thus, an individualistic telemedicine designer from the US with low power distance will dominate a collectivistic African who sees the American as 'in charge'. The low scores on long-term orientation for Tanzania convey a valuing for wisdom rather than knowledge and education. Importantly, the level of education is very low, with only a small percentage of people attending high school. This fact reinforces the African's view of Westerners as experts in telemedicine design. The scores for uncertainty avoidance are similar; however, the reasons are quite different. Tanzanians are comfortable with uncertainty because they tend to believe that what happens to them is due more to fate and chance than to their own ability to exert control and effect change. People in Tanzania tend to embrace feminine values such as looking after one another, and being polite and modest in behavior. A masculine approach to telemedicine design stresses the latest in gadgets and technology as being best. One might conclude that such a profile places Africans in a subservient position when dealing with Westerners on a design team. While oversimplified, many of the points raised in this cultural profile are a harbinger of the social norms uncovered in the next section.

The national healthcare system

The healthcare system in Tanzania is multi-leveled, and includes government-owned facilities, private hospitals and clinics, and traditional medicine practiced in the villages. The patient has the option of going to a government clinic or hospital, a private hospital, the village healer or some combination.

The government of Tanzania owns and operates a series of clinics and hospitals that operate on a Western, disease-oriented model. They were developed during the post-colonial socialist period and were heavily supported by development agencies. With the reduction in the level of aid, the quality of the government system of clinics and hospitals has deteriorated. The system tends to be substandard compared with comparable Western systems.

The government of Tanzania has a healthcare policy that also includes private hospitals. However, these hospitals serve specific constituencies and are generally not open to the ordinary Tanzanian villager. This is so because the lack of physical infrastructure, such as roads and public transit, prevents the villager from getting to the private clinic, and economics such as the cost of drugs and other resources, prevent them from being able to purchase the services that are uniquely available at private clinics.

At the village level, the primary healthcare system is administered by traditional healthcare providers using a magico-religious belief system. In the magico-religious approach, health and illness are closely linked to supernatural forces. Mystical powers, typically outside of human control, cause health and illness.[12] Traditional medicine consists of two broad categories of preventive/protective and curative activities. Oral treatments – what we in the West would consider magic – are combined with medicinal herbs to promote health and cure ailments.[13]

Family and gender roles in the healthcare context

The healthcare system in the US typically focuses solely on the individual patient as the source of a medical problem in need of a cure. In a collective and group-oriented culture such as Tanzania, the family assumes a large role in the functioning of the healthcare system and the interaction of the two systems can be the basis of serious problems and misunderstandings. Cultures that value the community or the extended family, for instance, may require the involvement and agreement of other family members, not just the patient. They also may influence people's willingness to keep important healthcare appointments.

Many cultures have strong expectations about modesty, and the bodily displays of women can make the medical examination itself a source of intercultural difficulties. In some cultures, role requirements governing appropriate behaviors for women do not permit undressing for an examination by male physicians or nurses.[12]

Conversational structures and language

Because of different interaction norms, the medical interview between caregiver and patient can be another source of intercultural communication problems. Some collective or high-context cultures may engage in extensive small talk before indicating their reasons for the medical interview. Similarly, direct and explicit discussions may cause the patient discomfort, while the use of indirection or other face-saving strategies may be preferred. In many cultures, doctors are perceived as authority figures with whom one must agree in the face-to-face medical interview. A patient may know that they will not be able to follow a proposed treatment plan but will be reluctant to respond to the doctor in a way that might appear to be a challenge to the doctor's authority.[12]

The healthcare scenarios – the social systems

In order to understand more clearly how the cultural environment would influence the behavior of individuals within the social system in the Tanzanian culture, a series of health scenarios was developed to test various hypotheses about how patients, doctors and nurses would respond to common healthcare situations. Each scenario envisions a fictitious patient living in an African village who is faced with different kinds of health problems of varying severity.

Interviews were conducted with African nationals studying in the US, who had experience with, and knowledge of, healthcare practices in their home countries. Their responses were analyzed for information to expand and enrich our understanding of the sociocultural environment. The issue for the respondents was to report what each of the participants in the scenario was thinking or doing, and how they would react based on the respondents' African heritage and the availability of healthcare choices. From the interpretations provided by the respondents, characteristics of the social system were identified and probable role expectations regarding the primary participants in the system – the doctor, the nurse and the patient – were deduced.

First scenario – different realities

The first scenario dealt with the treatment of common ailments, such as malaria. Respondents were asked to describe the steps a mother might take to obtain treatment for her child.

The respondents reported that, as the first line of defense, the mother or patient would use traditional medicines, such as herbs and barks, to treat the illness. They themselves were familiar with these traditional remedies, and viewed them as a basic requirement for daily life. It was suggested that the patient might go to a clinic if the treatment using the traditional approaches to the symptoms didn't work. The decision to go to a Western clinic, however, generally is made after consultation with other family members or parents, and frequently with input from the tribal elders.

When one person is ill, the rest of the village observes the treatment, which may be Western medications, traditional herbs or some combination of both. The knowledge gained, good or bad, becomes part of the collective wisdom of the village and will be used the next time someone contracts the same illness.

The decision regarding which combination of traditional and Western medicine to seek depends not only on the patient's predisposition towards traditional medicines and their effectiveness, but also on the patient's perception of how well he or she will be treated at the Western clinic and whether he or she can afford the cost. Generally, the patient will only go to a clinic for treatment:

- if the illness doesn't respond to traditional approaches
- if a clinic is available

- if the patient can afford treatment and medications
- if the medications are available at the clinic.

Since there are more clinics in the cities than in the rural areas, the probability that patients will access Western, clinic-based healthcare is greater in the urban areas.

The respondents discussed the deterioration of Western healthcare in many African countries over the past several years. As the healthcare capacity of these countries has declined, so too has trust in Western healthcare. As reported by the respondents, the general population does not have a very positive perception of healthcare workers. They are perceived as poorly trained and not well motivated. The perception of doctors is better, but the chronic shortage of doctors in most African countries makes this a moot point.

Several critical themes emerged from an analysis of the responses to the issues posed in this scenario. The most important was that most patients in a village setting within developing African countries hold different perceptions of reality when it comes to healthcare than do doctors and nurses. The patient is part of a village-based social system, which embodies a traditional view of healthcare, while doctors and nurses, trained in a Western tradition, are part of a different social system and see healthcare from a different reality. A way must be found to reconcile these two realities before a telemedicine system can be successfully introduced.

The second theme to emerge is the existence of economic and structural boundaries that make access to Western medicine difficult for the patient. Western-based healthcare systems in developing countries are often of poor quality and unevenly distributed between urban and rural populations. There is also the perception that nurses, and to a lesser extent doctors, are incompetent and poorly motivated, and corruption is rampant in the healthcare system. Both themes provide powerful barriers to the introduction of telemedicine in countries like Tanzania.

Second scenario – a stranger in a strange land

The patient in the second scenario has an illness that has gotten worse and hasn't responded to traditional remedies. She visits a local healthcare clinic, which is linked to a doctor using ICT. This scenario introduces the concept of a teleconsult or healthcare delivered from a distance, using technology.

The responses to the second scenario point out many of the communications difficulties that ensue when technology becomes the channel through which the patient in one social system is expected to communicate with a doctor in another. It was suggested that mediation of the communication process with an ICT system and an unfamiliar doctor would tend to confuse and frustrate the patient. Respondents felt that the patient would have a problem trusting a doctor who is seen for the first time on a TV screen. They also stated that trust and communication might improve if the doctor were introduced to the village people and if their picture were posted around the village as a way to become 'real'.

The scheduling aspects of telemedicine consults are more crucial than with face-to-face medicine because the patient and doctor must arrive at two different places at the same time. A precise schedule conflicts with the more casual concept of time held by Africans, who don't feel the need to keep track of it and manage it as Westerners do. This pertains not only to the patients but to the healthcare workers as well. In addition, the patient who lives far from the clinic will have difficulty arriving on time for an appointment because of the poor physical infrastructure in many African countries. Both of these issues may hamper enforcement of a strict telemedicine schedule.

It was generally felt that the presence of a camera in the exam room would be perceived as an invasion of the patient's privacy. In Muslim and some tribal cultures, taking pictures is considered rude and socially unacceptable; disrobing in front of the camera is even more unacceptable, particularly if the patient has not met the doctor face to face at some point.

Several themes relating to cross-cultural communications emerged from the issues posed in this scenario.

- High context versus low context cultures. Tanzania is a high-context culture where the communication between patient and healer typically entails a silent language that transmits shared meaning about the relationship, trust, time, collectivism and religion. In a telemedicine system, with technology as the channel of communication, the environment becomes low context and challenges most of the attitudes and behaviors inherent in the traditional system. Typically, when familiar cues are removed from the communication context, the person experiences anxiety and culture shock.
- Trust versus professionalism. A 'doc in a box' replaces face-to-face interaction between patient and healer. The trust in another person nurtured throughout a long-term relationship is replaced by distrust in strangers one has not met before.
- Time: monochronic versus polychronic. The polychronic pace of time in the village is replaced by the schedule of a Western organization. Lack of transportation and telephone systems militate against getting to an appointment on time. The more relaxed concept of time that ensues in most collectivist cultures, where primary importance is put on relationships, runs counter to the rules of scheduling that protect the valuable time of the doctor.
- Rules of modesty. Finally, the rules of modesty inherent in the religious beliefs are seriously compromised if the patient is expected to disrobe or bare parts of her body before a stranger. The issue of being photographed by a movie camera raises additional taboos.

Third scenario – an ethical dilemma

The third scenario deals with the treatment of a life-threatening illness such as HIV/AIDS, and raises the issue of moving a dying patient from one social system, the tribal village, to another, a Western hospital.

In this situation, as with the others, the predisposition of the patient is to consult with the traditional healer first. In this case, however, the family might seek help from Western medicine when the traditional medications don't work. The patient will still balance the advice of the doctor with that of the healer when deciding what combination of care to follow.

Traditional healers generally do not have the capability of diagnosing HIV; therefore, when AIDS develops, the traditional healer will often misdiagnose the illness as the flu or some other common ailment and treat accordingly. When the treatment doesn't work, the patient will likely believe he is cursed, which will be confirmed by the traditional healer. The healer will use magic to attack the curse that he perceives within the patient and his family. When magic fails, the patient is faced with two choices. He may give up and die or, he may go to a Western hospital for treatment. At the Western hospital, fear of the AIDS virus isolates the patient from other patients and the hospital staff, and because of lack of effective treatment, the patient dies, essentially alone.

The most important theme to emerge from this scenario is the ethics of taking the patient from a social system in which he is cared for to one in which he obtains medical care. A treatment that imparts fear, isolation and death seems far less humane than one in which the patient dies with support from family and tribal members. Neither cures the illness but the death that follows traditional medicine seems more humane than the one that results from Western medicine. If no cure exists, is it better not to know and die with hope or is it better to hope and die in isolation? The responses to the scenarios confirmed that the social system is far more complex than originally conceived.

Table 2.1 The health subsystems in Tanzania

Characteristics	Traditional health care	Western-based health care
Location of health care delivery	Village-based	Hospital and clinic-based
Concept of health and wellness	Magico-religious	Disease model
Treatments	Traditional medicines	Western medicines
Practitioners	Traditional healers	Doctors, nurses, technology
Family roles in health care	Patient and family are partners in decision making	Patient carrier of disease to be cured
Communication patterns	High context	Low context
	Trust	Professionalism
	Polychronic time	Monochronic time

The system consists of two health subsystems, traditional and Western, populated by people with two separate paradigms of health and wellness (*see* Table 2.1). Rather than being part of the same social system, the doctor and nurse are part of the Western subsystem while the patient is in the traditional subsystem. In order for telemedicine to work, the barriers separating these two subsystems must be bridged.

The technical system

The technical system should be designed to address the two primary criteria of the STS approach. It should be optimal for the cultural environment in which it operates and compatible with the healthcare-related social systems.

Designing an optimal system does not mean using the most advanced technology available, but rather using technology that is appropriate for the local environment. Generally, the key is that the technology should suit the level of development in the country, as well as the specific site at which it is installed. According to Field, the technology components of a telemedicine system should be off-the-shelf, rather than customized; have a low level of sophistication to learn and operate; and be individually upgradeable. Also, each component must be compatible with all other components.[14] In addition, the design team identified two further characteristics required for the technology to function in the national subsystems of Tanzania. The technology must be inexpensive to purchase and maintain, and it must be compatible with local telephone infrastructure and upgradeable if and when the infrastructure has improved.

The other consideration has to do with the joint operations of the technology with the social systems in Tanzania. The design team addressed the issue of compatibility with the healthcare social systems at MMH. The following are some of the preliminary design criteria that were identified:

- The patient and the doctor must be able to see each other in real time.
- Data, both text and pictures, must be able to be transmitted quickly and accurately, while the patient is still at the clinic.
- There must be a simple way of maintaining and accessing a patient record on both ends of the technology.
- Running counter to the above three requirements of the social systems, the technology must be complex and expensive enough so that the people using it *perceive it* as a valuable addition.

A demonstration system, using a hub-and-spoke technology design emerged from the process. Cameras, computers, the Internet and the local telephone infrastructure satisfied the basic requirements for an effectively functioning technology system (*see* Figure 2.2). The result was a combination system consisting of a camera at each site to transmit and receive live interactive video between sites, and a computer with a web cam to capture and transmit video clips and still pictures over the Internet as attachments to emails. Email was used as the vehicle to transmit written data with the pictures. A modified contact manager database was used as the patient record for the purposes of a demonstration, understanding that this part of the technology needs further refinement.

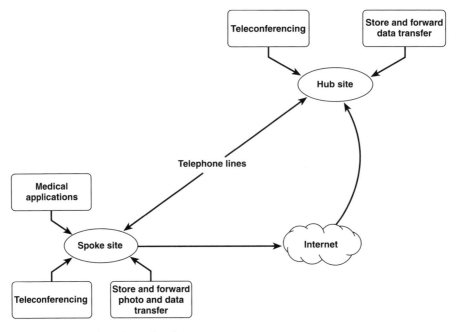

Figure 2.2 Hub and spoke technology.

The Kairuki Mikocheni Model (KMM)

The partnership forged between the Kairuki family and the North American team resulted in the development of a new consulting model which has been used throughout the intervening years to percolate innovation at Mission Mikocheni Hospital.[15] Placing a telemedicine system in a developing country such as Tanzania is far more difficult than first envisioned. It requires skill in negotiating the myriad sociocultural boundaries discussed earlier in this chapter, as well as technical knowledge and expenditure of energy over a significant period of time. Conventional consulting models haven't worked in Africa, primarily because they stress technical solutions to problems that have their roots in the cultural environment. The model that emerged from this partnership provides an altern-ative paradigm in which an international consulting team of both Western and local partners can collaborate to design and develop an effective telemedicine system.

The model is based on participative action research (AR), with several import-ant additions. Action research is a methodology by which meaningful work is performed and through which solutions to problems emerge. It is a process by which real-world problems in a society can be addressed by the people who have to live with the solutions they develop. Because of its emergent nature, new methods of practice and theory are brought into focus. The process of AR is cyclical and consists of five elements:

- diagnosis
- action planning
- action taking

- evaluation
- learning.

The researchers move back and forth through the elements in a somewhat messy process from which answers become apparent. In more complex social change processes, as described here, the learning that emerges from one solution often opens up new issues to explore. Thus, the KMM adds a linear component as well as the cyclical one, to the AR process (*see* Figure 2.3).

An international organization of equal partners, called the Client Consultant System Infrastructure (CCSI) is the cornerstone of the structure of the KMM. It is through this ad hoc organization that innovative work is done. Its defining characteristics, what Maturana calls criteria of distinction,[16] are as follows:

- an ad hoc, multinational, multicultural, social entity of equal partners
- oriented towards the goal of improving healthcare access and capacity
- structurally coupled to multiple environments with different cultures.

People may move in and out of the CCSI as needed, but the members are equal partners in the consulting process. In this model, the role of the consultant is significantly different from the expert model of consulting typically used in Africa. In the expert model, the consultant is assumed to be able to diagnose the problem and implement a solution that both the client and the consultant assume will work. The consultant remains separate from and outside the client system. In the KMM, by contrast, the consultant actually becomes a member of the client system, and fills different multiple roles as required, such as facilitator, teacher, resource coordinator and even dream weaver. Rather than being experts from afar, promoting inequality and dependence, the consultant becomes a participant in a group process.

The success of the CCSI is enhanced by a process of structural coupling. Maturana defines structural coupling as recurrent interaction that produces structural changes in the interacting entities.[16] The key activity in this concept is the mutual recurrent interaction that results in the structural linking of the parties. Practically, it means sleeping in your host's house, eating what he eats and developing empathy for the life he leads and the difficulties he faces. It means listening to his stories and telling him yours until you both create a common world. This recurrent interaction changes both participants, not only linking them to each other but to each other's environment as well. The process of structural coupling is the glue that holds the CCSI together and maintains its links to the various cultural environments.

The final component of the KMM, the interlude, is an outgrowth of the consultant being inside the CCSI as a participant, instead of outside as an observer. While an insider, the consultant can interact with other insiders, e.g. the client system, and facilitate the change within the AR model. In the process, however, the consultant gives up the privileged position as a researcher that allows them to understand the relationships between the client system and its environment. The interlude, a time between periods of activity when members of the CCSI are not working as a unit, is a period of reflection in which the participant/consultant withdraws from the system and examines what has been accomplished in the role of researcher/observer.[15]

The model described here addresses the cultural and social issues raised earlier in this chapter. Because the CCSI is an organization of equals who are structurally coupled to each other and to the multiple social systems and cultural environments that exist in an international telemedicine project, the barriers to communication and to cultural understanding are more likely to be overcome and the misunderstandings that result from individuals interacting from different cultural vantage points are lessened.

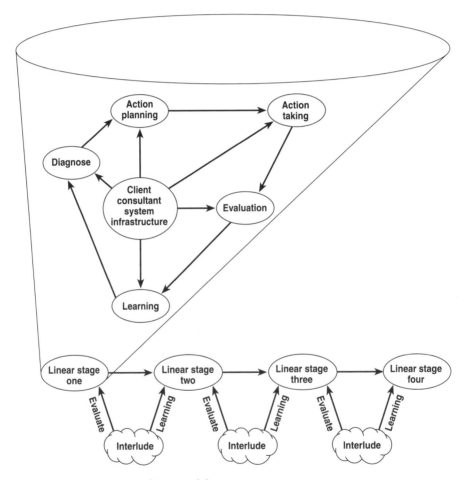

Figure 2.3 The KMM consulting model.

Summary and conclusions

This chapter shows that placing a telemedicine system into a developing country such as Tanzania is far more difficult than first envisioned. The cross-cultural interface between the Western technology and consultants and the local healthcare users of the telemedicine system presents enormous challenges that must be addressed if telemedicine is to succeed in developing countries.

Using the STS approach, we developed a cultural profile of Tanzania to describe what Hofstede calls 'the collective programming of the mind'.

An analysis of the cultural environment and the national values in Tanzania identified several critical differences between Western cultures and the culture of Tanzania. Subsequently, we developed a series of healthcare scenarios to provide us with additional information about the social system in which healthcare functions in Tanzania. Analysis of the responses of a group of African nationals to the scenarios indicated that significant differences exist between social subsystems. These differences serve as barriers to communication and cooperative efforts. In several important ways, the use of technology accentuates these barriers. Ways must be found to transcend these cultural and social boundaries if telemedicine is to work.

The second challenge addressed in this chapter is the complex role of the international design team. It was noted that telemedicine consultants are frequently from a different country and cultural background than the users. Unless they are aware of the cultural differences operating in the host culture, they unintentionally build failure into the system design. Compounding the problem is a national proclivity in many African countries to accept the superiority of the solution coming from outside experts. Finally, a telemedicine system is often expected to operate on an inter-country basis as well, where a consult may take place between a physician in a medical facility in the US and a physician in an urban hospital in Tanzania. A collaborative action research-based model, such as the Kairuki Mikocheni Model, provides a way for multiple social systems and cultures to develop a working relationship, potentially overcoming the barriers that isolate cultures and social groups. It empowers multinational designers and practitioners to structurally couple with the disparate cultural environments and health subsystems and stands the best chance of allowing an appropriate telemedicine system to develop.

In conclusion, telemedicine systems that attempt to function across national boundaries must integrate various understandings about differences in cultures, health subsystems, and paradigms of health and wellness. The system is vastly more complex than most design consultants envision. As Hofstede states in the companion article to this section, 'assuming that with so-called modern management techniques and theories outsiders can develop a country has proven a deplorable arrogance. At best, one can hope for a dialogue between equals with the locals, in which the Western partner acts as the expert in Western technology and the local partner as the expert in local culture, habits and feelings.'[2] The challenge in the development of telemedicine is to develop the dialogue among equals. The relationship between consultants and the funders who develop telemedicine on the one hand, and the users of telemedicine on the other, make the dialogue inherently unequal. Collaboration with local partners in development and implementation of telemedicine systems doesn't make the inequality disappear. The perception of inequality persists, institutionalizing the actual inequality. Hofstede emphasizes that cultural infrastructure cannot be pressure-cooked, it takes time to grow. In our view, however, cultural infrastructure will not grow by itself. It has to have a vehicle to transcend the boundaries that exist between cultures.

References

1   Coombs R and Hull R (1996) The politics of IT in organizations. In: Dutton WH (ed.) *Information and Communication Technologies: visions and realities*. OUP, Oxford.

2   Hofstede G (1993) Cultural constraints in management theories. *Academy of Management Executive*. 7: 81–93.

3   WHO Group Consultation on Health Telematics (1997) *A Health Telematics Policy: in support of the WHO's Health-for-all strategy for global health development*. WHO, Geneva, pp. 11–16.

4   Davis LE and Trist E (1974) Improving the quality of working life: sociotechnical case studies. In: O'Toole J (ed.) *Work and the Quality of Life*. MIT Press, Cambridge, MA.

5   Deresky H (2002) *Global Management: strategic and interpersonal*. Prentice Hall, Upper Saddle River, NJ.

6   Hall ET (1977) *Beyond Culture*. Anchor Books, Garden City, NY.

7   Harris PR and Moran RT (1991) *Managing Cultural Differences*. Gulf Publishing, Houston, TX.

8   CultureGrams (2004) *United Republic of Tanzania*. Axiom Press, Linden, UT.

9   Jensen M (2002) The African Internet: a status report. www3.sn.apc.org/africa/afstat.htm

10 Hofstede G (2001) *Culture's Consequences: comparing values, behaviors, institutions, and organizations across nations*. Sage Publications, Thousand Oaks, CA.

11 Theroux P (2003) *Dark Star Safari: overland from Cairo to Cape Town*. Houghton Mifflin, New York.

12 Lustig MW and Koester J (1999) *Intercultural Competence: interpersonal communication across cultures*. Addison Wesley Longman, New York.

13 Makinde A (1998) *African Philosophy, Culture and Traditional Medicine*. Ohio University Center for International Studies, Athens, OH.

14 Field MJ (ed.) (1996) *Telemedicine: a guide to assessing telecommunications in healthcare*. National Academy Press, Washington, DC.

15 Katzenstein J (2000) Developing an innovative international consulting model within a private healthcare system in Tanzania. PhD dissertation. Field Graduate Institute.

16 Maturana HR and Varela FJ (1987) *The Tree of Knowledge: the biological roots of human understanding*. Shambhala, Boston, MA.

Chapter 3

E-health for doctors in rural and urban India

CB Sridhar and Deena Suresh

The Information Age has made profound changes in society and is gradually penetrating the healthcare segment. The Internet, the World Wide Web (www) and telemedicine are some of the significant areas where rapid transition is occurring. Millions of physicians, healthcare providers and patients are accessing the Web daily for patient information, consultation and distance learning.[1]

Since India's independence from British rule in 1947, the country has made significant progress in the field of health and its delivery to the masses. For example, smallpox has been completely eradicated, the infant mortality rate has been brought down, life expectancy has gone up, pre and postnatal care has improved and there is overall progress in disease control and establishment of a modern health infrastructure.[2] A high standard of healthcare comparable to that occurring in developed countries is being offered to patients at affordable costs. There is room for improvement in practically every area of healthcare. Each day, the number of online medicine-related documents grow, and many can be accessed via the Internet. This powerful free-flow of information holds the promise of improving the standard of healthcare in many ways.[3]

Information technology has played a vital role in hastening the spread of healthcare to urban and rural areas in India. The Internet – 'an interconnection of networks' – has revolutionized the communications world like never before.[4,5]

Background to our projects

Medical advice through correspondence, letters, etc. has been in practice for several years. It is a routine system to communicate by letters to referring doctors. These letters used to be thorough, extensive and very informative pertaining to the care of the patients referred. The patients were encouraged to follow the guidelines given in the letter and keep in contact with the doctors as and when needed. In fact, this system of communication became so well established that all consultants were expected to follow this procedure. Failing to do so called for punitive measures from the hospital board. The busy resident doctors in hospitals are encouraged to discuss patient problems on the phone with senior consultants and put this in writing with the date and time on the case file. Thus it is possible to offer a high-quality service to patients on a regular basis (personal communication, CB Sridhar, 2002).

Other mediums used by doctors to provide tips on diagnosis or treatment of ailments include newspaper columns and/or radio and TV broadcasts. Tele-medicine through correspondence involved a considerable time lapse between the patient's query and the advice of the doctor, and protected the privacy of the patient. The response to queries through radio and TV broadcasts acceler-ated the spread of information and, like the newspapers, had the advantage of being both specific to the query as well as being shared by other members of the audience.

At present, e-health has a variety of purposes. Some of the more common purposes include:

- remote consultation
- second opinion
- interpretation services
- continuing education and exchange of clinical information
- home care
- online surgery in some very rare cases.

Of all these, the first three are common the world over.[2]

Doctors in India have various barriers to accessing medical information from the Internet. Various studies have elaborated these barriers.[8,9] The barriers and constraints include:

- lack of time to browse for medical information
- individual economic hardship
- poor infrastructure
- on duty/call most of the time
- population per physician is 1916.[7]

Looking into the cultural context, few countries in the world have such an ancient and diverse culture as India's. Stretching back in an unbroken sweep over 5000 years, India's culture has been enriched by successive waves of migration, which were absorbed into the Indian way of life. The Internet is proving to be a popular networking technology. The phenomenal advances in communications and information technology in India are resulting in a new look at how secondary and tertiary healthcare can be provided to the underprivileged masses. Following proof of concept validation, ISRO (Indian Space Research Organization) in conjunction with the Apollo Hospitals is ready to use satellite technology to provide specialist care not only within India but to other countries as well, by using the large number of highly qualified and trained specialists in urban India.[15]

Aware of the above limitations on access to medical information, Recon Healthcare Ltd, Bangalore, India, initiated a system of sending the required information quickly and in a cost-effective manner. This was done with the aim of spreading medical information to a large number of doctors in India. Two projects were taken and successfully completed. The two projects are discussed below.

Project 1: Internet as a tool to procure and spread medical information to doctors in India

Data procured in the year 2002 reported that there are 7 million Internet users in India.[6] In this paper, the percentage of requests by doctors for medical information from the Internet has been compiled for the period 1 July 1998 to 9 July 2002. The doctors consisted of physicians, surgeons, medical students and postgraduate trainees. Invariably, the information has been used by doctors to update medical care, emergency care, thesis/dissertation, publication of case reports, articles and presentation of data.

From the data on file regarding medical queries from doctors we separated medical information Internet requests from medical information non-Internet requests. Medical information from the Internet was pertaining to diagnostic techniques, conference details, withdrawal of molecules, surgical techniques, guidelines for treatment, abstracts of clinical studies comprising of efficacy, safety and tolerability, case reports and update on emergency care.

Exclusion criteria in this population were medical information not procured from the Internet and inclusion criteria were medical information procured from the Internet. Two hundred and seventy eight such Internet requests were received. These data were compared with information sought from non-Internet requests as procured from standard journals, textbooks and from our literature on file.

Results and discussion

Statistical analysis

Bar diagrams: annual increase in the number of Internet requests, Internet requests from India, Internet requests from south, west, east and north India, Internet versus non-Internet requests. Pie chart: the percentage distribution of Internet requests split into four regions in India is illustrated. The statistical analysis was done using the Student's 't'-test.

Results

The bar diagram in Figure 3.1 shows the gradual increase in the number of Internet requests. The year 2002 figure is requests made up to 9 July.

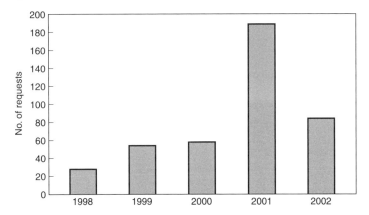

Figure 3.1 Annual increase in the number of requests.

The number of requests was segregated based on the four zones – east, west, north and south. The percentage request is shown in Figure 3.2. We observed that the maximum requests were from metropolitan cities – Bangalore (131), followed by Mumbai (23), Kolkata (14) and Delhi (25).

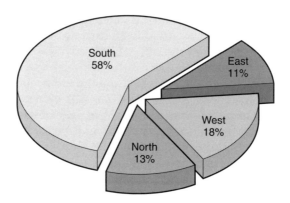

Figure 3.2 Percentage distribution of Internet requests.

An increasing trend in Internet requests was observed in this study.

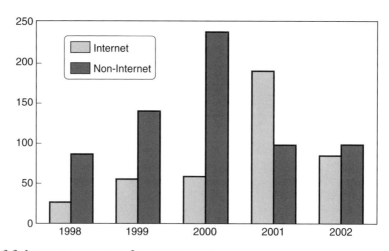

Figure 3.3 Internet versus non-Internet requests.

Figure 3.3 shows an interesting trend when comparing non-Internet requests with Internet requests through the years 1998, 1999, 2000, 2001 and 2002. During the first three years there were considerably more non-Internet requests than Internet requests and this was statistically significant for the year 1999 ($p > 0.05$) and 2000 ($p > 0.005$). From January 2001, the medical department sent regular emails to doctors informing them of the Internet facility being made available free of cost. It is clear that this approach of contacting doctors has paid dividends in the form of more Internet requests in the years 2001 and 2002, as shown in Figure 3.4. Added to this, continuing medical education (CME) programs were conducted and at these programs doctors were informed about the medical information services we offered. We saw a subsequent rise in the number of requests.

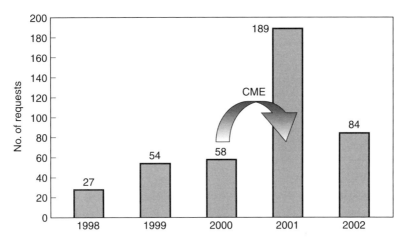

Figure 3.4 Increase in Internet requests following CME.

We are interested in assessing the impact of CME in rural cities. In this study we have defined rural as that area where a large percentage of people are dependent on agriculture for income and livelihood. We are aware that in today's world of globalization this might not be an appropriate criterion. For want of a better definition, we have taken this for our presentation.

Among the rural Indian cities, it was observed that Tumkur in Karnataka tops the list with 34 requests. This is a very encouraging trend and is sure to add to the knowledge of doctors in the field of medicine where the developments are occurring in an explosive way.

In a publication on Internet usage in training hospitals in Mumbai, India, it was revealed that among 182 medical students interviewed, approximately 40% surfed the Internet. Of those using the Internet, only 15% surfed for medical information. Of the 180 medical interns interviewed, at least 65% surfed the Internet. Of these, less than 25% used the Internet for medical information. Of the 106 resident doctors interviewed, almost 50% surfed the Internet. Of the 56 lecturers, only about 25% used the Internet to search for medical information. We would like to focus on the fact that of the 28 professionals, only about 25% found time to access the Internet on a fortnightly irregular basis. The above paper also informs us about access to Internet knowledge by the students, interns, resident doctors and lecturers in teaching hospitals in Mumbai and the inadequate usage of the same for furthering their knowledge.[8]

Geyoushi and Stones conducted a study to identify the constraints and facilitators to evidence-based practice, and the participants' perception about these barriers and facilitators. Forty-one doctors (28 from India and 13 from the Yemen) working in the field of reproductive healthcare, whether obstetrics and gynecology, general practice or family planning, participated in this study.

Barriers to implementation were lack of information sources, the paucity of resources, and difficulties in access. Economic institutional constraints due to a poor infrastructure and some cultural restrictions were identified as were lack of incentive and demotivation due to an inbred hierarchical system. Lack of time and individual economic hardships were also identified factors as was the irrelevance of some Western technology. Potential facilitators included medical family networking, teaching commitments and medical societies as a method of information distribution. The most important facilitator identified was the free availability of information through the Internet.

There are many barriers and constraints to implementing evidence-based reproductive healthcare in developing countries, whether on individual or institutional levels. Understanding these difficulties can help to overcome some of these barriers and offer practical solutions. Although the main problems revolve around economic and financial constraints, offering support from developed countries must go hand in hand with introducing, developing and maintaining a culture of evidence-based practice and mentality. This is essential if any of the solutions are to work.[9]

Our communication, in sharp contrast, is focusing on practicing doctors in India. More than 90% of our requests are from practicing doctors. In the Thakkar study,[8] the group had to access information themselves. However, in our study we received requests to access information for doctors. This difference can be explained by the fact that in the Thakkar study, residents reported few good facilities for accessing the Internet on campus, they were on call almost every other day and they had very little time to do more than check emails. No wonder a busy practicing doctor in an urban or rural area finds it impossible to spare his valuable time to browse the Internet for medical information. It is in this context that our communication assumes tremendous importance. We have shown that it is possible for us to communicate directly with doctors at their doorsteps, provided they have an Internet facility in their office or a cyber café near their area of practice.[10,11]

Project 2: Recon Healthcare Bangalore Model in spreading information from World Health Organization Reproductive Healthcare Library (WHO-RHL) to doctors in India

The WHO-RHL is one of the major sources of information pertaining to reproductive healthcare knowledge. It is the product of interaction between the WHO-RHL, research centers in developing countries and the Cochrane Collaboration. It is the first specialist database project for the Cochrane Collaboration, as well as for the WHO, and has followed evidence-based medicine. The information is stored on diskettes and CD-ROM, is updated annually and is available free to developing countries.[12]

The WHO-RHL contains systematic reviews of controlled trials on critical reproductive health topics, expert commentaries on the relevance of the findings for developing countries and practical advice on the management of reproductive health problems. The systematic reviews come from The Cochrane Library. The commentaries and practical advice are prepared by researchers from developing countries or by persons with extensive knowledge of the conditions and practice in those countries.

As this is in an electronic medium, one has to evolve methodologies by which this vast content of knowledge could be spread to doctors working in various parts of India – both rural and urban.[13] Doctors in rural India and many parts of urban India do not have easy access to this information. Therefore, it has become essential to come up with an effective system to achieve this. Academia usually has an enormous knowledge base without much of a facility to disseminate this rapidly. Industry, on the other hand, has facilities to communicate rapidly with doctors through their marketing executives, and via email. The combination of these two organizations becomes an effective method to spread knowledge rapidly to doctors whenever needed. When done this turns out to be a good example of academia–industry interaction (AII), with academia such as the WHO providing the knowledge base, and industry offering support for its dissemination. To the best of our knowledge, such an exercise in AII to spread medical knowledge in developing countries or developed countries has not been published.

Evidence-based healthcare involves deriving questions from clinical problems, searching systematically and thoroughly for the best relevant evidence, critically appraising the evidence and applying new knowledge in the clinical context. Although most clinicians support the notion of evidence-based healthcare in principle and wish to use this information generated by others, only a tiny fraction seek to acquire all the requisite skills themselves. A study in British general practice found that the commonest reason cited for not practicing evidence-based healthcare was lack of time followed by personal and organizational inertia.[14]

Materials and method

At Recon Healthcare, Bangalore, the medical department has taken the initiative to spread the information in the WHO-RHL to doctors, particularly gynecologists and obstetricians. This was done jointly with the marketing executives. Three topics were chosen from 18 topics after a consensus among the non-medical executives of the organization.

- Routine antenatal care for low-risk pregnancy.
- Routine iron and folate supplementation in pregnancy.
- Episiotomy policies in vaginal birth.

The titles were printed on a sheet and sent to 313 business officers of Recon Healthcare working all over India, with instructions to hand over the format to gynecologists and obstetricians in their area. Each business officer received ten such forms. The doctors were requested to enter their preferences and return their form to the officer, who would mail it to the Bangalore office. We expected responses from up to 3130 gynecologists and obstetricians.[11]

This study was initiated on 1 September 2001 and by 31 March 2002, 1346 doctors had responded and the faculty in medical department had received these forms. These were analyzed and the results are presented overleaf.

Results

The overall response in the four regions of India was as follows: west 58.04%, north 51.21%, south 32.62% and east 44.29%. To get feedback on the WHO-RHL information given to doctors, the questions in Table 3.1 were sent to the doctors (personal communication, Vishwanath Anantraman, 2002).

Table 3.1 Doctors' questionnaire

Questions	Answers (%)	
	Yes	No
Did you receive the WHO-RHL updates?	94	6
Was the write-up useful?	88.87	7.13
Did this help you in improving patient care?	83.73	10.7
Was the information applied in your practice?	78.48	13.4
Would you like to share this knowledge with your other doctor colleagues?	58.32	34.6

Discussion

The existing infrastructure being utilized for routine office work was used for the model. The postal charges amounted to Rs 32 520; stationery, including cartridge and paper, amounted to Rs 29 500. Hence, the total amounted to Rs 62 020. The expenditure incurred for disseminating medical information works out to Rs 46 per doctor (*see* Table 3.1). So, this model is a cost-effective one.

Table 3.2 Postal and stationery charges

Postal	Rs 32 520
Stationery (cartridge and paper)	Rs 29 500
Total	Rs 62 020 (= ~ $1240)
Cost per doctor	Rs 46

We have established a clear methodology by which knowledge could be disseminated, making use of already existing facilities such as Microsoft Windows 98, CD-ROM drive and a printer. Thus, no additional expensive infrastructure has been required. We named this model the Recon Healthcare Bangalore Model (RHBM) for disseminating medical knowledge to doctors in India.[15]

The following are the high points of RHBM.

- Making use of the available facility in the Corporate offices, which is used for other official work of the organization.
- Interaction with doctors, which is an already existing exercise.
- To this has been added dissemination of WHO-RHL information.
- 1346 doctors have been surveyed within a period of seven months at a cost of Rs 46 per doctor.

It is not possible for us to compare this with any other data, as such data are not yet available anywhere in developing countries. We are not aware of such data from a developed country either.

WHO-RHL information has been communicated to doctors across India. This is one of the primary objectives of WHO. Without any additional inputs, and with the methodology established in the RHBM, it should be possible for academia and industry to interact and spread the knowledge of WHO-RHL to a very large number of doctors in India within the shortest possible time. Our model has demonstrated that this is possible. Thus, making use of the already existing information technology in our country, we should be able to improve the standards of healthcare all over India. Similar models could be evolved to spread the health knowledge in other developing countries in all spheres of health knowledge.[13]

Usefulness of e-health in India

For e-health to be really useful in India it would have to reach the rural areas rather than merely enhancing the facilities of those who already have better means of obtaining medical services. If it is merely going to serve the needs of a few rich patients in cities like New Delhi and Mumbai, it will have little relevance. This is not to say that these segments should not have these facilities, but only to underline that they already have such facilities available and they could afford to have video conferencing not only within the country, but also even with the best of super specialists in any other part of the world.

Infrastructure

A certain amount of infrastructure and facilities are pre-requisites of an e-health program. These include minimal availability of:

- medical/paramedical staff
- electricity
- communication lines (telephone)
- clinical investigation facilities.

Looking at Indian conditions, if you look for a place with this minimal infrastructure, you will also find that there are doctors available. In other places you have neither doctors nor the infrastructure and facilities. This creates a peculiar condition. Efforts have to be made to overcome this contrasting situation.

Some hospitals, government, private or charitable trust owned, are available in any district town. A reasonable number of medical staff and associated medical facilities are also available in these towns. So telemedicine facilities (at the patient end) will have to be created in such district towns. Patients from the nearby villages visit these hospitals also. These patients can be linked to specialists in any other part of the country/world (where the best doctors would be available) and interaction can be established between these two ends. Telemedicine can be expensive in the initial stages, but over a period of time as the technologies develop, and people get used to using these facilities, the cost will gradually decrease.[16]

In a study,[17] it was found that an email link with the facility to send high-resolution digital images is a cheap and uncomplicated telemedicine method. The Swinfen Charitable Trust helped establish such a link in Patan Hospital, Kathmandu, Nepal, in March 2000. Over 12 months using these links, 42 telemedicine referrals were sent to specialists throughout the world. Referrals were: 36% respiratory medicine; 21% neurology; 21% dermatology; 14% cardiology; 5% nephrology; and 3% radiology. Twenty-eight had digital pictures attached, of which 96% were of high enough quality for specialists to be able to comment. Thirty-nine replies were received. The average time for a specialist reply was two days, and 45% were answered within 24 hours. All replies were judged by independent assessors to be helpful or very helpful for diagnosis, management and education. The assessors decided that in 50% of cases the advice, if acted upon, would have shortened hospital stay. This pilot study has shown that a low-cost telemedicine link is technically feasible and can be of significant benefit for diagnosis, management and education in a developing world setting.

There are super-specialty hospitals where telemedicine facilities are available and functioning very well. A few examples have been incorporated. No doubt, the benefits of technology are well known and acceptance is also good. Linking up to rural sectors is also progressing.

What interventions are appropriate to change the cultures for a successful program?

Web-based telemedicine solutions are gaining popularity owing to the Internet's low cost and almost universal availability.[18] The Internet is proving to be a very popular networking technology universally.

The development of the information superhighway presents a problem that will affect every person globally. This study explores how cultural and historical differences in countries influenced by British imperialism affect their integration into the global information infrastructure. Hofstede's models of cultural differences that define teaching and learning within an international culture are used as a theoretical framework to analyze data. The research strategy sampled electronically, explored, observed and drew conclusions in light of the country's history and culture. As information technology expands into a culture, elementary schools would be the last to be integrated. Forty-one of 156 elementary websites formed the Australian sample population. In India, the search reached the technical school and college level before encountering the infrastructure.

Historical and cultural explanations were explored for answers to the great disparity between the 'haves' and 'have-nots' in this country. There was evidence of a correlation between Hofstede's model of cultural differences and the growth of informational technology within Australia and India. Future implications of this framework would be to test whether Hofstede's model correlates consistently to integrating information technology in other countries. Integrating technology worldwide might be improved by considering differences in cultural learning characteristics within a country.[19]

Box 3.1   Success stories in telemedicine

Gujarat: The Online Telemedicine Research Institute (OTRI) provided telemedicine links for teleconsultation, thereby establishing 750 sessions in a period of 30 days in Bhuj after the earthquake in January 2001.

Uttar Pradesh: During the Kumbh Mela festival held every 12 years, which drew over 25 million pilgrims to the banks of River Ganga, the OTRI transferred data (cardiology and radiology data) of over 200 ailing pilgrims, as well as sending microscope images of microorganisms to monitor levels of cholera-causing bacteria in the river.

Bangalore: Asia Heart Foundation has successfully been practicing tele-cardiology between Bangalore and cities in eastern India. Paramedics are guided to save the patients suffering from acute myocardial infarction by performing life-saving procedures as per directions from doctors over video-conferencing.

Chennai: Apollo is providing expert opinion from its tertiary-level hospitals in bigger cities to those in the far-flung towns of India. In the period of around 27 months at Apollo over 4000 patients had benefited through teleconsultations and over 75% of those teleconsulted were treated in their respective cities.[20]

Are there core values that make the adoption of telemedicine successful?

The drivers for adoption of telemedicine could vary from country to country based on various factors. Some of the factors that would expedite the telemedicine revolution in India are:

Topography: think of a patient in Tinsukiya, Assam, or Aragonda, Andhra Pradesh, who requires a consultation with a specialist at Bangalore or Mumbai. The cost of travel and the travel itself could be a deterrent to the poor patient in these rural settings. Even if a specialist were available at the nearest town, reaching the interior of such a far-flung village would be a challenge. This is where telemedicine could be utilized as an effective medium for healthcare delivery. In India, with its diverse collection of landscapes with mountains and valleys and high altitudes, telemedicine could well be a boon for the patients.

Travel time/cost: there is a shortage of specialist/super-specialist professionals in India, especially in rural areas. It might not be good time management on the part of the specialist to travel all the way to the rural areas without having enough patients to attend to there. Travel time can be cut down dramatically while the expertise is made available in real time via technology. The specialist's physical presence becomes necessary only when a surgical procedure is planned. In reality, even surgical procedures are being conducted with guidance from specialists at remote locations. For a patient, cost of travel is a major worry, especially if they have to fly in to a specialist care center in a city.

Pressure to reduce costs: cost of healthcare and questions on who will bear the burden of care are issues across the world, developed countries included. The incidental expenses related to patient care, i.e. the cost associated with factors other than the actual medical care such as travel, accommodation for relatives, food, etc, also contribute substantially to the cost of treatment. In a country where health insurance is yet to catch up, the cost of care is borne by patients, in many cases by selling property and livestock. If hospitals can reduce the costs associated with treatment it would go a long way towards reducing the burden of care on the patient. Telemedicine seems to be the answer.[21]

Given the scarcity of medical facilities in rural areas, efforts will have to be made to take this technology to rural areas. There will have to be a planned intervention program dedicated to this end. The Development and Educational Communication Unit (DECU) of the Indian Space Research Organisation (ISRO) is now trying to set up a need-based telemedicine project in different parts of the country. ISRO has recently initiated a GRAMSAT ('satellite for villages') program. It is aimed at reaching out to the villages for development and educational purposes. A variety of satellite-based technologies/applications will be used for this purpose.[2]

In a study carried out over an 18-month period, teleconsultations were conducted by email between a neonatal intensive care unit at an urban teaching hospital in western India and a rural primary care center 40 km away. There were email consultations about 182 newborn babies; these consultations comprised 309 messages sent from the primary care centre and 272 messages from the teaching hospital. The average reply time was 11.3 hours. Thirty-eight babies were referred to the intensive care unit at the teaching hospital after these consultations. The remaining 144 babies were managed at the primary care center. Telemedicine helped in the diagnosis, referral, treatment and follow-up of patients. The cost of the email service was estimated to be Rs 12 000 and the savings in avoided transfer were estimated to be Rs 546 000, a cost-benefit ratio of 1:45.[22]

Conclusion

This chapter highlights our attempt to improve the spread of health information in the area of healthcare in rural and urban India. Our country, with its diverse culture and large population, definitely has to look increasingly into such technologies to acquire and spread knowledge in the health field very rapidly. Adequate infrastructure facilities are available in our country. It is a question of channelling this in a proper direction by establishing methods to disseminate health knowledge into rural and urban India. We have worked towards establishing a model called Recon Healthcare Bangalore Model. Without incurring additional expenditure, the existing infrastructure was effectively harnessed and a good, cost-effective model was established. Developing countries must become interested in establishing such models. If they do, the world will definitely move one step forward in improving healthcare facilities very rapidly.

A practicing doctor in rural India does not have access to the Internet and a doctor in urban India does not have time to access the Internet. Due to these constraints, doctors appreciate the information provided to them when they request it. From this, we understand that doctors are definitely interested in getting the latest information to update their knowledge base.

With the increasing availability of Internet facilities and usage, we can be confident that the medical knowledge of doctors at all levels can be enhanced very quickly. This confidence stems from the fact that our trend analysis over the years shows that there is an increasing need for up-to-date medical information as evidenced by the increase in the number of requests. Necessarily, such rapid transmission of knowledge, especially to doctors in rural areas, will be of great benefit to patient care. The private sector, by directly communicating with the doctor as a part of its service and commitment to patient care, can make a very significant contribution in building up its knowledge base and apply the same to patient care.

References

1   Angood PB (2001) Telemedicine, the Internet, and World Wide Web: overview, current status, and relevance to surgeons. *World J Surg.* **25**: 1449–57.
2   Subhash J (2001) Telemedicine: what, why and for whom. www.orbicom.uqam.ca/in_focus/columns/en /archives/2001_juil.html; accessed 10 April 2003.
3   Akatsn H and Kuffner J (1998) Medicine and the Internet. *West J Med.* **169**: 311–17.
4   Glowniak JV (1995) Medical resources on the Internet. *Ann Intern Med.* **123**: 123–31.
5   Leiner BM, Cerf VG, Clark DD *et al.* (2001) A brief history of the Internet. www.isoc.org/internet-history/brief.html; accessed 4 August 2001.
6   The World Fact book 2002, CIA Publication. www.cia.gov/cia/publications/factbook/geos/in.html; accessed 15 April 2003.
7   Population and Vital Statistics. http://w3.whosea.org/eip/annex1ind.htm; accessed 14 April 2003.
8   Thakker N. Internet usage in India. *The CyberMed Catalyst.* www.amip.org/catalyst/cc_thakker2_html; accessed 4 August 2001.
9   Geyoushi B and Stones W (2001) Pathways to evidence based reproductive healthcare in developing countries. 9th International Cochrane Colloquium, Lyon, France, 9–13 October. *Cochrane* 2001 1:op048.
10   Sridhar CB, Suresh D and Gowda RN (2001) Internet: a powerful tool in disseminating medical knowledge in urban and rural India. *Karnataka Journal of Medical Sciences.* **4**(4): 9–13.
11   Sridhar CB and Suresh D (2002) Paper presented at the XVIII Asian and Oceanic Congress of Obstetrics and Gynaecology, 5–10 September, Bangalore, India.
12   The Cochrane Collaboration. www.update-software.com/RHL; accessed on 26 September, 2002.
13   Suresh D and Sridhar CB (2002) Paper presented at SSGRR 2002s International Conference on Advances in Infrastructure for e-business, e-education, e-science, e-medicine on the Internet, July, L'Aquila, Italy.

14 Greenhalgh T, Hughes J, Humphrey C *et al*. (2002) A comparative case study of two models of a clinical Informaticist service. *British Medical Journal*. **324**: 524–9

15 Sridhar CB and Suresh D (2003) Model for Bangalore helped disseminate information to doctors in India. In Letters, *British Medical Journal*. **326**: 337.

16 Ganapathy K (2002) Telemedicine and neurosciences in developing countries. *Surg Neurol*. **58**: 388–94.

17 Graham LE, Zimmerman M, Vassallo DJ *et al*. (2003) Telemedicine – the way ahead for medicine in the developing world. *Trop Doct*.**33**: 36–8.

18 Sood SP and Bhatia JS (2002) Internet as the backbone for telemedicine: how far/ close are we? Presented at All India Seminar, Challenges ahead with Information Technology, 19–20 January, Longowal.

19 Plowman TS (1999) The information superhighway: a comparative look at the growth of informational technology in Australia and India. *International Journal of Educational Telecommunications*. **5**(2): 93–110.

20 Srikanth RP. Telemedicine: emergence of the virtual doctor. www.express-computer.com/20030310/focus1.shtml; accessed 10 April 2003.

21 Salam S. Telemedicine: hype vs reality. www.expresshealthcaremgmt.com/20020630/medtech1.shtml; accessed 10 April 2003.

22 Deodhar JJ (2002) Telemedicine by email – experience in neonatal care at a primary care facility in rural India. *Telemed Telecare*. **8** (Suppl. 2): 20–21.

Section 3

Technological innovation in e-health

Structures surrounding e-health systems: effects of legal and administrative structures on development of IT in healthcare services – focus on Finland

Ville Harkke and Mikael Collan

Introduction

During the latter half of the 20th century and the beginning of the 21st century developments in information technology (IT) and automating work have changed the work processes in most information-heavy fields of human activity, resulting in gains in productivity and reducing the effects of human error.[1] This has generally not been the case for the healthcare sector, except for automating some financial and administrative tasks. The technologies necessary for reorganizing work even in this sector have existed for some time, but wide adoption of these technologies has been slower than one would expect. As world economic growth has slowed down since the end of the 1990s, healthcare systems in most of the industrialized world are facing increased pressure towards enhanced efficiency due to diminishing public financing and an aging population.[2] The need for increased use of new technology and new work methods is clearer than ever.

Introduction of new technology does not, of course, solve the problems of the field as such; proper implementation and wide enough use of the systems are important requirements. The use of semi-automated processes and partially implemented systems can even have adverse effects on efficiency and quality of care, as suggested by Lederman and Morrison.[3]

There is an observable difference in IT usage between public and private healthcare institutions, at least in Finland. The private clinics have a direct financial incentive to cut costs and to maximize the satisfaction of their customers, whereas the public institutions are constantly struggling with financing problems and understaffing, and generally lack the ability to invest in the newest technology. The health service providers are, however, not the only players in the field of healthcare. Insurers, pharmacies, laboratories and regulating bodies all have their stake in the structure of healthcare systems, and cooperated efforts are necessary for truly beneficial changes. It seems that the private healthcare enterprises are embracing disruptive technologies to enhance their efficiency just as discussed in the classic article, but the public organizations are more prone to use new technology to support existing processes thus limiting the scope of organizational change.

The critical changes of the processes and implementation of better systems will not even be possible until the information systems in different organizations are able to function together and the critical information flows between the organizations are automated. Technological innovations as such will only function as catalysts of required organizational change, but as such catalysts these are invaluable. This is clearly visible in the layered presentation of the problem field presented in this book. Technological innovation can only thrive where the underlying cultural and organizational contexts allow and encourage it, and even then the level of success depends on management of change, cooperation between the stakeholders and, fundamentally, on changes in the mental models about healthcare processes.

In this chapter, first we describe the organizational framework in Finland within which the e-health services exist, and look at administrative issues within the framework that are not supportive of advancement in the sector. Second, we elaborate some issues particular to e-health from a legal perspective. Third, we address the discussed issues from the point of view of some of the actors in the sector. We base the third part on a small (non-representative) survey sent to actors in the field of health services in southwestern Finland. Finally, we draw some conclusions and summarize.

Organizational environment in Finland

In Finland, healthcare is basically organized around publicly financed organizations and supported by private institutions in larger cities. The universal health insurance provided by the Social Insurance Institute of Finland (SIIF) covers use of the public healthcare services fully and a percentage of the privately produced services,[4] for example 60% of the private doctor's fees.[5] A certain level of healthcare is guaranteed by law for every Finnish citizen. The primary administrative units, the municipalities, have since the 1990s had the right to choose how the services demanded by law are produced, including buying the services from private service providers.[6]

The private service providers act as a catalyst for restructuring even the public systems, by showing in practice that the same services can be produced with a smaller use of resources.

Despite the existence of universal health insurance, citizens tend to be insured by private insurance companies as well, either through their own home insurance healthcare packages (covering mainly accidents, etc.) or by their employers. This complicates the administrative processes in cases of work-related illnesses, acute injuries and other situations where a patient is insured by several organizations.

Due to the independence of the municipalities, the health systems in different parts of the country are very different from each other, all naturally providing the level of service required by law. In most districts there are organizations for everyday illnesses, for special care, inpatient wards, etc., that have all been founded at different times, and there is no generally applied organizational structure even within the municipalities or health districts. The existence of different organizational cultures within the bigger healthcare structures causes some administrative problems of its own, but also makes development of information systems difficult due to differences in work processes and information requirements.

Information systems compatibility is a major issue in developing functional healthcare systems.[7] In Finland, the fragmentation of information systems has been a major obstacle on the road towards systems that would significantly alter the processes of the healthcare system, increasing efficiency and effectiveness. This situation has been noted by the governing authorities, and the Ministry of Social Affairs and Health has started a project for preparing a nationwide electronic health record system. The project is organized as a workgroup and the main objective is to define the contents and criteria for a national electronic health record system and to maintain a cooperation network for implementing the system. The workgroup presented a strategy to the Minister of Social Affairs and Health in January 2004. This strategy contains standards for data structures, data communication protocols and data security that are to be implemented by all health centers and hospitals by 2007.[8] This provides the public sector with not only a more secure environment for investing in information technology but also with a direct incentive to do so.

Some examples of IT use in the Finnish healthcare system

Electronic prescriptions

Delivering drug prescriptions electronically has been possible in principle since the 1995 Ministry of Social Affairs and Health regulation for delivering prescription drugs. The regulation allowed for electronic data transfers on a general level but provided no specific guidelines as to how the system should work.

There have been two major publicly financed pilot projects around electronic prescriptions in Finland: the SIIF smart card project in 1989–93 and the healthcare cooperation project in the Satakunta region 1998–2000, called Satakunnan Makropilotti. The smart card project used personal health cards as data storage for prescriptions. It was a limited success, but the system was never intended to be the default system for the whole country.[9] The Makropilotti project had as its main goal the development of information technology (local information system, reference database, secure email and local service portal) to support service development in health and social services. A special law was enacted to enable patient data transfer between the different organizations within the seven municipalities partaking in the pilot. The electronic prescription service never got to wider pilot use and the project was terminated in 2000. The project cannot be described as a success as such, but it unveiled a number of obstacles in the way of developing health systems. There is:

- no clear structure for service development
- unclear limits of responsibilities
- no authority governing the whole customer service process.[10]

Based on the previous experiences, in November 2003 the Ministry of Social

Affairs and Health initiated a more extensive pilot for testing electronic prescriptions. The pilot covers four public healthcare districts and a number of private pharmacies, and is based on a central prescriptions database maintained by the SIIF. The serious involvement of the SIIF will relieve the users of the pilot system from most of the insurance-related paperwork, thus enabling true process improvements. The pilot project is legally based on a special decree of the Ministry of Social Affairs and Health (771/2003) and will run until the end of 2004. Should the results of the pilot be positive, the permanent legislation around the subject is likely to be changed rapidly.

One of the central obstacles in developing electronic prescriptions has been the absence of clear norms and standards about, among other things, electronic signatures which verify the identity of the describing doctor.[9] The law governing electronic signatures was passed in the Finnish parliament on 24 January 2003, and defines the acceptable forms of verification for electronic interaction with public servants and government organizations.[11] This alone will not remove all of the problems, but now there is at least basic jurisdiction on which future guidelines can be built.

Telemedicine

There are a number of telemedicine applications in use in Finland, especially in northern parts. The Finnish Office for Health Care Technology Assessment (FinOHTA) together with Northern Ostrobothnia Hospital District, organized a project to assess the effectiveness and the cost-effectiveness of telemedicine, focusing on applications in radiology, psychiatry, surgery and ophthalmology. The personnel using the systems learnt the new methods fast, but usability of the systems was not deemed perfect. The main advantages lie in reduced travelling of the personnel, making telemedicine applications financially viable only over considerable distances as in Northern Finland.[12] Telemedicine applications have to struggle with the same legal and organizational problems as the rest of healthcare informatics: the electronic connection is understood as an extension of the presence of the doctor/patient and transfers of medical data between organizations is still subject to several data secrecy laws and regulations.

Electronic patient records and image processing

There are several different electronic patient record systems in use, as well as different image processing systems. One of the main tasks of the work group mentioned above is to create guidelines for nationwide compatibility. Most of the electronic imaging systems in use in Finland are compliant with the DICOM (Digital Imaging and Communications in Medicine) standard, and the EHR (electronic health records) systems built today are following HL7 (health level 7) structures. There are functioning region-wide radiology information systems (RISs) in the Turku and Helsinki regions, enabling remote consultations and digital archiving of the images, and similar systems are under development in other regions.[13] These systems will probably not be fully compatible as the regulation governing them is very vague, and the systems are, naturally, developed by competing systems development companies each trying to add features their competitors did not include. The basic structures do, however, follow the international standards, so a general mishmash like the one created in the hospitals of Finland in the 1970s by a large number of in-house development projects could be avoided.

Legal issues affecting e-health implementation

E-health services consist of parts that are not unknown to legislation. However, as a combination of electronic and physical transactions, e-health is unique, and there are very few laws that are specifically drafted to answer to the special circumstances of e-health, or cyber medicine. The major parts that make e-health are telecommunications, information technology and health services. Each one of these is governed by a set of laws, which are specific to each one of the parts. E-health is therefore governed by a combination of the laws governing its parts. This means that there are a number of regulatory and other legal issues that govern e-health directly or indirectly.

Below we present some issues that are specific to e-health, and are known to hinder the implementation of e-health services.

Medical data and patient data enjoy a high level of protection of privacy in many legal systems. For controlled substances identification of the buyer is important

When patient information is transmitted between doctors within a company, usually there doesn't seem to be any problem with regulation and jurisdiction, as in-house systems are perceived as closed systems. However, when patient data is transferred from one service provider to another (e.g. public to private or vice versa) there may be problems of compatibility between systems and different security measures in place. The systems of the public organizations are required to keep archives of every document connected to their actions.[14] Archives do not need to be on paper anymore, but in some organizations most of them are. This causes some administrative problems in trying to create seamless information flows. It is not unacceptable to think that from the point of view of security, the systems used in the private sector are at least of the same quality as, if not of higher quality than, those in the public sector. However, as the legal requirements are different or carried out differently, systems compatibility between private and public sector systems is not easily achieved. It seems that protection of anonymity of patients and the secrecy of information is not an issue that creates obstacles; however, the discussion is about what kind of cryptography and other security measures need to be in place for growing flows of patient information.

The marketing and selling of controlled substances (e.g. certain medicines) brings forth another issue: validating the identity of the buyer is necessary to ensure that the substances are not ending up in the wrong hands. If, for example, medication is sold through the Internet, it is plausible to think that the service must at some point include an identity check – how this is accomplished is not clear. Another issue, although connected to selling of controlled substances, is the issue of electronic drug prescriptions. If a doctor electronically transfers information to pharmacies (or to a database, where pharmacies can check prescriptions for patients), problems with counterfeit prescriptions can be circumvented, providing that the practitioners using the service operate according to the law, and can be identified. Now the new law governing electronic signatures is in place in Finland the communication between doctors and pharmacies could be arranged. As the SIIF is involved in most of the medication transactions and there was no paperless system (or even precise guidelines for developing one) for delivering insurance claims to the SIIF prior to launching the pilot project mentioned above, the systems development was slow. Development of fully paperless systems is still hindered by the National Agency for Medicines (NAM) requirements. NAM requires paper records of all the delivered drugs as well as ten-year archiving of prescriptions (original paper documents) of certain drugs affecting the central nervous system, as well as drugs classified as narcotics.[15]

There is no universal licensing system for medical practitioners that would govern international medical consultations made through the Internet

Because there is no international community for medical practitioners that would or could give licenses to practitioners that ensure quality of the service, it is difficult for a user of e-health services offering medical consultations to be sure of the quality of the product. If there is a risk that someone is posing as a medical practitioner (doctor) it jeopardizes the credibility of e-health.

Another issue that may play an important role in the acceptance of e-health services is the position that different patient insurance systems take towards them. If insurance will cover consultations made through the Internet, or perhaps a mobile device, there is considerably less hindrance for adaptation by users. In the case of private insurance, the step to accept at least some selected e-health services may be low. However, in cases of public insurance (e.g. Finland), the process of acceptance may be a long registration and regulatory process.

Issues of contracts between parties in transactions made through the Internet may in some cases resemble transactions not made through the Internet. However, in cases of litigation, the Internet presents problems

Important questions arise, like where a transaction, or in the case of e-health a consultation, has taken place when a patient resides in a different location from the service provider. In other words, which country's jurisdiction is applied in, for example, malpractice suits filed on consultations made over the Internet? This type of problem is avoided if services operate within national borders. However, as the Internet is global it is not hard to imagine problems arising from enforcing and litigating contracts signed only on the Internet.

The number of issues that do not have a clear answer is large; this means that there is considerable uncertainty as to what can (and what cannot) be done by providers of e-health services. This translates to management decisions about investments in the sector, and means that investments can be postponed because the companies do not wish to find themselves in situations where their investments are suspended by regulatory decisions. Paradoxically it seems that it is not possible to get binding pre-investment information about the regulatory status of projects, or getting such information will take so long that the investment is no longer worthwhile and getting the information is a very exhausting process. The initial answers from the Finnish regulatory bodies concerning a number of possible projects have been ex-ante negative, which means there have been very few stakeholders who have even begun to explore innovations other than those they know to be possible.

Views of stakeholders about the administrative and judicial framework governing IT in health services

In order to understand better the feelings and thoughts of the actual stakeholders in the field of health services production, an exploratory survey about the use of e-health was prepared in cooperation with students from the Turku School of Economics and Business Administration in 2002. The survey was sent to approximately one hundred companies providing healthcare services, ranging from pharmacies and individual private doctors to large healthcare centers. Answers were received from 25 companies, usually from managers responsible for investments in IT in the company. The questions on the survey varied from basic questions about the readiness of the respondents to utilize different e-health innovations (in connection with the Internet) and what their attitudes are towards e-health as an addition to their business generally and specifically. One of the issues taken up in the questionnaire was the interest of parties to engage in using e-prescriptions. The reason for this was that the authors were aware of the difficulties in the development of systems regarding e-prescriptions and the administrative hindrances that are slowing the progress of using e-prescriptions. The authors wish to point out that the survey is not a representative survey and the results are only exploratory. Therefore they can only be used in creating a basic understanding of the attitudes of the community of health service providers in Finland.

In the following sections we will go through the results from the survey in four phases, according to issues that were thought relevant by the authors.

1   It seems that stakeholders are positive about the use of IT and feel that it has potential for enhancing their productivity

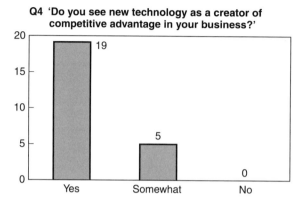

Figure 4.1 Opinions on new technology as a source of competitive edge.

Three-quarters of the respondents (75%) indicated that they were either ready immediately or would be ready within 1–3 years to use e-health services. Only one respondent answered that it would take them more than three years. The rest were not sure how long it would take. More than 86% of the responses indicated that the respondents already have the required infrastructure and readiness for launching e-health services. More than 87% of the respondents reported that they feel that new technology gives at least a possibility to gain competitive advantages in the field. The term 'e-health' is not very commonly known to the companies in the field; however, on the basis of their readiness and attitudes most companies are ready to adopt e-health services very quickly.

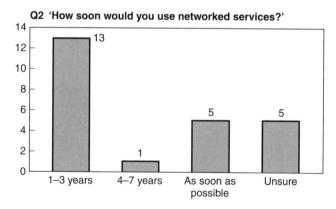

Figure 4.2 Readiness to use e-health (networked) services.

2   In-house tasks are often already done with IT solutions and there are positive experiences

All the answers indicated that the respondents feel that an information system is or would be important to their operations, and more than 86% stated that they have a functioning information system at work in their business. Roughly 54% of the respondents said that they either were thinking about using the Internet as a marketing channel for their products, or are already using it ($\sim 21\%$). The number of answers that were negative about using the Internet as a marketing channel has partly to do with the fact that seven of the responding firms were pharmacies. Pharmacies are highly regulated in Finland, and it seems that even if regulation is not prohibitive in all aspects of marketing via the Internet, it is a hindering factor. It is probable that marketing alone is not perceived as a sufficient justification to build new systems. For those respondents who have already been using the Internet as a channel for their marketing, their experiences have been mostly positive. Twenty-five percent of the respondents indicated that they have plans to sell their products on the Internet, but only one indicated that it had actually sold its products via the Internet. Pharmacies had positive experiences due to the enhancements in ordering and delivery procedures for customers who were using the Internet service. The comments made by pharmacies that had not sold their products on the Internet specified that this was due to administrative and regulatory hindrances; selling drugs on the Internet is not presently allowed. Further comments stated that the actual delivery of the drugs would have to be realized by a credible and trustworthy company. One response suggested that the products that would most likely be sold over the Internet would be products already most well known to the customers (at least in the case of retail customers). On a further note, some of the respondents are actually service providers and do not concentrate per se on selling any products. Attitudes towards the Internet as a way to enhance business varied from mildly reserved to very positive. Also a concern over the truthfulness of information mediated through the Internet was voiced in one answer.

3   On a number of occasions it was mentioned that the administration by the Social Insurance Institution of Finland (SIIF) and the National Agency for Medicines (NAM) are hindering development

From the limited material at our disposal we could detect a feeling of frustration among the respondents. It seems that there is a wall that the service providers and especially pharmacies are facing when trying to launch innovations in the level of preliminary acceptance from the administrative bodies. It seems to us that as companies' internal information systems do not fall under the jurisdiction of the governing bodies, they seem to be experiencing constant development and are used to enhance the operational efficiency of the companies. The thought just expressed is not based on any extensive research material, but is rather derived from the loosely structured information and based on the survey results.

4   Most of the respondents specify that incorporating electronic drug prescriptions would be an important step. This is, however, not possible due to administrative hindrances

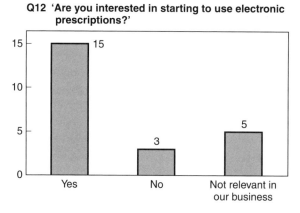

Figure 4.3 Interest in electronic prescriptions.

Nearly 80% of the answers stated that the businesses would be interested in using electronic drug prescriptions. One answer stated that based on observations from a longer period of time it seems quite hard to expect any changes in the near future due to lack of cooperation from administrative bodies.

In general, it can be said that most of the respondents have an information system in use and that they have a positive picture of IT in the production of health services. This indicates that there is interest within companies to develop their information systems to further enhance their productivity and services. However, it was quite obvious that stakeholders feel uncertain about pursuing development in IT as the administrative and legal frameworks are not transparent.

Discussion and conclusion

We have introduced the main setting of the Finnish administrative framework for healthcare services and seen that service production is divided into the services provided by private companies and those provided by the public services. There is a gap between the productivity of private services and public services and we feel that one of the reasons for the existence of this gap is more advanced use of IT. One factor hindering the development in the public sector – and indirectly even the private sector, as the systems will need to communicate with each other – is the existence of administrative and legal barriers that do not take into account the possibilities offered by the technologies available today. Legislation and administration have not been able to develop in pace with technical innovations. This has caused a bottleneck in areas such as production of healthcare services that have a strong focus on privacy and customer (patient) protection.

The lack of up-to-date governance (laws and administration) of IT in healthcare is a major source of uncertainty and a serious hindrance for development in the sector. The obvious conclusion is that in order to work optimally from the point of view of all stakeholders, the legislation and administration of IT in healthcare service production should be brought up to date with the technological advances, otherwise we will most likely see a stagnation in the development of such systems. Companies operating in the field of health services provision need proof of cooperation from the regulators to invest in and fully embrace new technology.

The legislation, of course, has as a main goal to secure the quality and accountability of care, and laws in the health field cannot be changed radically overnight as the organizational structures are built around the existing ways of practicing medicine. But without proper standards, guidelines and legislation, even incremental changes may be deemed impossible. The processes within tradition-bound and complex healthcare organizations are difficult enough to change due to organizational inertia and resistance to change, so every hindering factor from the surrounding society may turn into a major obstacle.

The very slowly diminishing uncertainty about the legal and administrative issues in implementing and designing IT infrastructure in Finland has been felt by companies operating in the sector. Our survey found that companies would be interested in implementing new systems but are sometimes unable to do so because of institutional constraints. A fast pre-approval procedure for healthcare systems by regulators or a set of clear rules and principles of conduct would promote acceptance and implementation of IT in the healthcare sector. The latest developments in legislation and the numerous government projects aimed at developing guidelines for IT in healthcare do manifest a commitment to change in the highest levels of administration, but the healthcare sector will probably nevertheless remain a few years behind the rest of our society in the field of information technology usage.

References

1   Brynjolfsson E and Hitt LM (1998) Beyond the productivity paradox. *Communications of the ACM.* **41**(8): 49–55.
2   Hurst J and Jee-Hughes M (2000) Performance measurement and performance management in OECD health systems. *DEELSA/ELSA/WD*(2000)8 OECD 2000.
3   Lederman R and Morrison I (2002) Examining quality of care – how poor information flow can impact on hospital workflow and affect patient outcomes. *Proceedings of the 35th Hawaii International Conference on System Sciences.*
4   Suomen terveyspolitiikasta, *STM Esitteitä* 1999: 13 (Ministry of Health and Social Services pamphlets 1999: 13) www.vn.fi/stm/suomi/vastuual/vast01fr.htm
5   SIIFinland homepage. http://193.209.217.5/in/internet/english.nsf/NET/150502164636EH?openDocument; accessed 25 May 2002.
6   Suomi R and Tähkäpää J (2002) The strategic role of ICT in the competition between public and private health care sectors in the Nordic welfare societies – Case Finland. *Proceedings of the 35th Hawaii International Conference on System Sciences.*
7   Harkke V and Landor P (2002) Mobile e-health: the challenge of eight obstacles. *Proceedings of International Conference on Decision Making and Decision Support in the Internet Age.*
8   Ministry of Social Affairs and Health (2004) Bulletin 21/2004. Ministry of Social Affairs and Health, Helsinki.

9   Ministry of Social Affairs and Health (2002) Sähköistä reseptiä koskeva esiselvitys (report on electronic prescriptions). Ministry of Social Affairs and Health, Helsinki.

10 Jukka Ohtonen (toim.) Satakunnan Makropilotti: tulosten arviointi (Result evaluation of the Makropilotti project). *FinOHTAn raportti 21/2002*. FinOHTA.

11 Laki sähköisistä allekirjoituksista 24.1.2003/14 (Law about electronic signatures). Finnish Law 14/2003, 2003.

12 Telelääketieteen arviointi Pohjois-Pohjanmaan sairaanhoitopiirissä (Evaluation of telemedicine in the Northern Osthrobotnia region). *FinOHTAn raportti 20/2002*. FinOHTA.

13 IMPAKTI 4/2001: Tietoa terveydenhuollon menetelmien arvioinnista.

14 Arkistolaki 831/94 (Archives Act), Finnish Law 831/94, 1994.

15 NAM order(MÄÄRÄYS) 10/2002 LÄÄKKEIDEN TOIMITTAMINEN (on delivering drugs) NAM, 18.12.2002.

Chapter 5

Secure, remote, ubiquitous access of electronic health records

John Fulcher

Background

The provision of healthcare necessarily involves the generation, collation, storage and access of patient data, in an ethical and legal manner. Furthermore, both patients and managers need to be assured that whatever system is in place is inherently confidential, secure and accountable. The latter implies some form of audit trail to assist in dispute resolution. Traditional paper-based records rely on physical security measures, such as safes, locks and controlled office and/or building access. Moreover, access to patient data belonging to other healthcare providers at remote sites necessarily involves copying, transmitting and securely storing third-party patient records.

The following summarizes the security needs (so-called trust issues) which must be satisfied within any system, be it healthcare or otherwise.[1]

- **Authority** – in any particular domain, a trusted authority must exist who issues not only their own identity, but also the identities of individuals further down the chain of command.
- **Identity** – procedures need to be put in place to ensure identities are only issued to individuals who *should* have access to the system; traditionally, paper-based identities are often protected by way of photographs, holograms and/or lamination.
- **Authentication** – involves the positive identification of an individual, for example by way of paper-based IDs (such as birth certificates, driving licenses, passports), signed written letters of authority or fingerprints.
- **Authorization** – the process of granting permission to authenticated users. In the medical field this could take the form of licensing doctors to practice in various states and territories. Alternatively a hospital administrator may be authorized to create new patient records, but not to alter the medical information contained therein.
- **Confidentiality** – only authenticated, authorized people are allowed access to their data stored in the system in question.
- **Integrity** – information cannot be modified by unauthorized users.
- **Non-repudiation** – is the ability to guarantee that a specific transaction occurred on a particular date and/or time. Traditionally this often takes the form of a public notary witnessing signatures on a document.

In this chapter we concern ourselves with the transition currently underway within the healthcare industry towards electronic health records (EHRs) and the repercussions this has for the secure, remote access of patient data.

The move towards EHRs

Access, ownership and privacy of medical records are fundamental considerations in any e-health application.[2–6] Indeed, social, political and/or legal concerns – rather than technological ones – often dictate the final deployment of e-health systems in the field.

It would appear that most stakeholders agree that e-health (health informatics) is inevitable, despite there being a lack of consensus on its implementation details. For example, the European Union views e-health as showing promise for improving quality, cost and access. At the same time, they cite the following barriers and pitfalls: the need for organizational change, cross-organizational cooperation and adherence to standards.[7] The eEurope 2005 Plan identifies several promising fields, including health cards which contain basic patient data, connectivity of healthcare providers and points of care, as well as online information, all of which would be supported by 'broadband networks and a culture of security, which lie at the heart of many future electronic services'.

In the US, security is viewed as paramount to the success of e-health systems, although the Health Insurance Portability and Accountability Act (HIPAA) does not go beyond a motherhood statement touting a 'commonsense' approach for implementing security for internal systems and processes.[1] An alternative model of healthcare, in which the public is becoming increasingly more participatory, has been proposed in Canada.[8] The Canadian Institute for Health Informatics has observed individuals increasingly requesting access to their own health data, and storing it electronically using 'my health record' software, which is becoming increasingly more available on e-health websites.

Within this context, numerous authors cite the potential advantages of moving from paper-based to electronic health records, one of which is the reduction of errors contained therein. A recent US study, for example, found that the annual toll from preventable errors exceeds the combined number of deaths and injuries from road and air crashes, suicides, falls, poisonings and drownings.[9] Given this, the widespread adoption of EHRs is therefore seen as having potential for significantly increasing consumer safety. The irony with electronic storage of patient health (medical) records, however, is that while most stakeholders agree on the general principle, there is no consensus on *specific* formats.

EHRs contain their own inherent risks; first and foremost, digital records may be read, modified and/or copied by (unauthorized) hackers. A common misconception is that the chief risk to privacy and confidentiality is from intruders breaking into the system from outside. In reality, accidental or malicious disclosure (by disgruntled employees, for instance), insider curiosity or uncontrolled secondary usage (such as on-selling to unauthorized third parties) can often render systems much more vulnerable.[10–12] To take but one recent example: a Florida state health department worker recently compiled a list of 4000 people infected with HIV and forwarded this information to the *St Petersburg Times* and *Tampa Tribune*.[1]

We now revisit the security trust issues cited earlier in the chapter. *Identity* in the digital age often takes the form of personal identification number (PIN) or username/(encrypted)password. These are quite vulnerable to intruders, and as such cannot be considered sufficiently secure. Numerous anecdotes abound in the IT industry which indicate that users' behavior patterns can negate what little security is inherent in the system. Consider for example, the following: using 'password' as the password, or 100% of doctors in one particular practice using 'doctor' as their password, or, perhaps worst of all, affixing post-sticks on which the passwords are written to the computer monitor! In a digital environment, *integrity* can be assured through the use of digital signature (hashing) algorithms, which, when combined with (secure) time stamping, can reveal subsequent attempts to alter the data. Last, digital transactions ensure *non-repudiation*, since they utilize digital signatures by strongly authenticated and authorized users.[1]

As already stated, security, confidentiality and privacy are ensured in computer systems by way of encryption, common industry standards being Public Key Infrastructure (PKI) and Pretty Good Privacy (PGP). One-time (volatile) passwords guard against *re-use* of valid passwords which may have fallen into the hands of unauthorized system users. Hardware tokens, such as smart cards or USB iKeys, can also be useful in this regard. Systems can be rendered even more secure by incorporating biometrics – those physical characteristics which 'uniquely' distinguish humans from each other (*see* Future directions, p. 91). However, the bottom line is that because all the above techniques store information in digital form, there remains the possibility, however slight, of an intruder hacking into a system and stealing this information (even to the point of committing identity theft, as occurs with paper-based systems).

Duty-of-care principles dictate access to medical records within the Australian context. The Federal Department of Health and Aged Care acknowledges that the increased computerization of doctors' general practice is occurring in an *uncontrolled* environment. Likewise, the Australian EHR Task Force acknowledges that more work needs to take place with both messaging standards and security (PKI). They further suggest that (a) HL7 be adopted as the messaging standard, and (b) XML be adopted as the preferred technology medium for health information interchange (www.noie.gov.au/projects/ecommerce/ehealth/index.htm).

The linking of various EHRs cannot proceed without the confidence of the public, especially as regards compliance with privacy and other similar legislation.[6] With this in mind, the federal government recently conducted trials in two Australian States, with the longer-term aim of developing a national e-health information network (www.healthconnect.gov.au). One of these trials was conducted with remote indigenous (Aboriginal) health services in the Katherine region of the Northern Territory, and the other with an aging population residing in Hobart, Tasmania.

Access, ownership, confidentiality and ubiquity

In April 2003, the US Department of Health and Human Services (HHS) introduced comprehensive federal legislation that gives patients sweeping protections over the privacy of their medical records. In the words of HHS Secretary

Thompson: 'Patients now will have a strong foundation of federal protections for the personal medical information that they share with their doctors, hospitals and others who provide their care and help pay for it' (www.hhs.gov/ocr/hippa). Under this privacy legislation:

- patients must first give specific authorization before entities covered by the regulation can use or disclose protected information
- covered entities need to provide patients with written notice of their privacy practices and patients' privacy rights
- pharmacies, health plans and other covered entities must first obtain an individual's specific authorization before sending them marketing materials
- patients will be able to access their personal medical records and request changes to correct any errors.

The legal position in Australia is that medical records are *jointly* owned by both doctor and patient. The key aspects of the recently enacted Guideline on the Private Health Sector (www.privacy.gov.au) are access, collection, disclosure and use, with particular emphasis on 'voluntary, informed consent'. The Australian Privacy Commissioner is of the view that we must 'ensure all consumers can confidently take maximum advantage of the information economy while allowing them to protect their privacy with minimum inconvenience'.[14]

There are widely differing views as to whether the addition of biometrics would be privacy enhancing or privacy restricting.[14,15] Such privacy concerns override questions of access and ownership, which in turn override the technical issues surrounding remote access and security. What are the consequences of unauthorized eavesdropping on confidential medical records? For example, 'outing' of people's specific medical problems could have dire consequences, even in the case of de-identified data. We shall return to consider biometrics in the discussion of future directions (p. 91).

On the issue of ubiquity,[16,17] it has been observed in Canada that the geographic location of health services is becoming less of an issue. Perhaps the 'anywhere, anytime, anyplace access to patient medical records' – unrealized a decade ago in the then 'age of increasing mobility within the global economy'[18] – is beginning to emerge. The access model reported on pp. 87–91 goes part of the way to enabling ubiquity in relation to the secure, remote access of EHRs.

Unique Patient Identifiers (UPIs)

As is the case with EHRs, most stakeholders regard unique patient identifiers (UPIs) as holding potential benefits in an e-health setting, for instance the enhancement of privacy, confidentiality and security.[8] Unfortunately, just as with EHRs, there is a lack of agreement on exactly how 'uniqueness' is quantified in this regard. The practice of assigning random digits, as with 16-digit credit card numbers, or four-digit automatic teller machine (ATM) personal identification numbers (PINs), is the de facto standard in some jurisdictions.

In the case of the US, social security numbers serve as a de facto identifier, while in New Zealand and Malaysia, true national identity cards have been in use for some time. By contrast, there is considerable opposition to the introduction of a National ID Card in the US (for example, see '5 Reasons Not to Create a National

IDS Card', www.aclu.org/Privacy/PrivacyMain.cfm). In Australia, an attempt to introduce a similar national identity card came unstuck during the late 1980s.[19] France and Germany have both been using health smartcards for some years now.

In the wake of the public hysteria surrounding the failed 'Australia Card', people's tax file numbers have come to serve a similar purpose. Birth certificate, passport or driver's license numbers are alternative potential 'unique' but non-ideal identifiers. The Australian national Medicare number is not in fact unique, and doctor's practices, hospitals, pathology companies and so forth use incompatible identifiers and formats.

In an attempt to progress towards a UPI, in 2002 the NSW State Government commenced the roll-out of a local government (regional) UPI, which was later expanded statewide. Choice of UPI was left to individual area health services, but was essentially random-number based. It is interesting to note in passing that in this state-based UPI roll-out, an earlier proposal to use a 'health smart card' as a means of increasing consumer control over information was dropped.[20,21]

For the Diabetes field trial (*see* p. 89), the small number of participating doctors and patients meant that the (divisional) random-digit identifiers generated previously for the IDGP Diabetes Program sufficed. By contrast, The Canadian Institute for Health Information considered two possibilities: (i) expansion of an existing number, versus (ii) using a biometric identifier.

Ultimately, the problem with randomly assigned digits, just as with credit card numbers or PINs, is loss or theft. A *truly* unique identifier is not possible with the assignment of random digits, but *is* possible if patient biometrics are incorporated. Generally speaking, the most secure systems are based on a threefold approach, namely by utilizing (a) something we are (a physical characteristic or biometric), (b) something we possess (such as a physical key or token) and (c) something we know (for example, a password or PIN).[22] Focus on (a) would ensure both uniqueness and permanency, and thereby enhance patients' security and privacy.

Smart_ID field trial

Responsibility for healthcare in Australia is spread across local (regional), state (NSW in this case) and federal governments. The federal government oversees primary care (community health, aged care, nursing homes and the like), while state governments look after secondary healthcare (hospitals).

The conclusions reached in this section are drawn in large part from a three-year (2000–02) Smart_ID R&D project undertaken in conjunction with the Illawarra Division of General Practice (IDGP), and funded by the Australian government under its Strategic Partnerships with Industry Research and Training (SPIRT) scheme (nowadays known as Linkage Grants). Divisions such as IDGP correspond roughly to local government areas.

The collaborative Smart_ID project built on a pre-existing relationship between the university and the industrial partner – IDGP.[23] More specifically, it expanded on an IDGP Diabetes Program which commenced at the end of 1999, and involved collecting patient HbA1C, cholesterol, triglyceride, weight, height and blood pressure from individual doctor's surgeries, and subsequently storing this information back on a centralized server at the division. The underlying premises of this project were:

- data needed to be not only accurate, but also comparable
- the system needed to be automated
- patients could move around between surgeries, in the knowledge that this data would follow them.

By the end of the 12-month trial, a total of 40 general practitioners (GPs) and 540 (type-2) diabetes patients were enrolled in the program. Of these, six GPs and 13 patients proceeded onto the Smart_ID field trial. It should be noted here that the latter group were essentially computer-literate and pro-technology.

To place this Smart_ID project in context, it should be emphasized that IDGP was primarily interested in issues to do with access – namely currency, portability and ability to be informed. These were seen as facilitating the movement of patients around the region and providing them with a means for accessing their own medical (diabetes) records.

Preliminary surveys

In between the 1999 introduction of the IDGP Diabetes Program and commencement of the 2002 Smart_ID field trial, both GPs and patients were surveyed.[13,24] Basically, both groups indicated a willingness to use smart devices, for relevant organizations to also have access to patient EHRs and, moreover, for biometrics to be incorporated onto the smart device. Furthermore, approximately half the patients surveyed believed that UPIs would lead to improved healthcare, while two-thirds expressed concern over their associated risks – namely the possible compromising of privacy and security.

USB iKeys versus smart cards

Smart devices – such as smartcards and iKeys – offer a limited amount of on-board storage (encrypted and/or compressed as necessary) and can provide ready access to remotely stored EHRs in non-emergency situations.[25] Furthermore in emergency situations – such as cardiac or diabetes episodes – vital patient data can be read on any suitably configured computer (i.e. smartcard reader or, even more readily, in-built USB port).

In the past, smart cards have been used primarily *within*, rather than *across* organizations (such as hospitals, health insurance companies and medical groups).[26] One factor that has hindered the more widespread adoption of smart cards in a health environment is the plethora of (incompatible) protocols and Application Programming Interface standards; another is that 'more research is needed on privacy and security'. Nevertheless, 80 million smart cards are currently being used within Germany's healthcare system.[27] Once again, the observation is made that 'of course privacy, technology, legal and cost issues must be addressed before such health-related applications become widespread'.

Storage of complete medical histories and vital records on smart cards has been advocated for Hong Kong – more specifically, record management, security and authentication, and clinical alert system.[26] This is in direct contrast with the

Smart_ID project, where the smart device was used *solely* as the secure access mechanism to medical records stored remotely on a secure server.

In the future, we could witness the mergance of smart device and Internet technologies, thus enabling anywhere/anytime/anyplace access (in order to cater for increased patient mobility). Significant technical challenges remain however: 'the exchange of electronic medical data requires the establishment of a canonical medical structure with supporting data abstraction processes, to provide unified views of medical information'.[26] Moreover, the social, legal and ethical obstacles are even more daunting, as outlined earlier. Imagine a scenario, for example, whereby a citizen's driving record could be updated within minutes of committing a parking violation, say, where smart devices are used for authentication: 'such an application could present some interesting legal issues, depending on which country or state issued the license' (sic).[27]

An even more pertinent scenario is the use of smart devices for authorization in a healthcare setting. More specifically, 'configuration for dialysis equipment, as well as medical information, could be stored on smart cards and inserted into a smart card-enabled dialysis machine anywhere in the world. Of course, privacy, technology, legal and cost issues must be addressed before such health-related applications become widespread'.[29] Once again, we come up against social, legal and privacy issues potentially overriding any technical ones.

Over the past few years, the Australian Health Insurance Commission (HIC) has been conducting a 'Digital Certificate' scheme, whereby participating GPs are issued with unique (random number) identifiers, residing on either smart cards or USB iKeys (most in fact have opted for the latter in recent times). We chose iKeys in preference to smart cards for the Smart_ID field trial; both media exhibit similar storage capacities, PKI security capability and access times. Since most modern-day computers come fitted with USB ports, this obviates the additional cost associated with external smart card readers, despite the cost per card being considerably lower than USB iKeys if purchased in bulk. We selected the same type of iKey used by the HIC (Rainbow Technologies iKey1032 www.rainbow.com/ikey1000_sw.html) for our project. We further observe that USB iKeys are becoming more accepted by the general public, as general purpose, portable storage devices – in fact since the completion of the Smart_ID project, they have become ubiquitous in the computer industry.[28]

Similar issues exist regarding loss or theft of either type of smart device (i.e. re-issuing of smart cards/iKeys). On occasions during the Diabetes field trial, patients forgot to bring their iKey with them to the doctor's surgery. There is the additional problem with either device of a 'plan B' back-up – what happens in the case of a collapsed patient, for example? If they have their smart card or iKey on their person, then it may be feasible to insert this device into a nearby computer, provided the smart device is not password-protected, especially if a biometric has been encoded onto the device.

Field trial set-up

A communications link is established initially between the doctor's computer and the IDGP server via dial-up modem. Programs running on both machines then enable the transfer of patient data. This does not happen until first the GP, followed by the patient, insert their respective iKeys into the GP computer USB port. Access to a specific patient's diabetes record is granted only if *both* doctor and patient have been previously enrolled in the Diabetes Program (which, by the way, facilitates movement of patients between different doctors' surgeries). Note that no patient data are stored on the iKey itself – it is simply used as the secure access mechanism. In earlier, similar (cardiac) trials at other sites, smart cards rather than iKeys were used (www.smartcard.com.au).

The software running on the GP's computer searches for new data entered into Medical Director (the de facto case management software package used in the Illawarra region), then transfers the patient's record to the IDGP server. A Web interface has also been developed which enables patients to access this data consistent with the NSW (State) Government's Health Clinical Management Guidelines for type-2 diabetes.

Thus in this three-year Smart_ID project, the technical solution revolved around the use of USB iKeys to access patient records stored remotely from the doctor's surgery, on a central data repository.[30,31] This resulted in a more comprehensive diagnostic tool than that afforded the doctor by way of Medical Director clinical software running on their local PC alone.

Field trial results

Now while the use of iKeys per se proved relatively straightforward, it became apparent that the overriding factors affecting widespread adoption are more likely to be non-technical: GP workflow processes, EHR formats, UPIs and, more especially, privacy legislation impact significantly in this regard.[25]

Perhaps an even more significant outcome from this Smart_ID project was the development of a technological model to define remote, ubiquitous access to EHRs.[32]

Despite some technical and operational glitches early in the 2002 Smart_ID field trial, coupled with the low numbers of participants, we were nevertheless able to draw some significant conclusions, these being:

- both GPs and patients agreed that the Smart_ID system had the potential for improving information management in medical practices (all six GPs and 20 patients surveyed)[30,31]
- the use of iKeys did not significantly impact on consultation times (10–12 minutes typically, the additional time being that necessary to load the Smart_ID system),
- all expressed a preference for iKeys over smart cards,
- patients viewed computer-based medical records as being an essential technology for healthcare in the future; likewise the adoption of a UPI (roughly half of the GPs and patients surveyed prior to commencement of the 2002 Diabetes field trial).[13,24]

Videotapes of consultations revealed that use of the iKey engendered more discussion between GP and patient, since it allowed access to remote patient data not normally available when a patient visits a different doctor from their usual GP (but who nevertheless is also registered in the Illawarra Diabetes Program).

Doctors were less enthusiastic than patients, with non-participants citing lack of available time to be trained in system usage, and participation in enough projects already (sic), while nevertheless expressing confidence in using computing techno-logy in their medical practices. The key consideration from a busy GP's perspective, however, is the impact on consultations – time is money, after all (i.e. efficient workflow processes). Patients were more enthusiastic, but recall that only com-puter-literate members of the public participated in this Smart_ID field trial.

Last, the effectiveness of the Smart_ID system used in the field trial was evidenced by an unexpected side benefit: some patients who accessed their diabetes records on the IDGP website were able to report back to their GP that certain entries were in error. Not surprisingly then, patients on the whole regarded the iKey as an empowering tool.

Now to the question of access, which we can view from three different perspectives, namely: (i) currency; (ii) portability; and (iii) ability to be informed, as previously discussed. By *currency* we mean detection of a registered iKey in the USB port of the consulting doctor's computer. In other words, access to EHRs stored on the remote server is only possible while the iKey is connected. *Portability* refers to the ability of patients to move around the region and consult with *any* doctor registered with the Diabetes Program. *Ability to be informed* relates to a patient's right to determine who is granted access to their EHR. By requiring *both* iKeys to be inserted in sequence before access is granted, patients are able to monitor doctor(s)' access. In other words, the process is self-informing – and once again empowering from a patient's perspective.

To sum up, the two critical findings from the Smart_ID field trial were: (i) both GPs and patients agreed that Smart_ID devices had the potential for improving information management in medical practices; and (ii) the use of iKeys did not significantly impact on consultation times. This experience of a certain (com-puter-literate, pro-technology) cross-section of the public should be contrasted with more global public attitudes: only between 10% [30,31] and 42%[14] previously indicated they would be in favour of using biometrics for accessing EHRs (and in the case of the latter, 25% for both biometric and smart device together; and 22% for smart device only).

Relevance to telemedicine

The unifying concept of this telemedicine book is that new technologies have not been widely adopted because of human and organizational factors. In Section 3 of this book, Technological innovation in e-health – we consider questions such as the role that innovation plays in successful telemedicine, the proof needed for healthcare professionals to embrace new technologies, and the actions and structures that can promote high acceptance of new technologies in healthcare organizations (we will revisit these issues in Section 7). Suffice to say at this stage that as a result of the Smart_ID project, we have developed a technological model which enables the secure, remote and ubiquitous access of EHRs.[32]

Future directions

The access mechanism commonly employed with both smart cards and iKeys is user name/(encrypted)password, similar to the PINs used on more primitive, yet ubiquitous, magnetic stripe ATM cards. PINs are essentially random digits, whereas passwords are alphanumeric, with security further enhanced by use of PKI.

The advantage of biometrics is that they are universal (everyone has them), unique (no two people have exactly the same characteristics), permanent (they don't change over time) and collectable (readily quantifiable).[33]

Now rather than use (random) digit identifiers, patient biometrics have the potential of facilitating a much more secure access mechanism – in other words, by comparing freshly captured biometric identifiers with those stored on the smart device. This potential is due to the fact that we always carry our biometric identifiers with us – they cannot be forgotten, lost or stolen (and subsequently misused by an impostor), as can cards.[33–40] Biometrics do not eliminate the possibility of a security breach, but they do lead to systems which are difficult to compromise.

Incorporation of biometrics onto smart devices offers another potential advantage, in relation to lost or misplaced iKeys (or smart cards). In the eventuality of a patient losing consciousness, it may be possible to compare (certain) stored biometric characteristics with freshly captured versions. This is feasible for fingerprints, iris, hand geometry and perhaps face, but obviously not for voice or handwritten signatures. However, the responsible hospital staff/health professional would need to: (a) be able to access the health computer system; and (b) override any inbuilt security on the iKey (smart card).

Some vendors have opted for so-called 'two-factor authentication'. For instance, WiseKey combine iris recognition with public key cryptography (PKI) (www.wisekey.com/pages/health.htm), whereas ActivCard combine PKI and biometrics (or digital certificates – e.g. one-time password) to provide 'true security and portability' with their smart card (www.activcard.com/activ/services/library/ehealth.pdf). In the Parkinsonpas (Dutch Parkinsons) Project (www.prisma-eu.net/deliverables/SC2ehealth.pdf), biometric templates were stored in a smart card which featured an integrated (Siemens) fingertip reader.

In a report on the use of smart cards in the Canadian medical sector it was concluded that technical adequacy is a necessary yet insufficient condition for adoption.[41] More critical was that an obligation be placed on patients to actually *use* them – only then would we see the widespread adoption of such smart devices and in due course advantages flow to the health professionals concerned.

The overriding considerations for both health professional and wider public acceptance of biometric systems are accuracy, efficiency, non-intrusiveness, confidentiality (such as on-forwarding of information to unauthorized third parties) and cost – in particular the amount of additional computer equipment needed to implement them. In regard to the latter, in-built microphones can be used for speech recognition, and commonly fitted peripherals such as Web cameras can be used for iris and face recognition; handwritten signature and fingerprint recognition, however, require more sophisticated peripheral devices (graphics tablet and/or scanner, respectively), although some USB iKeys now come fitted with in-built fingerprint scanners.

This begs the question as to whether the field has matured to the point where biometrics can be effectively employed for secure access of EHRs. Industry proponents appear to take it for granted that it has; others, such as the American Civil Liberties Union (ACLU), err on the side of caution.

One industry observer has stated: 'The biometrics industry needs to provide wide education on biometrics; for example, that verification systems cannot, in general, be used for forensic purposes, or that their civil liberties are not being eroded or threatened. Until this is widely understood there will be public pressure against biometrics'.[42] The most active vertical market for biometrics is viewed as being healthcare. Moreover, healthcare providers in the US are being driven by the recently introduced Health Insurance Portability and Accountability Act (HIPAA), which mandates both the privacy of electronic medical records and limits access to only those people authorized to view them (www.hhs.gov/ocr/hipaa). Biometrics are viewed as a key technology for achieving HIPAA compliance, namely by means of strong authentication of remote users over a network.

By contrast, the American Civil Liberties Union opposes the use of face recognition software at airports, due to its ineffectiveness and also to privacy concerns. The ACLU further observes that several US government agencies (such as Immigration & Naturalization on the US–Mexico border) have abandoned facial recognition systems after finding their performance failed to match claimed levels, with unacceptably high levels of both false positives and false negatives being reported (www.aclu.org/Privacy/PrivacyMain.cfm). Sydney airport, by contrast, used face *verification* rather than face recognition per se in their SmartGate system (i.e. fresh facial capture versus passport photo) (www.anu. edu.au/people/Roger.Clarke/DV/SmartGate.html). Some other airports have chosen alternative biometric techniques (e.g. London Heathrow and Amsterdam Schiphol have opted for iris scanning, whereas Kennedy, Los Angeles and Miami use hand geometry).

Apart from privacy and security considerations – and to an extent cost – the bottom line from a consumer's (the public's) point of view, is accuracy and reliability. In relation to the former, accuracy rates vary with biometric type. False acceptance and false rejection rates (FAR and FRR) are commonly used to measure accuracy. The most accurate biometric features are, in decreasing order: iris (0% FAR; 2% FRR), followed by fingerprints (0.001% FAR; 6% FRR), with both face and signatures being much worse.[40] By contrast, current biometric usage rates vary from fingerprints (39%), hand geometry (37%), speech (16%), face (7%), iris (4%) and signatures (3%) (*Economist*, September 2000). The ultimate biometric is most likely DNA, but at this point in time would be far too intrusive to be of practical use.

The other major impediment to the widespread adoption of biometric systems is lack of standardization – either formal or de facto (industry) – although BioAPI (www.bioapi.org/BioAPI_home.htm) has been making inroads in recent times.

It should be emphasized here that it would take only *one* disastrous field trial to sway public opinion against using biometrics. The importance of pilot system trials cannot be overemphasized. Positive outcomes can include the resolution of potential interoperability problems, whereas negative outcomes (in other words, poor experience which doesn't match expectations) can set the entire field back for decades. Indeed, an unrealistic build-up of expectations can be quite counterproductive (witness the effect of the dotcom crash in the early years of the 21st century on the IT industry generally, or the perpetual non-delivery in the field of artificial intelligence).[43,44] To an extent, this has already occurred with regard to face recognition for airport security (see, for example, the *Boston Globe* of 18 July 2002, reporting on the Logan Airport experience).

Conclusion

Now to return to the issue of lack of adoption of new technologies in e-health. Based on our experience with the Smart_ID system developed for diabetes patients and their doctors, we are able to draw some general conclusions in regard to such matters.

First, a precondition to patients participating in the Smart_ID field trial was that they be enrolled in the Illawarra Diabetes Program. These diabetes patients were invariably computer literate and pro-technology. Furthermore, they were all favourably disposed towards the use of EHRs and UPIs, including in the case of the latter incorporation of biometric identifiers. Patients left the field trial even more favourably disposed, having had positive experiences of both the USB iKeys and the ability to view their own EHRs via a Web browser.

Doctors enrolled in the Smart_ID field trial were likewise technically literate, and most (but not all) were willing to undergo the minimal training required in the use of the iKeys. Impact on consultation times was considered minimal.

Both patients and doctors could see the benefits which flow from being able to access patient data during consultations – more informed and engaging discussions often followed as a result of this.

Since the field trial, the USB iKey system has been expanded to *all* doctors enrolled in the Diabetes Program in the Illawarra region (not just the six who participated in the field trial). Likewise, iKeys are subsequently being used to link patient data stored on the IDGP server to diabetes health professionals connected to the Illawarra Area Health Service Local Area Network. In summary, the IDGP and IAHS both continue to advocate for the adoption of iKeys. Once doctors experience their ease of use and access to EHRs, they invariably embrace the new technology – in other words, they learn from their own (positive) experience. Fear of the unknown, and/or an unwillingness to change from the way things have always been done (in other words, inertia) can easily impede the adoption of new technology, unless the resulting benefits are immediately obvious.

Furthermore, we are not talking about a *radical* step up in technology here, but rather a simple procedure involving the insertion of an iKey in the computer's USB port, followed by accessing files stored on the remote server. Asking healthcare providers to take *too* big a leap with new technology could well be a deterrent to its adoption (i.e. taking them too far out of their 'comfort zone').

Another point worthy of note is that use of USB iKeys is consistent with the Australian government's Digital Certificate Scheme, by which participating GPs are issued with unique identifiers on either smart cards or iKeys. The long-term goal of the Health Insurance Commission is to facilitate online reimbursement of doctors thus registered. By extension, the government could foster widespread adoption of such technology if financial incentives (i.e. rebates) were added to the mix.

Finally, publicizing successes such as the Smart_ID project – both nationally[23,24,30] and internationally[2,13,25,31,32,40] – also plays a significant role in the future adoption of such technologies.

To return briefly to biometric systems – is the public willing to accept 95% (99%, 99.5%) accuracy? In practice, it comes down to a balance between security and accessibility to achieve an acceptable level of risk – more specifically, are patients willing to sacrifice some privacy for greater security? Operation and system integration are other challenges which, if not adequately addressed, can render biometric solutions unworkable in real-life deployment. Further, there are limitations due to background lighting for face/iris, background noise for speech, and so forth. It should also be pointed out that there is nothing to be gained by combining different biometrics, since this leads to diminishing accuracy overall (the whole being *less* than the sum of the individual parts).[45]

So what are the key considerations for the acceptance and widespread adoption of this new technology within a healthcare context? In a nutshell, the best catalyst for acceptance would be successful practical demonstrations and field trials. To date we have established the viability of using iKeys (smart cards) for remote, secure access of patients' EHRs.[31,32] More specifically, we have devised a technological model for secure, remote and ubiquitous access of EHRs.[32] Further field trials are needed to confirm the benefits to be gained from incorporating patient biometrics onto such smart devices.[40] Apart from providing a technical solution, it is suggested that biometrics could provide true 'uniqueness' – in the sense of UPIs – for secure access of EHRs. Last, incorporation of biometrics has the potential for *enhancing*, rather than reducing, patient security and privacy.

Acknowledgements

This work was funded by the Australian Research Council under its Strategic Partnerships with Industry Research and Training (SPIRT) scheme – grant number C00001904. The permission of the Illawarra Division of General Practice to publish this work is gratefully acknowledged.

References

1   Hedges G (2000) Establishing Accountability in e-health Technologies. Statement of Industry Representative Arthur Andersen LLP to the House Committee on Science Subcommittee on Technology (available online at: www.house.gov/science/hedges_033000.htm).

2   Fulcher J (2002) Privacy issues arising from a Smart_ID application in e-health. *Proceedings International Conference on Advances in Infrastructure for eBusiness, eEducation, eScience and eMedicine on the Internet*, 29 July–4 August, L'Aquila, Italy.

3   Win KT, Croll P, Cooper J *et al.* (2002) Issues of privacy, confidentiality and access in electronic health records. *J Law & Information Science.* **12**(1): 24–5.

4   Song H, Croll P and Win KT (2003) A prototype patient eConsent in access control to electronic medical records. *Proceedings of the Asia-Pacific Association of Medical Informatics Conference – APAMI*, 20–22 October, Daegu, Korea.

5   Win KT, Croll P and Cooper J (2003) Engineering pragmatic patient consent in electronic health record systems. *Proceedings of the World Congress on Medical Physics and Biomedical Engineering*, 24–29 August, Sydney, Australia.

6   Kara A (2001) Protecting privacy in remote-sensing monitoring. *IEEE Computer.* **34**(5): 24–7.

7   Ligtvoet A (2003) Prisma Strategic Guideline 2: e-health. *Stitching RAND Europe, The Netherlands* (available online at: www.prisma-eu.net/deliverables/SC2ehealth.pdf).

8   Canadian Institute for Health Information (2000) Unique identifiers for health services recipients in Canada: a background paper. Ottawa, Canada (available online at: www.secure.cihi.ca/cihiweb/en/downloads/infostand_unique_e_recipients_backpaper.pdf).

9   Kohn L, Corrigan J and Donaldson M (1999) *To Err is Human, Building a Safer Health System.* National Academy Press, Washington, DC.

10 Simpson R (1996) Security threats are usually an inside job. *Nursing Management.* **27**(12): 43.

11 Rindfleisch T (1997) Privacy, information technology and health care. *Communications ACM.* **40**(8): 93–100.

12 Carter M (2000) Integrated electronic health records and patient privacy: possible benefits but real dangers. *Medical J Australia.* **172**: 28–30.

13 Bomba D and DeSilva A (2001) An Australian case study of patient attitudes towards the use of computerised medical records and unique identifiers. *Proceedings of the World Medical Informatics Conference*, London, UK, pp. 1430–4.

14 Crompton M (2002) Biometrics and privacy: the end of the world as we know it, or the white knight of privacy? *Proceedings of the Biometrics – Security and Authentication Conference*, 20 March, Sydney, Australia (Keynote Address).

15 Tomko G (1998) Biometrics as a privacy-enhancing technology: friend or foe of privacy? (available online at: www.dss.state.ct.us/digital/tomko.htm).

16 Hansmann U *et al.* (2003) *Pervasive Computing: the mobile world.* Springer-Verlag, Berlin, Germany.

17 Thomas P (ed.) (2000) *Personal and Ubiquitous Computing.* Springer-Verlag, London, UK.

18 Kohl D (1995) Crossing the privacy minefield. *Health Management Technology.* **16**(9): 50.

19 Clarke R (1987) Just another piece of plastic for your wallet: the 'Australia Card' scheme (available online at: www.anu.edu/people/Roger.Clarke/DV/OzCard.html).

20 Privacy Committee of NSW (1995) Smart cards: Big Brother's little helpers. (available online at: www.austlii.edu.au/au/other/privacy/smart/index.html).

21 NSW Health Council (2000) *A Better Health System for NSW – The Menadue Report.* NSW Government.

22 Pfleeger C (1997) *Security in Computing.* Prentice Hall, Upper Saddle River, NJ.

23 Cromwell D, Bomba D, Tu H *et al.* (2002) Dividends for care coordination from investments in information technology: lessons from the Illawarra Coordinated Care Trial. In: *The Australian Coordinated Care Trials: recollections of an evaluation*, pp. 249–61. Commonwealth Department of Health and Aged Care.

24 Spinks K, Fulcher J and Dalley A (2001) Survey of GP Attitudes to smartcards. *Proceedings of the 10th Health Informatics Association of NSW Conference*, 17–18 February, Hunter Valley, Australia.

25 Fulcher J (2003) The use of smart devices in e-health. *Proceedings of the International Symposium on Information & Communications Technology*, 24–26 September, Dublin, Ireland.

26 Chan A, Cao J, Chan H *et al.* (2001) A Web-enabled framework for smart card application in health services. *Communications ACM.* **44**(9): 77–82.

27 Sheifer K and Procaccino J (2002) Smart card evolution. *Communications ACM.* **45**(7): 83–8.

28 Bretz E (2002) Tons of storage on a key ring. *IEEE Spectrum.* **39**(11): 49.

29 Fancher C (1996) Smartcards. *Scientific American* (available online at: www.sciam.com).

30 Bomba D, Fulcher J and Dalley A (2002) Lessons learnt from the UoW-IDGP Smart_ID Project. *Proceedings of the Health Informatics Conference*, 4–6 August, Melbourne, Australia.

31 Bomba D, Fulcher J and Dalley A (2004) An Australian case study of a patient-GP diabetes I-Key innovation project. *J Information Technology in Healthcare* (in press).

32 Dalley A, Fulcher J, Bomba D *et al.* (2004) A technological model to define access to electronic clinical records. *IEEE Trans Information Technology in Biomedicine* (in press).

33 Hong L, Jain A and Pankanti S (2000) Biometric identification. *Communications ACM.* **43**(2): 91–8.

34   Bolle R, Jain A and Paqkanti S (eds) (1999) *Biometrics: personal identification in a networked society*. Kluwer Academic Publishers, New York, NY.

35   Lockie M (2002) *Biometric Technology*. Heinemann, Oxford, UK.

36   Wayman J (ed.) (2002) *Biometric Systems: technology, design and performance evaluation*. Springer-Verlag, Berlin, Germany.

37   Zhang D (ed.) (2002) *Biometric Solutions for Authentication in an e-World*. Kluwer Academic Publishers, Boston, MA.

38   Chirillo J and Blaul S (2003) *Implementing Biometric Security*. Wiley, Indianapolis, IN.

39   Woodward J, Orians N and Higgins P (2003) *Biometrics*. McGraw-Hill, New York, NY.

40   Fulcher J (2004) The use of patient biometrics in accessing electronic health records. *Intl J Health Technology Management* (in press).

41   Benoit A and Hamel G (2001) Adoption of smart cards in the medical sector: the Canadian experience. *Social Science & Medicine*. **53**(7): 879–94.

42   Hamilton W (2002) Markets and regions for biometrics. *Secure Computing Magazine*. **March**: 15 (available online at: www.scmagazine.com).

43   Fulcher J (2001) Practical (Artificial) Intelligence. *Proceedings of the 5th National Thai Computer Science & Engineering Conference*, 7–9 November, Chiang Mai, Thailand (invited Keynote Speech).

44   Fulcher J and Jain L (eds) (2004) *Applied Intelligent Systems: new directions*. Springer-Verlag, Berlin, Germany.

45   Daugman J (2002) Combining multiple biometrics (available online at: www.cl.cam. ac.uk/users/jgd1000/combine/combine.html).

Chapter 6

Using ICT to better support the fragmentary nature of healthcare

Lynne P Baldwin and Malcolm Clarke

Introduction

Patients are, obviously, central to any national healthcare service. As we live in an age where people are living longer and demanding a better quality of life in terms of health throughout their lives, the demands placed on any healthcare service are therefore great. The financial burden on either the patients themselves or the government to keep patients in hospital or in institutions such as care homes for the elderly, the mentally impaired or others who require full-time care and assistance is great. Such care cannot, at present, be provided in their homes, although it is hoped that when or if technology is installed in our homes, this will allow the healthcare service to deliver the same (or better) quality of care but without the enormous costs involved.

It is not, however, just a matter of financial cost. Involving us more in our own healthcare at an earlier age or stage has two advantages. One, being at home or, at least, as near to home as possible, has psychological advantages that positively impact on our mental, and thus physical, health. Two, there is the possibility that, as we feel more comfortable with the technology and/or our confidence grows in approaching healthcare professionals or health issues (many people fear both), we might take a more proactive role in our own healthcare and thus either delay the need for intervention or, at best, manage a potential problem away.

It might be argued, however, that while those of us who work with computers regularly are thus both confident and, it is hoped, competent with such technology, the same is not necessarily true of the general public, the very people the healthcare service aims to support. Technology is often viewed by those without such exposure as impersonal, adding to, not bridging, the communication gap between those engaged in the interaction. While such lack of empathy and personal contact might be expected, and acceptable, in, say, sending off a tax form to the relevant authority, in the case of healthcare we, as patients, expect exactly the opposite, that is, we wish to be treated with every sympathy and with due regard to our emotional as well as physical needs. We expect (although we do not always get) a warm welcome from those that we come into contact with in the healthcare sector, and we want to be given sufficient time and attention to express our needs, fears and the like in the most supportive environment possible at a time when we may feel vulnerable and scared and in need of support. For the patient with little or no experience of the technological wizardry surrounding computers (and there are many more than we like to think), not to mention the technology of the healthcare world (scanners, probes and all manner of equipment whose purpose is not necessarily immediately apparent), and with the additional fear engendered by those with serious or potentially serious medical issues, the hospital, clinic or wherever can be a pretty scary place.

However, it is not only the *patients* who are fearful of the seemingly negative impact of technology in mediating the dialogue between patient and healthcare professional; those working in the healthcare sector are similarly voicing their concerns with regard to the use of computers. This is, perhaps, somewhat surprising given that healthcare is, of all the professional activities, most likely to be 'technology-rich'. While healthcare professionals seem very keen indeed to have the latest scanner, imaging equipment or instruments (what surgeon would proudly claim 'Yes, it's a very old model/tool that I use to carry out this complex procedure' when trying to reassure the patient that they are shortly to operate on!), there does not appear to be the same enthusiasm for using the computer in a similarly supporting role. Computers, in healthcare and elsewhere, are sometimes viewed akin to humans, and with the same human powers. The popular press seems to suggest that teachers, doctors and others might well find themselves out of a job in the not too distant future given the sophistication of the technology to do what has/had hitherto been regarded as activity only possible by humans. There are mutterings along these lines in the professions themselves, which might in part explain a reluctance to embrace computer-centered technology. Whether patient or healthcare professional, the computer is seen as something which can only negatively impact the personal contact that each expects of the interaction between the humans involved. It seems that for those of us engaged in promoting computer-supported interaction, we have much to do to persuade those involved that the computer, appropriately used, is as much of value as the other 'tools of the trade', so to speak.

Discussion of e-health is, as the above demonstrates, a complex business, as the editors of this publication rightly acknowledge. In their study of human factors at the beginning of this publication, they present a six-layer onion, with organizational learning and success, as the goal, at its heart. They argue that it is only by looking at each layer that we can hope to make sense of the whole, but that the complexity of the interactions makes this problematic. This chapter of the book encapsulates various aspects of all six outer 'rings' of this onion, namely that organizational learning and success is dependent on us exploring the cultural and institutional context, technological innovation, change management, actors, network and alliances, and mental models with clinical perspective. As you will see from the seven sections of this publication, Chapters 2 to 7 are each devoted to discussion of these six rings of the organizational learning and success onion. Presented in this chapter is the technological innovation layer of this onion, although as you will see, this cannot be divorced from the other layers which together make their contribution to organizational learning and success.

Every country claims that the needs of patients come first, and the UK is no exception. The National Health Service (NHS) in the UK published its NHS Plan in July 2000,[1] saying that patients and people were central to its radical reform of healthcare and that although this included more hospitals and beds, shorter waiting times and improved care for older people, an essential element was that patients should have more power and information. The NHS Plan is permeated with words and phrases that emphasize the need to involve patients more in their own healthcare. Although it would seem difficult to see how patients could be anything other than involved given that it is their body/mind that is being seen, treated or managed, this suggests that patients are currently viewed more as 'cases' rather than as individuals, as people. That is, that they come into the doctor's surgery with a problem, and that it is the problem, rather than the patient, that is being seen. While in some sense this is naturally necessary, as patients want the health problem 'solved' in some way, as in the case of, say, a broken finger being mended or a minor injury being treated, not all patients present things which might be seen as a 'problem to be solved'. Indeed, it might be argued that much cannot be 'solved' anyway; asthma, psoriasis, mental health conditions and the like do not, and cannot, go away, and it is more that these need to be managed, as effectively as possible, by both the patients themselves (who are, after all, dealing with their healthcare day in and day out) and, on occasion, with the assistance of various healthcare professionals. However, healthcare is as much about dealing with a wide range of 'everyday' issues, such as helping a first-time mother with her new baby or helping someone deal with the death of a loved one. Whether borne out or not, there is a perception, at least, that doctors and consultants, in particular, are viewed by their patients as somewhat distant, over-authoritative and dispassionate. Indeed, the word 'clinical' does not only mean 'relating to health' but also detached, lacking in empathy. Whether stated explicitly or implicitly, there seems to be a call for healthcare professionals to engage more fully with their patients, and to see them more as some kind of 'partner' in their healthcare rather than someone 'in authority'. Patients are somewhat in awe of doctors and, in particular, consultants, and this raises issues with regard to the patient/healthcare relationship.

The UK health service

It is first necessary to provide some background as to how healthcare is organized in the UK, as this varies from country to country. One vital aspect of healthcare in the UK is that for the vast majority of the population it is paid for not via private medical insurance but instead through the system of taxation. It is thus seen as 'free', in some sense, by patients as they do not need to pay for any treatment direct to either the local doctor/GP or any other healthcare professional. While patients may regard it as 'free', it is nonetheless extremely expensive for the government to provide, particularly in a country where the number of taxpayers is decreasing in relative terms, the population of those over 65 is significantly greater than in previous generations and the fact that healthcare 'solutions' such as drugs or surgery are now that much more expensive. In addition, patients expect and demand more of the healthcare services these days, and with the advent of the Internet are much more informed as to the choices available. In other countries, both in Europe and elsewhere, patients can see a specialist/consultant in a hospital without needing to be referred there by their own local doctor, and may enter the health system directly at the secondary or tertiary care level (*see* Figure 6.1). In the UK, this is not possible; a patient must enter the system at the primary care level and first see their own doctor, known as a general practitioner (GP), whose surgery/clinic is normally located close to the home of the patient. As in many states in the US, there is little evidence that the healthcare system is moving towards 'enabling less expensive professionals' (such as nurses) to do 'progressively more sophisticated things', as Christenen *et al.* (p. 106)[2] argue that we should be considering if we are to use what they call 'disruptive innovations' to radically alter, with a view to improving, healthcare at both a local and national level. The local doctor/GP is, then, a kind of 'gatekeeper'[3] to other services should these be needed. In the US this would correspond to managed care.

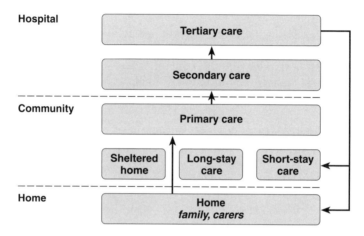

Figure 6.1 Healthcare structure.

The health service provided at this level is known, in general, as primary care. It is the responsibility of the doctor/GP to refer the patient on to what is known as secondary care, usually a hospital, where more specialized equipment, and specialists/consultants are on hand. Where secondary care is unable to provide a solution, referral is made to the more specialized tertiary care centres, either by primary care directly or from secondary to tertiary care. As with any healthcare system, there are potential drawbacks, and these have implications for the speed and accuracy of the treatment both at primary and secondary care level. Referring the patient from primary care to secondary care normally involves a lengthy process of letter writing between the doctor/clinician and the specialist/consultant in the hospital in trying to book an appointment. The specialist/consultant in the hospital then has to contact the patient to tell them of the time and day of the appointment. It goes without saying that this is a lengthy process, and time, for those with serious illness, may be in short supply. The doctor/clinician is somewhat divorced from what happens from that point on and, given the problems associated with relying on a postal service (normally efficient enough, but the UK has suffered from postal strikes in recent years) to relay communication between consultant/hospital and patient, there is the danger of information either arriving late or, worse, not arriving at all. A patient referred to secondary care may have moved house in the time between first seeing their doctor/GP and the first consultation with the specialist/consultant. Although this may seem trivial, cases have been reported in the media where this new information has not been conveyed, and that this has adversely affected the healthcare of the patients concerned. Patients themselves are unaware of the processes going on behind the scenes, so to speak, and so it is not difficult to see that they would not necessarily realize the importance of informing anyone of their change of address. Moreover, although they may consider reporting such information to their own doctor/GP at primary care level, they would not know whom to contact at secondary care level as the name of the specialist/consultant or their place of work would likely not be known. It might be argued that the organization of healthcare in the UK is not very patient-centered; once the patient presents themselves to the doctor/GP at the primary care level, and it is decided that intervention at secondary care level is required, then the patient plays a relatively passive role in the management of their healthcare, or the processes associated with it.

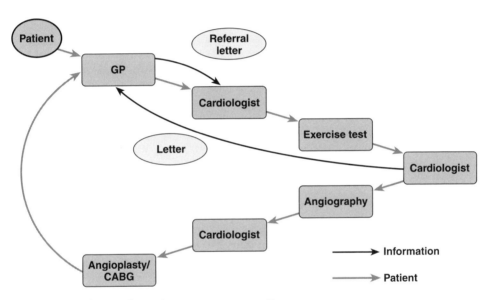

Figure 6.2 Pathway of care for coronary artery disease.

Patient care pathways provide a useful insight into many of the factors that affect the perception of the standard of service and care that the patient may receive. Figure 6.2 might represent a typical patient care pathway for a patient presenting to the doctor/GP with chest pain. In the UK, the doctor/GP will refer the patient to the cardiologist. The referral is made in the form of the 'referral letter', which should include a medical summary of presenting symptoms, history, relevant existing conditions, drugs, results of tests and any other pertinent information. However, information content may be very limited. In this case, it is the patient that moves around the system. At the first consultation with the cardiologist, it is likely that the tests necessary to make an unequivocal diagnosis, such as a stress exercise test and an echocardiogram, will not have been performed and the information will not be available. The patient must return for these and return on a further occasion to see the cardiologist. Only at this point is there the information that can be used to make the diagnosis. A positive exercise test will result in angiography and likely treatment such as angioplasty or coronary artery bypass graft (CABG).

The patient care pathway highlights where delay is experienced, which is a significant cause of dissatisfaction for patients. National Service Frameworks in the UK (NSF – Coronary Heart Disease) outline targets for specialities. However, the analysis of Figure 6.2 clearly highlights the distinct lack of information that is exchanged between the doctor/GP and cardiologist. Even when the patient returns from hospital following treatment and is rehabilitated, the doctor/GP may have little information on the procedures that were carried out and on the management that must follow to maintain the patient. It is the role of technology and information and communication technology (ICT) to improve what information is gathered, where it is gathered and how it is exchanged between the key players responsible for the management and care of the patient. The structure of the health service in different countries differs, often in quite fundamental ways. However, the pathway of care can be seen to offer assistance in many ways and offers an important analysis tool for considering factors. It provides an abstract view of the desired pathway against which existing services may be compared and changes may be identified. It also offers a tool that allows alternatives to be considered. This may include changes to the pathway of care experienced by the patient, for example steps may be eliminated, added or replaced. New pathways may be created, especially those which might improve gaining, management and movement of information.

Current role of technology

Information and communication technology can (and does) play a role in both primary care and secondary care. And with the move to involve patients further in their care, in the future patients themselves may well make their own contributions in some way, both passive by searching information or active by contacting health workers perhaps from their home computer. That information systems are becoming increasingly more sophisticated is uncontested. Indeed, Rodger and Pendharkar[4] describe a variety of fascinating technological developments used by the Department of Defense in the US. However, whether it is sophisticated, which somehow carries with it the assumption that it is somehow 'better' or, at least, 'good' in comparison to whatever was in place before, is of little value, particularly in terms of healthcare. As a report by Payton and Brennan[5] on a phone-accessible Web-based computer network that was developed for the use of those caring for patients suffering from Alzheimer's disease demonstrates, an 'unsophisticated' response answered the needs. It revealed that what carers actually wanted was 'someone to converse with and share ideas' (p. 88) and that access to an encyclopedia into the disease or even a decision-making utility was not regarded as useful by this particular set of users. This has important implications for those developing information systems, namely that when we are ill or request intervention of one sort or another from healthcare professionals, we do not ask for sophistication but rather that we receive an appropriate, timely and accurate response. They want such a response to be personal, sensitive and with due regard to their emotional as well as physical needs; a tall order indeed for healthcare professionals working in an emotionally charged and often fraught environment.

Whatever the role that technology will play in the modernization of the NHS or any other global, national or local healthcare system, none can doubt that it is perceived as vital to its success. Quick to grasp this have been the technology multinational companies, eager for business. Huge multinational organizations involved in producing computer technology for industry, particularly in a financial climate where competition is fierce and there has recently been a significant downturn in business, are keen to promote any service as, naturally enough, they are in the business of selling technology. They would understandably claim to be in the business of improving the health of patients, although the cynical among us might recall the very many horror stories of extremely expensive information systems that not only took far longer to build than their designers said at the outset but that also did not deliver what their customers expected; some did not even work at all and had to be shelved. That said, the future of technology looks bright, as illustrated in the following story. Recounting the speech made by Bill Gates, founder of the world's most well-known software company, Microsoft, Hawkes[6] reports that Gates, who is currently actively seeking to develop new products for the NHS in the UK and likely elsewhere, tells a story of how things might be in the future technology-led and managed health service. In this wonderful technology-enriched future, a businessman is knocked down by a cyclist, but is not so seriously injured that he cannot use his mobile phone to gasp 'Call my doctor now!'. The mobile phone, upon recognizing his voice, dials Dr X's surgery, and the female receptionist somehow verifies his identity, locates him (from the mobile phone signal) and calls an ambulance. While on his way to hospital, the receptionist sends his medical records electronically, so that the Accident and Emergency team have them to hand upon his arrival. The businessman's own doctor calls up the record of the treatment online, offering his patient reassurance that he has had the best possible care and treatment.

As Baldwin et al. note,[7] the businessman has been very lucky on at least four counts. One, the accident happened during normal opening hours of the surgery. Two, the technology worked perfectly. Three, the ambulance was able to reach the spot quickly. Four, the patient records were correct and up to date. This seems to be an excellent example of how such technology could be successfully used. However, for such a scenario to play out, it would seem that the context in question is not beset by the practical difficulties that, we suggest, permeate our professional and personal lives.

This scene is based on the premise that either such accidents happen only during normal working hours (while we have no research to back up our view here, common sense leads us to conclude that this seems highly improbable) or that in this new NHS, the clinic/surgery of our local doctor is open 24 hours a day. Given budgetary and other constraints, clinics/surgeries of local doctors in the UK are open for only a few hours in the morning and a few hours in the late afternoon/early evening Mondays to Fridays (and not at all at the weekend), for the most part. It would also be difficult, if not impossible, at least for those of us who use technology extensively, to imagine an environment where technology worked perfectly, all of the time. Indeed, some would likely be grateful if it worked reasonably well some of the time! Until the advent of technology which functions so wonderfully, relying on technology alone should surely not form part of any vision of a healthcare system.

Ambulance services in many countries in the West are very good indeed, so perhaps we do not need to suspend our disbelief too much when envisaging the speedy arrival of an ambulance. That said, however, the patient must live in a reasonably urban setting; ambulances cannot respond so quickly (if at all) in a rural one, and it is not peak time. Luck must also play a part; good weather conditions and little traffic in this scenario. Correct and up-to-date records are yet another aspect of the world of work which is a worthy goal but rarely (if, indeed, it is possible) achieved. However careful, professional or whatever we are with administration, errors are made and/or things are not entered in a timely fashion.

Imagining ourselves as that businessman (we are by nature fairly selfish; something well understood by image makers enticing us to buy), it is easy to see how we might be seduced by such a picture of healthcare in the future. The message to the taxpayer/government is, then, invest heavily in (very expensive) technology and we will all get the right treatment at the right time and, it would follow from this, though of course the point is not explicitly made, that we would all live long, healthy and happy lives. On a slightly less optimistic note, we see that some things in life will not change that much according to the example given. The doctor is male. The receptionist is female. The patient, chosen as someone worth saving, is a businessman. There is a crumb of comfort in this, however; we will not need to suffer the mental anguish associated with the task of altering our mental models of the stereotypical healthcare professional or who is valued more highly in our Western society.

While there is plenty of information about healthcare available in print or, increasingly, on the Internet, when faced with a healthcare issue that requires intervention, in the vast majority of cases, today at least, we need to deal with a healthcare professional face to face. The importance of the doctor/GP in primary care is clear; it is, at least in the UK, the first port of call for the patient. Although the appropriate response may not require further intervention, the doctor/GP and (normally) specialist/consultant are key. For the patient, who may well have built a good relationship with their doctor over a long period of time, being referred to a specialist/consultant in a hospital is not without its difficulties. Among these is the fact that the patient has never met the specialist/consultant; building a new relationship with a stranger is, for many, not easy. This is made more problematic by the fact that they are probably very anxious or upset, and thus not at their best in terms of expressing themselves well, clearly or, importantly, accurately. Yet the value of that initial visit depends not only on what the specialist/consultant knows about that particular illness or disease but on the quality of the information provided by the patient. And patients, naturally enough, do not necessarily know what is, or is not, relevant information that would help the specialist/consultant in their diagnosis and subsequent treatment or care.

One of the most vital aspects of effective and efficient care is an accurate (as is possible) record of patient care up to the time when the specialist/consultant sees the patient. It is at this time that the specialist/consultant makes the vital decision as to what treatment is or is not appropriate, and when this needs to be carried out. The decision(s) made at that time are crucial to the patient's subsequent care and health, and it is clear that the knowledge and information available to the specialist/consultant needs to be as accurate and as full as is possible. As

Summerton notes,[8] inefficiency and/or inaccuracy can adversely affect not only prognosis but also the nature of any intervention(s), and the earlier those choices (that is, decisions) are made, the better.

Such information is stored in three (at least) different places. One, informally, by way of the knowledge and experience gained by the doctor (and/or, perhaps, another clinician in the primary care surgery/clinic, such as a nurse) who has been involved in the care of the patient up to that time. Two, formally, by way of the records that are kept in the primary care surgery/clinic, which in many places are still kept in handwritten form only. Within primary care in the UK, computerization is almost 100% and there is a high level of use of electronic records within the consultation. However, secondary care is not computerized to this extent, and almost all communication between primary and secondary care is by paper. Three, informally, by way of what the patient knows about their own health, history and experiences.

As described earlier, the information currently available to the specialist/consultant when meeting the patient for the first time is limited to only two of the three sources available. One, formally, by way of the information that is forwarded by primary care and which is sent before (hopefully) the patient arrives (although in many cases this may be limited). This is commonly known as the 'referral letter'. Two, informally, by way of what the patient knows about their own health, history and experiences. Gaining information by way of only these two sources means that there is the potential for a breakdown (at worst) or a lack of richness in information sharing between those working in primary care and those working in secondary/tertiary care, and, vitally, between patient and healthcare professional.

Effective communication both *among* healthcare workers and *between* healthcare workers and their patients in both primary and secondary care is vital. Information in the current NHS is stored in various places and access is restricted; there is no central, complete patient record that is accessible to all healthcare professionals at the various levels of care. There is also no mechanism for allowing the patient to interact both with their local nurse and/or doctor/GP (at primary care level) while at the same time engaging with the specialist/consultant (at secondary/tertiary care level). At the same time, there is a reluctance for primary care to gain diagnostic information on the condition and any such tests are deferred to the hospital. It is not unusual for these tests to be performed *after* the first visit to the specialist/consultant, restricting further the knowledge/information that could be available. The knowledge/information that the specialist/consultant has to hand during the first consultation is shown in Box 6.1 (*see* p. 108). Also shown is what is *not* currently available across the healthcare sector in the UK to assist the specialist/consultant in their decision making.

> ### Box 6.1 Information available at the specialist/consultant–patient consultation
>
> ---
>
> Knowledge/information currently available to specialist/consultant
> - a brief letter of referral from the doctor/GP
> - information gleaned from the patient during the consultation.
>
> Knowledge/information that specialist/consultant does *not* have
> - full, formal written/other patient record from the doctor/GP
> - information gleaned from the doctor/GP other than that contained in the formal written/other patient record
> - information gleaned from any other healthcare professional (such as a nurse) who has been engaged in the care of the patient.
>
> Knowledge/information that specialist/consultant *may not* have
> - information from diagnostic tests
> - information from previous visits to the hospital.

The AIDMAN platform

In this section we describe a clinical ICT system called AIDMAN that has been developed and is now successfully used in the UK. The system is designed to re-evaluate the relationships that exist between all sectors of healthcare and, by use of ICT, can provide the third, vital, source of information lacking in consultations that are not telemediated. The 'virtual' consultation is able to bring together patient, healthcare professional from primary care and the consultant/specialist. In this scenario, the patient may bring knowledge of symptoms and previous history, the primary care healthcare professional brings informal knowledge of the patient gained from significant period of care of the patient up to that time, and the full formal, patient record held by the healthcare professionals at primary care level. AIDMAN (Advanced Informatics Distributed Medical Access Network) was designed to offer the patient the advantage of a 'virtual' consultation.[9–14] Face-to-face consultation offers particular advantages over other channels of communication, and although AIDMAN is in essence a clinical ICT system involving video-conferencing, its success has come by obtaining diagnostic information at the primary care level and forwarding that information, such as high-definition images, ECG and ultrasound, in advance of the consultation. Using a computer-based video-conference system (Proshare V5.2) also enables shared access to data applications and other peripherals or medical systems that might be considered useful in presenting clinical data during the consultation. AIDMAN has been designed to be communication technology independent and in the UK uses ISDN, but may easily use a network connection in its place. Within the project, satellite technology was evaluated to determine its capability to support Web-based tools and video-conferencing; vital if the infrastructure in a particular region or country is not able to provide the links required by more conventional means.

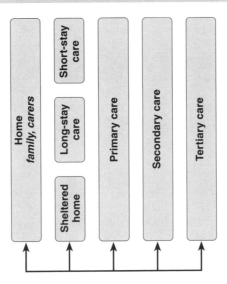

Figure 6.3 Healthcare structure of the AIDMAN platform.

Part of the novelty of the approach is that much of the healthcare is nurse-led, rather than doctor/GP-led at primary care level and it brings together the isolated 'islands' of knowledge and information held by both the patient and healthcare professionals involved in their care. During the consultation, the patient has at their side a medically trained person; this person can therefore use their hands or nose to provide the information gained by way of touch and smell, and can also operate the camera should the specialist/consultant wish to view a particular aspect of the body in order to aid diagnosis and determine the extent and severity of the problem (*see* Figure 6.4). In this example, the patient has had leg ulcers for some months and there is no healing. The district nurse (right), will have visited the patient's home on a regular basis in order to change dressings, etc., and established a rapport and trust. Having the same district nurse in the consultation gives the patient a sense of support, and the clinical knowledge built up by the nurse can facilitate the consultation; the nurse can answer questions succinctly and fully, and other aspects of the clinical background can be included. The consultant and nurse, together with the patient, would use the pre-intervention teleclinic to agree the procedure to be carried out, in this case to operate on the vein. They would also describe the forthcoming process to the patient. The postoperative teleclinic is used for follow-up and to deal with complications. One of the major benefits of this collaborative approach is that when complications are detected, they can be dealt with much more quickly.

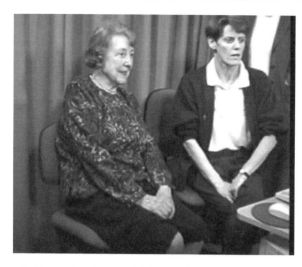

Figure 6.4 Patient (left) and local nurse (right) during a dermatology teleclinic. There is a digital camera which gives real-time analogue video and can capture very high-resolution digital images of the same scene. A second camera on top of the monitor is used for 'talking heads'.

It is important to realize that the AIDMAN system is a total approach that is based on the use of technology to support health delivery and communication between all key players. Although video-conferencing is used to support the virtual consultation, high-definition images, reports, results from tests, shared access to data applications and other peripherals or medical systems might be used at any time during the consultation to present clinical data to either the medically trained person at one end, or the specialist/consultant at the other. It is an end-to-end solution and impacts on process at each stage of the pathway of care. Figure 6.5 shows a screenshot from a typical telecardiology session with both ends viewing the result from a stress exercise ECG test and accessing the clinical notes through the general practice database in order to review the drug therapy. The example highlights how the video-conference window is shrunk to a small size as the session becomes an exchange of information.

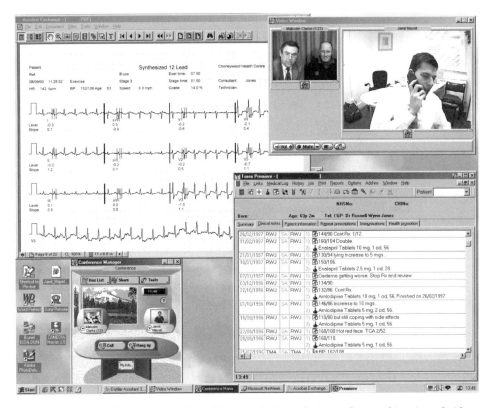

Figure 6.5 Screenshot of a typical cardiology teleclinic showing the combination of video-conference, test results, data and application sharing.

Figure 6.6 shows how the pathway of care for cardiology might be modified by the use of technology. Stress exercise ECG testing is performed locally. An electronic referral, which would include the ECG report, and any other relevant medical history is forwarded to the cardiologist. The cardiologist now has the information that allows diagnosis to be made and a virtual consultation can be scheduled on the basis of need and urgency. A severely abnormal test might result in a virtual consultation within days, otherwise it would be scheduled as normal priority, whereas should the ECG be normal, no consultation would be needed. It is also clear that the first outpatient appointment in the original pathway of care is eliminated. Estimates of the number of patients referred inappropriately to the consultant can often exceed 50%, but by having information these may be eliminated. The most significant difference is the increase in the flow of information between each sector of healthcare. Also note that management information is bidirectional, which reinforces the new model for healthcare structure. The ICT allows key health professionals from all sectors to collaborate, and bring each of their specialist skills to the problem. Here the pathway of care has been used to show the effect of altering the position of a test, the order of processes and the introduction of new flows of information. Eliminating half the outpatient appointments and removing 50% of inappropriate referrals, the new pathway of care could reduce the number of appointments by 75%.

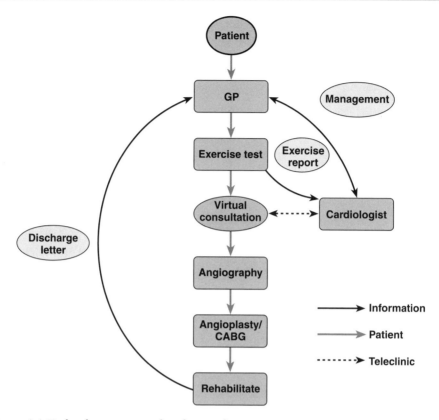

Figure 6.6 Technology-supported pathway of care.

Communication technology is general and TCP/IP networks are used. However, satellite links have been tested to successfully deliver to remote regions of Greece and, more recently, to cruise ships in the Mediterranean as part of the Medaship project. AIDMAN was initially set up to investigate the provision of digital telemedicine in an area of the world where patients find themselves remote from consultants/hospitals in some way, in this case four hospitals in Greece; one in the capital, the KAT Hospital in Athens, and the other three in healthcare centres in Corfu, Mykonos and Mytilini (all 'remote' islands off the coast of mainland Greece). Its use in the UK has also been investigated. In this case it has been introduced in Chorleywood Health Centre, close to London and four neighbouring hospitals. Figure 6.7 illustrates its application and use in the primary and secondary care sectors at the current time.

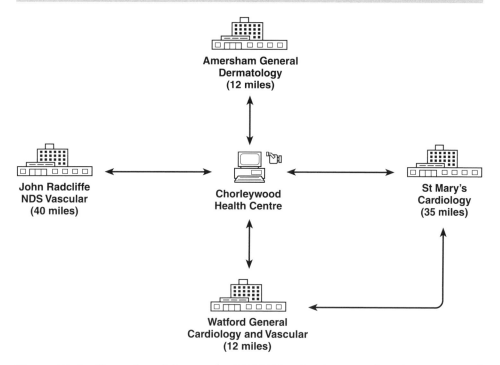

Figure 6.7 An illustration of the current AIDMAN project between the primary care and secondary care levels.

The major difference between the UK and Greece is that the AIDMAN system in the UK is not serving remote or rural communities and thus, for success, the system must be shown to deliver extra benefits to the patient other than overcoming distance, time and travel. The benefits for the rural community are well known, with many successful projects such as the AFCAN service in Alaska, the Centre for Telemedicine in Tromso, Northern Territories network in Australia, and UC Davies, in California, to name a few. The goal for changes to any healthcare delivery system must be better health outcome for the patient. If at the same time it makes it more convenient, improves access and reduces cost, then these are extra benefits. It may be argued that reducing costs means that more services can be afforded, and so the global health system benefits, and this is a good thing. Such systems can provide access to health systems for those that would otherwise have severe difficulty. Many telemedicine programmes are established to serve the needs of remote communities that are isolated and may be cut off for weeks due to weather conditions. Such communities are often small and cannot support even a full-time doctor, and instead may have a nurse. For these situations, telemedicine may be used to support the local health professional in the diagnosis and best management of the condition. The intention would be to keep the patient in the community and to avoid travel, which would be expensive and may not be possible.

These projects have experienced an increase in the type and use of diagnostic equipment that is used and supported in the remote location. Digital equipment to perform a wide variety of tests is available and more are released on the market each year. Costs are also falling. Digital equipment for ECG, blood pressure, temperature, SpO$_2$, digital images, retinoscopes, ophthalmoscopes, ultrasound, spirometry and stethoscopes are available and affordable. The information from these devices can be recorded and forwarded to whoever requires it. In the AIDMAN project, the initial design for the virtual workstation was based on a Pentium II machine and includes desktop video-conferencing (Proshare Version 5.2), a digital video camera for simultaneous analogue video and high-resolution digital still image, flat-bed scanner, soundcard and hands-free speaker phone. Figure 6.8 provides an illustration of its architecture.

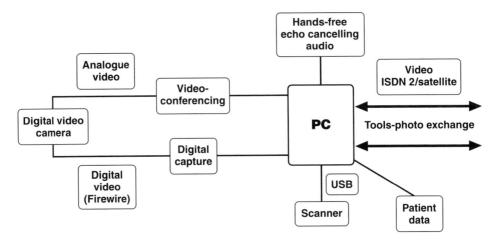

Figure 6.8 The architecture of a teleclinic in an end-station.

Many consultants appreciate diagnostic information in advance of the consultation, so that they can consider their diagnosis and then use the time with the patient more effectively. They also have the opportunity to ensure the quality of the information and that it is complete. This allows them to be able to request further information before the consultation. The system can access data from sources such as digital images, ultrasound, ECG or digital or digitized X-rays or computer tomography (CT scans) for use in the consultation. These can also be transmitted by other means in advance, for example attachments to email or DICOM. There is, naturally, scope to install all manner of other diagnostic equipment in order to support the interaction between the patient/medically trained person and the consultant.

The technology described here is unique in that it combines both 'store and forward' and 'real-time video' to bring all of these together, virtually speaking, by way of teleconsultation.

Experience with AIDMAN suggests that there are many benefits that are not currently provided by way of the traditional management of healthcare. They may be physical in nature, or more psychological. The benefits not only for the patient but also for healthcare professionals more generally are now outlined.

For the patient

- They are seen quickly on an as-needed basis.
- No time is wasted if there is a negative result.
- By the end of the teleconsultation, they know whether, or when, they will be referred; the decision is made at that point.
- The advantage of being diagnosed both quickly and with minimum disruption to everyday life and work.
- No need to wait (and worry) about when the letter from the hospital with an appointment will arrive.
- The patient has 'met' (in a supported manner) the specialist/consultant, and has started the initial, important, process of building a relationship with the person who will play an important role in their future treatment and care.
- The patient has the opportunity to ask questions ahead of any face-to-face meeting with the specialist/consultant. This helps to manage their expectations and reduce anxiety about the unknown, i.e. what is likely to happen.
- The patient can be given advice on preparation for a forthcoming procedure which may involve cooperation with the local health professionals.
- Changes to current medication and care can be implemented.
- As the patient is sitting in a familiar clinic, with a familiar doctor/healthcare professional, the psychological and physical trauma associated with the sub-sequent visit to the specialist/consultant is alleviated.
- It may help patients to better understand consultation *before* they undertake it, and thus to better prepare for it, as well as to help to 'de-mystify' what are, to many, the unknown processes involved in their healthcare.
- It provides added reassurance, as they have been closely involved in the dialogue between the doctor/healthcare professional and the specialist/consultant, and can thus have confidence that both share a common view of their care and treatment.
- Management of the case is negotiated and agreed by all parties, i.e. consultant, doctor and patient, thus the potential to make consultation more effective for all participants.
- It may help change the current perceptions that patients have of healthcare, namely that they are relatively passive participants in the process. This brings with it the notion of 'advocacy'. Teleconsultation is a physical (at least) demonstration of the central role that *they* play in the process, and that they are (or should be) *active* participants who engage in the management of their own health.

For the specialist/consultant and the doctor/healthcare professional

- They are in the same room (virtually speaking) at the same time with the patient
- It is interactive; the consultant and/or doctor can ask the patient as many questions as is necessary to get the information needed to make the correct diagnosis and determine the most appropriate management.
- As full a history as is possible is available from the patient, the health professional (doctor, nurse or other) and the medical records.

- The patient may feel or be unable, or unwilling, to explain their symptoms or feelings. The doctor/healthcare professional (who will have had a longer and closer relationship with the patient) will thus have greater insights into the patient with regard to both their physical and mental state which may be of use to the specialist/consultant.
- Diagnostic information has been sent in advance of the meeting with the specialist/consultant so that an initial diagnosis can be made, which permits prioritization of seeing each patient and saves significant time within the consultation.
- The opportunity to call up/bring in new information as the teleconsultation progresses. For example, an old X-ray which, until that point, was not seen as significant/useful.
- By the end of the teleconsultation, they know whether, or when, the patient will be referred; the decision is made at that point.
- Arrangements for further tests, investigations or procedures to be performed in advance of admission to hospital can be arranged and confirmed.
- Confidence that the patient has received the message about referral.
- The specialist/consultant has 'met' the patient, and has started the initial, important, process of building a relationship.
- The specialist/consultant asks questions ahead of their meeting with the patient. This provides an opportunity for the specialist/consultant to help the patient to manage their expectations and reduce anxiety about the unknown, i.e. what is likely to happen.
- As the patient is sitting in a familiar clinic, with a familiar doctor/healthcare professional, it provides an opportunity for the specialist/consultant to alleviate the psychological and physical trauma associated with the subsequent visit.
- It provides an opportunity for the specialist/consultant to help patients to better understand consultation *before* they undertake it, and thus to better prepare for it, as well as to help to 'demystify' what is, to many, the unknown processes involved.
- It allows for the doctor/healthcare professional and the specialist/consultant to have confidence that both share (or not!) a common view of their care and treatment.
- Management of the case is negotiated and agreed by all parties, i.e., consultant, doctor and patient, thus the potential to make consultation more effective for all participants.
- It may help change the current perceptions that doctors/healthcare professionals and specialists/consultants have of patients and/or healthcare, namely that patients are relatively passive participants in the process. This brings with it the notion of 'advocacy'. Teleconsultation is a physical (at least) demonstration of the central role that *they* play in the process, and that patients are (or should be) *active* participants who engage in the management of their own health.
- An opportunity for doctors/healthcare professionals and specialists/consultants to learn from each other more about patients, disease, treatment and related aspects of the management of healthcare.
- An opportunity for doctors/healthcare professionals and specialists/consultants to 'bridge the gap', psychologically speaking, that is seen to exist between primary and secondary/tertiary healthcare.

- Encourages and supports collaborative working between health professionals in different sectors of healthcare.
- The patient can be prepared by the local nurse in advance of the actual consultation (for example, change into a gown), which saves significant time in the actual consultation.

Human and organizational factors

As is the case with the adoption of any information system, there are the difficulties associated with using technology in the workplace. Although research demonstrates that patients welcome teleconsultation as a medium for communication and decision making about their health, experience shows that rolling out platforms such as AIDMAN for use in other surgeries/clinics or other healthcare settings is not just a matter of installing the equipment, although there are technical issues which might limit its uptake on a national scale. One of these limitations is the cost, not only of installation, but also of maintenance and, as anyone who uses computers and related technology knows, a high level of ongoing support is required given the inevitable breakdowns. If there are too many breakdowns, then doctors, nurses and other healthcare professionals will not want to use it, however useful it might be to their clinical work.

Another limitation to a system such as AIDMAN is that it necessarily changes the relationships between all involved. Although the teleconsultation brings the doctor/GP (and/or nurses, for example) and the specialist/consultant together, virtually speaking, it has to date been used with healthcare professionals who are positive and enthusiastic, who have (or feel that they have) the necessary interpersonal and other skills to carry out the interaction effectively and who do not mind having their own weaknesses exposed to others, in particular, to the patient. So, for example, a newly qualified doctor/GP might feel threatened by having to discuss, in front of the patient, an aspect of healthcare with which they are unfamiliar, or admit that they have not carried out certain checks or administered certain treatments before, and so would be reluctant, or even refuse, to use AIDMAN. On the other hand, installing a system such as AIDMAN provides an opportunity for all concerned to learn from each other more about disease, treatment and related aspects of management of care; but some are more resistant to change (which is what learning is all about) than others.

Christensen et al. (2000) also report several interesting examples of resistance to 'disruptive innovations' in the healthcare sector and, quite rightly, say that this can be found at all levels of any organization, either local or national. There is thus the need for further research into the perceptions of a range of healthcare professionals in a variety of healthcare settings in order to ascertain the types of organization, and people within them, who will be more (or less) likely to embrace such technology. It is also necessary to find out how, precisely, such technology should be brought onstream in a new setting. It has been installed over several years at Chorleywood in the UK and installing and using it elsewhere will likely need new, and perhaps different, methods and approaches. An information system such as AIDMAN does, of course, cost money. In order for other healthcare professionals to consider its use in their own healthcare settings, there will be a need to provide further explanation as to what particular clinical issues are likely candidates for teleconsultation and which are not. So, for example, although teledermatology has been used with much success, there are some dermatological cases that do not lend themselves to such intervention; the doctor/GP should instead immediately refer the patient to the specialist/consultant.

Experience from many sectors has also shown that introducing technology to the workplace brings its own problems and appropriate management techniques must be adopted early if a project is to be successful. Technology can be notoriously difficult to introduce where existing practice is well established and there can be considerable reluctance to adopt and use unfamiliar technology. This can soon turn to a refusal, and the few 'die hard' users can quickly affect discontent among others. A few breakdowns or problems will rapidly add fuel to the argument to continue with old practice and it may become difficult to convince users to continue their use of the new system. The benefits of the new system must be constantly emphasized and demonstrated (why bother to do more work if there is no benefit?). Christensen *et al.*[2] argue strongly that 'disruptive technologies' are 'precisely what are needed to reform healthcare' and that it is in the interests of doctors/GPs and/or specialists/consultants to do so (p. 109). The authors of this chapter, committed as we are to introducing such technology across the sector, could not agree more. Users should be encouraged and supported, and their problems and views must be listened to. Success comes when they start asking for more and new ways of working with the system. Sometimes hard decisions must be taken for the sake of the success of the project. Some people may never accept new practices and the time may come to part ways.

The majority of telemedicine projects span aspects of healthcare as diverse as mental health, diabetes or foetal monitoring. Each system is designed differently, is unlikely to be compatible with others and needs different technical support and user training. While such individual systems have proved useful in a particular context,[15–20] the implications for a national healthcare system mean that each clinic, hospital or other healthcare setting would need to purchase a different technological device for each particular healthcare issue. So, a system for diabetes, another for mental health and yet another for foetal monitoring, and so on. In addition, each device would need different technical support and different user training and would, naturally, take up a great deal of space in the workplace. Maintaining such systems would be problematic and expensive, particularly given the rapidly changing nature of information systems today. It would also be very expensive. In a country such as the UK, where (scarce) financial resources for healthcare come from the taxpayer, it is difficult to see how those managing the healthcare budget would justify the cost in investing in such single, one-issue systems. Another difficulty of such one-issue systems is that a great deal of effort would have to be made in persuading doctors/general practitioners or specialists/consultants to use such systems; only around 12% of these healthcare professionals have computers on their desks and, like many, may not embrace technology with the same enthusiasm as their designers.

The significance of the telemedicine platform

The significance and value of AIDMAN is that it can be applied/used for *every/any* healthcare issue. Indeed, one of the limitations of other systems is that they will not be cost-effective if health service providers have to buy separate systems for different healthcare issues. Doing so would not only be more expensive but it would likely mean a clinic/surgery cluttered with technological devices, each of which would require different training and support. It is difficult to see how, in a healthcare climate where technology is little used, healthcare professionals would be tempted to invest in such a seemingly bewildering array of technological 'kit' – systems must be designed to be general purpose and be reused for many health areas. Of course this also matches the philosophy of primary care, and it would seem inevitable that a system aimed at supporting this sector will need to be designed to match such requirements.

It is also clear that technology can stretch the boundaries for healthcare and monitoring, and there will be an increasing use of technology to monitor the patient in their own home, or close to home, or even as they go about their daily life, with appropriate data or alarms being sent to the healthcare professional for advice or intervention. In such a way, changes to a person's state of health might be detected even before they themselves are aware of it, and early intervention can prevent further deterioration which may well result in the need for admission to hospital in order to manage an exacerbation or acute attack of the condition. It is likely primary care will become increasingly responsible for managing chronic illness in the community, and platforms such as AIDMAN offer an excellent means of support to the primary healthcare team and the patient.

Our experience leads us to conclude that AIDMAN has demonstrated its use and efficacy across a variety of healthcare issues as diverse as dermatology, cardiology and vascular surgery; oncology is soon to join these and AIDMAN offers an interesting tool to support patients through a difficult time and in making difficult decisions. It has proved a versatile platform, and as such should prove cost-effective when used in this way. The physical and psychological benefits of AIDMAN to both patient and healthcare professional are such that it allows for richer communication between the patient and the specialist/consultant and between doctor/healthcare professional and the specialist/consultant involved in the health and care of their patient. The roles of both the doctor/healthcare professional and the specialist/consultant differ from the traditional ones, in particular, the role taken by the doctor/healthcare professional in primary care. Here, they act more in the role of 'advocate' for the patient during the consultation.

E-health, as our use of AIDMAN demonstrates, has the potential (in the right hands) to allow patients to engage more fully in their own healthcare and to feel more empowered in the process. Patients want an empathetic approach from healthcare professionals and to feel that what they say is not only 'data' for the healthcare professional to use in decision making but that they, as individuals, are valued. They want their voice to be heard, and to feel as much of an equal partner in the relationship and any decision making. AIDMAN demonstrates that such technology is a powerful tool in helping to bring about a more personalized, empowering interaction for the patient and, importantly, that such interaction has similar benefits to the healthcare professional. So, rather than the technology 'taking over' and making the human interaction *less* personal, as many inside and outside the profession might fear, it instead has the potential to do just the opposite, that is, to enrich and strengthen the human to human communication that is so essential to successful interaction and, in this case, help to ensure that the decision making is the best that it can be.

Our future research agenda includes looking at how, precisely, the consultation process is changed and, importantly, to explore the impact of this on health outcome. Further research and analysis of teleconsultation sessions so far carried out will reveal to what extent these do, or do not, mirror more 'traditional' consultations and whether such a model varies according to clinician, illness or any other factor(s). In order to roll out AIDMAN for use in other surgeries/clinics or other healthcare settings, there is a need to find out the technical, social and other issues which might limit its uptake on a national scale. Another is to explore to what extent AIDMAN can be used by healthcare professionals to learn from each other more about disease, treatment and related aspects of management of care, and how this affects the quality of their decision making.

Referral to a specialist is an important aspect of healthcare, regardless of how healthcare is organized at local and/or national level. That said, there are important differences related to context. By way of example, Forrest[3] reports that patients in the US are twice as likely as patients in the UK to see a specialist within any 12-month period, although rates of keeping appointments are almost identical. This makes discussion of the role of innovation in successful telemedicine somewhat problematic as what is 'successful' in one context may be regarded differently in another.

Telepsychiatry in Canada[21] is regarded by patients as highly successful for a variety of reasons. It would likely be reasonably easy to find plenty of studies in telepsychiatry that could be used to provide evidence that 'telepsychiatry is good', and that given these success stories healthcare organizations around the world should put into place such a service as soon as they can. However, on closer examination of the study, the success, as measured by patients, can be attributed to the fact that the alternative is no psychiatric service at all, or at least not without travelling considerable distance, as the patients live in the remotest regions of Canada. For such patients, *any* service, even if the level of service provided is regarded as poor (by clinicians) when measured against psychiatric services elsewhere, will be rated highly. Geographical location is but one factor that complicates discussion of what is meant by 'success'. Another is who is being asked.

Having said that 'success' is problematic in that it does not exist per se but is instead dependent on context and who we ask to gauge any telemedical intervention, innovation is another such issue. Technology plays a vital part in all of our lives these days, and this is as true for the healthcare services as anywhere else. What is important, of course, is that we, as humans, do not allow ourselves to be so seduced by the technology that we lose sight of what it is, that is, a tool. And, like all tools, it is not useful or 'good' in itself. A spoon is, for instance, a great tool if you want to eat ice cream but useless if you want to speak to someone in another country. People, in this case patients, do not want innovation, they want to be made better, and as efficiently and effectively as possible. And governments or organizations that pay for healthcare want it done as cheaply as possible. Cost, however, is problematic. It can be measured (with difficulty) in terms of dollars perhaps, with low cost being seen as synonymous with 'success'. Indeed, Whitten et al.[22] make it clear from their study of 612 articles that attempted to measure actual cost benefit data of telemedicine services that there is absolutely no good evidence that such benefits exist. We might conclude from this that telemedicine on a wider scale, nationally and internationally, might thus be doomed.

However, one of the difficulties with this evidence is that it is naturally gathered only from small-scale projects, in one location, for one particular healthcare issue. Given this, it is unsurprising that these have not proved cost-effective; they are measured as stand-alones, and contrasted with normal practice for a particular cohort of patients undergoing a particular type of treatment or path. It may also be the case that the telemedicine is being used to deliver the same healthcare, only by a slightly different method, and that within the global economy there will be little benefit as only one small component is being affected. Indeed, the most often reported outcome of a telemedicine pilot is a reduction in the number of referrals on to the next higher level of healthcare, and post analysis normally shows that this has come about because of the *educational* aspects that the telemedicine system delivers. Furthermore, as the pilot progresses, there is often an accompanying reduction in the use of the telemedicine system as the remote healthcare professional becomes confident to make the decisions themselves and unsupported.

The conclusion is that AIDMAN offers much more than a simple referral tool, and we need to examine the further potentials. Instead, we need to envision something far more radical: the AIDMAN system (if it can be called that) as *the* system, on a national scale. Unfortunately, a randomized clinical trial, so often seen as the only reasonable and/or reliable method of testing a new service or drug in healthcare sector journals, is clearly not going to be possible. What is proving, to us at least, far more difficult to model is the cost (economically and otherwise) of having such a system operating across the whole healthcare sector in the UK. We are working on it, however!

This chapter presents the technological innovation layer of the six-layer onion described earlier, although as this conclusion demonstrates, this cannot be divorced from the other layers which together make their contribution to organizational learning and success. As for whether there is enthusiasm for such 'disruptive innovation' at all levels of the healthcare system in the UK, the answer is, as ever, dependent on who is being asked. There are fervent supporters of such innovation at all levels, but innovation always has its critics. That said, it is our view that the UK is ready to embrace a system that Christensen et al. would call a 'disruptive innovation'.[2]

It would seem to us that implementing a local, national or even global information system, in this case a healthcare one such as AIDMAN, is not about healthcare per se but instead about the ability to successfully manage change. As Christensen et al. rightly note,[2] improving healthcare by introducing 'disruptive innovations' involves a complex mix of people, from governments through to an individual in a particular healthcare setting. While exhorting the leaders at national and local levels to work more closely together, Christensen et al.[2] rightly recognize that effective leadership is key. However, as Fitzgerald et al. note,[23] effectively managing change cannot be reduced to a set of 'critical success factors'; human behaviour (and that is what we are talking about with information systems) is far more complex than that. However, successful information systems might be characterized as having the following:

- driven by the business need rather than the technology
- clear backing and commitment from many within the organization
- any project, big or small, must have its champions, and at different organizational levels. Such 'movers and shakers' must be prepared to carry their vision through and to be accountable for its implementation
- teamwork within the organization more generally
- teamwork at the level of the development itself
- humour and common sense (this is in extremely short supply in any organization, unfortunately!)
- involve the users of the ICT when designing it
- project management is clearly a vital factor in ensuring a project's success. However, 'project management' is as much about 'people management' as managing the actual product, the system, itself
- central to the success of any new system, whether an ICT one or otherwise, is the management of people's expectations.

In the end, all systems development, or indeed any change, is about the management of risk. Do those 'movers and shakers' exist in the NHS and the government in the UK? Do they have a vision and the skills and abilities to make it work in practice? The cynics among us would perhaps doubt that such organizations, loathe to change as they are, have such people. As patients, we can only hope that they do!

References

1 *The NHS explained.* www.nhs.uk/thenhsexplained; accessed: 24 January 2002.
2 Christensen CM, Bohmer R and Kenagy J (2000) Will disruptive innovations cure healthcare? *Harvard Business Review.* September/October: 102–12.
3 Forrest CB (2003) Primary care gatekeeping and referrals: effective filter or failed experiment? *British Medical J.* **326**: 692–5.
4 Rodger JA and Pendharkar PC (2000) Using telemedicine in the Department of Defense. *Communications of the ACM.* **43**(3): 19–20.
5 Payton FC and Brennan PF (1999) How a community health information network is really used. *Communications of the ACM.* **42**(12): 85–9.
6 Hawkes N (2001) Gates unveils vision for online NHS of the future. *The Times.* 7 December: 10.
7 Baldwin LP, Eldabi T and Paul RJ (2002) Clinical information systems: augmenting case management. Proceedings of the *Seventh Annual Conference of the UK Academy for Information Systems,* 10–12 April, Leeds, UK.
8 Summerton N (2000) Diagnosis and general practice. *British J General Practice.* **50**: 995–1000.
9 Clarke M and Jones RW (2001) What route to viability for telemedicine in the UK? *Proceedings of the Healthcare 2001 Conference,* March, Harrogate, UK, pp. 190–5.
10 Clarke M, Lioupis D, Kanellopoulos N, Jones RW and Nassiopoulos A (2000) AIDMAN – Advanced Informatics Distributed Medical Access Network. *Proceedings of the Geomark 2000 Conference,* April, Paris, France, pp. 203–6.

11   Clarke M, Jones RW and Lioupis D (2000) The AIDMAN project: a practical investigation of some of the challenges in telemedicine. *British J Healthcare and Information Management.* **17**(5): 24–6.

12   Clarke M, Jones RW, George S and Cairns D (1999) Teledermatology – the UK experience of setting up an integrated teledermatology service. *Proceedings of the Medical Information and Education 1999 Conference*, August, Ljubljana, Slovenia, pp. 274–7.

13   Clarke M, Jones RW, Kanellopoulos N, Lioupis D and Nassiopoulos A (1999) AIDMAN – Advanced Informatics Distributed Medical Access Network. *Proceedings of the Medical Information and Education 1999 Conference*, August, Ljubljana, Slovenia, pp. 625–30.

14   Jones RW, Clarke M, Kanellopoulos N, Lioupis D and Fowles R (1999) The AIDMAN project – a telemedicine approach to cardiology investigation, referral and outpatient care. *Proceedings of the Telemed 1999 Conference*, November, London, UK, pp. 32–4.

15   Gilmour E, Campbell SM, Loane MA, Esmail A, Griffiths CE, Roland MO, Parry EJ, Corbett RO, Eedy D, Gore HE, Mathews C, Steel K and Wootton R (1998) Comparison of teleconsultations and face-to-face consultations: preliminary results of a UK multi-centre teledermatology study. *British J Teledermatology.* **139**(1): 81–97.

16   Jones DH, Crichton C, Macdonald A, Potts S, Sime D, Toms J and McKinlay J (1996) Teledermatology in the highlands of Scotland. *J Telemedicine and Telecare.* **2**(1): 7–9.

17   Lesher JL, Loretta S, Davis FW, Gourdin DE and Thompson WO (1998) Telemedicine evaluation of cutaneous diseases: a blinded comparative study. *J American Academy of Teledermatology.* **38**(1): 27–31.

18   Loane MA, Corbett R, Bloomer SE, Eedy DJ, Gore HE, Mathews C, Steele K and Wootton R (1998) Diagnostic accuracy and clinical management by realtime dermatology; results from the Northern Ireland arms of the UK Multicentre Tele-dermatology Trial. *J Telemedicine and Telecare.* **4**(2): 95–100.

19   Lowitt MH, Kessler II, Kauffman CL, Hooper FJ, Siegel E and Burnett JW (1998) Teledermatology and in-person examinations: a comparison of patient and physician perceptions and diagnostic agreement. *Archives of Dermatology.* **134**(4): 471–6.

20   Oakley AM, Duffill MB and Reeve P (1998) Practising dermatology via telemedicine. *New Zealand Med J.* **111**(1071): 296–9.

21   Bishop JE, O'Reilly RL, Maddox K and Hutchinson LJ (2002) Client satisfaction in a feasibility study comparing face-to-face interviews with telepsychiatry. *J Telemed and Telecare.* **8**(4): 217–21.

22   Whitten PS, Mair FS, Haycox A, May CR, Williams TL and Hellmich S (2002) Systematic review of cost effectiveness studies of telemedicine interventions. *British Med J.* **324**: 1434–7.

23   Fitzgerald G, Baldwin LP, Klecun-Dabrowska E and Siddiqui F (2000) IT at the heart of business; a strategic approach to information technology. In: *The IS Management Series* vol. 1. The British Computer Society, Swindon, UK.

Section 4

Change management in e-health

Chapter 7

Do healthcare professionals use IT?

Ton AM Spil, Roel W Schuring and Margreet B Michel-Verkerke

Introduction

Information technology (IT) is emerging in healthcare,[1] but successfully implementing information systems in healthcare organizations appears to be a difficult task.[2] Information Technology is seen as an enabler of change in healthcare organizations.[3] Southon[4] suggests that (information) technology adoption decisions in healthcare are complex because of the uncertainty of benefits and the rate of change of technology.[5] This book tries to unravel this complexity, and in this chapter we look at successful change management from a user perspective. Determinants on other levels may also be important, such as the level of project management, the level of the organization or even the level of the society.[6] On a system level, reimbursement structures, regulations and the existence of standards may have an explanatory role. On an organization level, the previous strategic choices, strategic priorities, size and location of the organization, and many other factors may play a role. Similarly, Kimberly and Evanisko discuss such factors.[7] On a project level, resources, project management, etc., will play a role. No explicit attention will be given to these factors in this chapter.

Thornett[8] describes benefits as improved quality of care, disease prevention and disease management of chronic physical illnesses. Why then, do these systems not diffuse into the health organizations? The adoption of IT in healthcare has increased, which underlines the importance of user requirements.[9] In later work Beuscart-Zéphir links the adoption to the activities of the healthcare professionals.[10] Fleisner and Hofkircher refer to the same problem when they conclude that relevant information will not be improved unless additional requirements are met.[11]

A multiple case study among 56 general practitioners (GPs) on the influence of resistance, relevance, requirements and resources on the introduction of an electronic prescription system (EPS) demonstrates that the EPS is not used in at least 72% of cases. First, a broad background of the model is given. To explain the non-use of the system we combine the notions of information usage of Delone and McLean[12] and Davis,[13] and the notion of innovation from Rogers.[14] We use the semantic ladder from Stamper[15] and information levels from Shannon and Weaver[16] to straighten them out (social, pragmatic, semantic and syntactic levels). To explain relevance we will build on the notions of Saracevic.[17] This will be described in the definition and framework section. Together these concepts build up a framework for an interview model that we used in all cases as described in the case study method (*see* p. 139). Finally we make conclusions for every determinant of the model.

Background

We can use a wide range of sources that discuss user perspectives in the introduction of IT. This section gives a short overview of intriguing literature. The aim is to demonstrate that 'requirements' is not the *only* user-related determinant of user adoption. Rather, it is an important determinant among other factors. One of the ultimate goals of our research project in this field is to propose a model that neatly balances the role of such factors.

First, we present the dimensions of the USE IT model to predict and evaluate innovation and diffusion of information systems: the innovation-dimension and the domain-dimension, which make four determinants for success: relevance, requirements, resistance and resources (Table 7.1).

Table 7.1 The USE IT model[18]

USE IT model	User domain	Information technology domain
Product	Relevance	Requirements
Process	Resistance	Resources

By process, we mean the innovation process, similar to the process defined by Saarinen and Sääksjärvi[19] and the innovation process structure of Larsen.[20] The product is the result of this innovation process. This corresponds with the definition of the product by Saarinen and Sääksjärvi and the artefact structure in the framework of Larsen. Also the IT domain is part of the artefact structure; the user domain represents the organizational structure in Larsen's framework. The time horizon structure can be part of the requirements and the knowledge structure can be considered as an element of the resources.

Resistance is the personal attitude of all stakeholder groups towards the introduction of an information system (IS).[21] The main IS-quality aspect of resistance is the attitude and the willingness to change. Pare and Elam[3] also focus on the attitude of the professional when they assess clinical information systems. The end users have an important role because their norms and values determine the effectiveness of the information system.

Expectance of reduced quality of work life satisfaction, high complexity and the lack of trialability can result in resistance.[14,22] Observability reduces resistance.[14] Leavitt[23] introduced four domains in which these risks will occur: tasks, structure, technology and people. Offenbeek and Koopman connect people with resistance potential because they can feel that the quality of their working life will be decreased.[24] Mumford observed that user participation contributes to effective organizational change.[25] When we focus on IT introduction more specifically, we again see a number of interesting literature sources. Thong and Yap discuss the user satisfaction approach to IT effectiveness.[26] They mention the debatable operationalization, poor theoretical construct and misapplication as a result of the approach. On the basis of their review, they conclude that attitude is the construct that lies at the root of user-satisfaction, and suggest ways to improve operationalization and measurement of attitude. Paré and Elam studied attitudes, expectations and skills in relation to physicians' acceptance of IT systems.[3] Physicians with formal training on computers were more knowledgeable about informatics concepts and reported that computers would be more beneficial to healthcare, although it is not clear whether the training causes this attitude. Venkatesh *et al.*,[27] however, make the hypothesis that 'attitude toward using technology will *not* have a significant influence on behavioral intention'.[27]

We argue this hypothesis in this chapter with previous results that resistance was found to be the cumulative effect of the other three determinants.[28] But attitude, permission and capability of the end user will influence the adoption apart from the other dimensions.

The *relevance* determinant is defined by Schuring and Spil as: 'the degree to which the user expects that the IT-system will solve his problems or will help to realize his actually relevant goals'.[29] The word 'expects' expresses that relevance is a factor that is important in the course of the adoption process, not only in evaluation. The word 'actually' is crucial in their view of relevance. Relevance is not to be confused with the degree to which the user considers outcomes as being positive. The set of outcome dimensions that someone considers 'positive' is larger than the set of outcome dimensions that are relevant.

Imagine a physician, who basically considers IT outcomes of a computer decision support system, such as assistance in diagnosis, disease prevention or more appropriate dosing of drugs, as 'positive'. This does not automatically imply that the IT adoption is relevant to him; it is only relevant if these dimensions are high on his 'goal agenda'. Relevance defined in this way comprises relative advantage,[14] net benefits,[30] perceived usefulness[13] and job relevance,[31] and results in task support satisfaction, which is a criterion for user satisfaction.[22] Also, it becomes clear that user priorities regarding IT innovations vary strongly.

The functional uncertainty is often described in information systems literature. It occurs in the task domain of Leavitt. In each situation, the interpretation and the meaning can be different. Therefore, it is necessary to establish a functional specification with users and providers of the information systems. Henry and Stone[32] state this to be information quality. Larsen[20] notes, however, 'the quality of the IS/IT product is a necessary but not sufficient prerequisite for IS innovation success. The *people* within the organizations determine the outcome.'

Within the healthcare sector, Walley and Davies conducted a study of the internal barriers to technological IT advancement in the healthcare sector.[5] The involvement of stakeholders is arguably one of the most distinctive characteristics of IT projects. In their study on the implementation of an electronic prescription system, Schuring and Spil found that lack of relevance was the major determinant that explained the failure of the implementation.[28]

The *requirements* determinant evaluates the meaning of the information system. Requirements are defined as the degree to which the user needs are satisfied with the product quality of the innovation.[33] This includes such aspects as the functional capability, the ease of start-up and the ease of use.

Meeting the end-user's requirements results in high information quality, system quality,[30] high interface satisfaction[22] and high compatibility.[14] There are instruments to identify user needs, but Walley and Davies question whether they are actually used.[5] Van der Pijl shows that there is more to say about people than just resistance or user participation.[34] Both users and providers of information systems have their own targets, not necessarily going hand in hand. A central question is whether the provider intention is the same as the user interpretation.[35] We think that a requirements contract between user and provider can help to bridge the information gap.[36]

Resources are defined as the degree to which material and immaterial goods are available to design, operate and maintain the information system.[33] The main focus of the determinant resources will be on the people and on the costs these people cause. Next to that the reliability of the IT and the information systems are considered. Resources defined in this way refer to service and system quality,[30] management support and mature IS function.[19] Resources (human, physical and monetary components[37]) are needed to implement the new information system into the organization. The human resources can be insufficient in both time and experience (risk of technology). Insufficient material resources will have a limiting influence on the other three risk domains.[24]

To measure the determinants the USE IT tool consists of structured interviews. In this way a more precise insight can be obtained into the nature and relevance of problems and solutions, before implementation and this insight can be tested with the same tool during the evaluation of the implementation. In the next section we will elaborate each determinant of the USE IT model.

USE IT: definition and framework

Resistance

The tendency of human beings to resist and fear new and unknown things and the willingness to stick to the familiar procedures has been studied widely.[38,39] Attributing the rejection of innovations only to anxiety and fear of change, however, is an oversimplified view of the process of technology transfer.[40] Carey[41] finds a correlation between acceptance of change and variables such as previous use (experience), education and current usage of a new system.[41] She also reports commitment, exposure to change and preparation for change as being important for successful implementation of new technologies and systems. So a much broader view on the subject of resistance is appropriate. We position it on the social level of the semantic ladder.[15]

We start with the first known published reference to research on resistance to change in organizations by Coch and French.[42] They were early explorers in the world of resistance when they concluded 'by preventing or greatly modifying group resistance to change, this concomitant to change may well be greatly reduced'. Besides taking the notion of resistance influencing successful change, they state that it can be different on group and individual level. Later change management literature categorizes into the individual, group and organizational (structure) levels.

On the group level, Lewin refers to 'group standards' when looking for reasons for resistance to change.[43] He concludes that the more individuals take group standards of their environment, the greater will the resistance to change of an individual group member be. Lewin further continues that group standards with social values are often referred to as 'social habits'. The way to reduce the level of resistance may thus be either to diminish the strength of the value of the group standard or to change social habits themselves.

Both Lawrence[44] and Zuboff[45] conclude that resistance is not simply an irrational phenomenon to be overcome.[46] Zuboff sees positive and negative aspects to resistance. More authors describe this healing effect of resistance.[47–49] Insightful and well-intended debate, criticism or disagreement do not necessarily equate to negative resistance, but rather may be intended to produce better understanding as well as additional options and solutions. Rogers[14] also explains that it is perfectly rational for later adopters to be more hesitating about the introduction of an innovation; they do not have sufficient resources to overcome the consequences of adoption failure.

Kotter and Schlesinger[50] diagnose resistance from the negative viewpoint as:

- parochial self-interest (fear of loosing something worthwhile[51])
- misunderstanding and lack of trust
- different assessments (belief that change is worthless[51])
- low tolerance for change.

Fuller also discovers different levels of concern regarding resistance.[52] Self-concern can be seen in awareness, personal commitment and personal consequences. Task concern is related to controlling the change, and cooperation concern sees both concerns in collaboration and reengineering. Schmidt et al.,[53] whose study was a mirror of control for this study, refers to Zmud,[54] who adds a fourth environmental category. Lapointe et al. applies these categories in explaining the dynamics of IT adoption in healthcare.[55] She based her theory on the theory of reasoned action where 'individual behaviour is directly determined by one variable intention which, in turn, is determined by two variables: attitude and subjective norms'. In line with Scott,[56] Prasad and Prasad[57] make the distinction between formal and informal (routine) resistance. Strebel[58] already described this as personal compact, formally a job description and appraisal, but informally psychological (mutual expectations) and socially (cultural values). This brings us back to the notion that change is intensely personal[59] and therefore our empirical material is gathered very close to professionals coping with the change.

Kotter and Schlesinger are mainly interested in the self-concern. Mittelstaedt et al. adds the inability of either individual or group to cope with the change.[60] Also the situation can call for postponement. The situational factors we see as mainly emerging on organizational level are:

- not for them (reject)
- unwilling or unable (accept)
- postpone (time and situation) (accept).

Gatignon and Robertson[61] and Szmigin and Foxall[62] use sort-like distinctions: the latter introduce opposition instead of unwilling or unable. Ram and Sheth[63] call this habit resistance and also relate to Rogers,[14] when they state that often an initial resistance has to be overcome. Please note that most of the literature in this paragraph is based on resistance of consumers. It might not always apply in a healthcare environment.

Offenbeek and Koopman introduce the resistance potential and make a distinction between change-ability of the problem system and desired change.[24] This potential of resistance would be people-determined resistance according to Markus.[64] System-determined resistance is handled in the technical determinant of IS success but the interaction-determined resistance, which is mainly political (inter)organizational resistance, can only be seen within the reasons to postpone of Mittelstaedt *et al.*[60]

Other publications on the subject of resistance challenge or enhance the 'accepted' concepts.[65] Piderit suggests that resistance to change is a complex, multidimensional response with emotional, cognitive, and intentional components.[48] For example, no participation or not enough communication may result in an emotionally resistant attitude to the changes, even though the changes make good business sense (cognitive). Alternatively, initially enthusiastic (emotional) and clearly seeing the need for change (cognitive), people give up (i.e. our intentions change) because they are not given the support they expect and think they'll need in order to make the changes happen. It is rare that employees are all negative or all positive across the three dimensions. It is important to remember that resistance to change is normal and frequently functional.

'Moving too quickly toward congruent positive attitudes toward a proposed change might cut off the discussion and improvisation that may be necessary for revising the initial change proposal in an adaptive manner.' In other words, discussion, disagreement and experimentation can lead consistently to more successful change, whereas effective communication and participation are powerful tools for overcoming and avoiding misunderstandings.[49]

Zaltman and Duncan's[66] resistance framework discusses four categories of barriers, 'cultural, social, organizational, and psychological', that can obstruct change.[66] These categories are in turn broken down into a total of 18 resistance factors, which disrupt change efforts and distort adopter perceptions of innovations. This framework can be useful because it explores change from the opposite perspective to most other models. By focusing attention on factors that erect barriers to change, Zaltman and Duncan help to recognize such obstacles as they arise or even to identify and address their underlying issues before they arise. It is important to note that a given individual can harbor intense pro-change and pro-resistance sentiments simultaneously.

Though detailed in its 18 factors, this framework is not suitable for the goal of this study. More appropriate is a model with its roots in change management, educational and training literature, structuring resistance and affection into three categories: ability, attitude and opportunity. Metselaar *et al.*[67] describe this used in training against (negative) and with (positive) resistance based on a concept from the social psychology.[68] Lanning[39] comes with the same result in an empirical study for a planned change approach. We adopt these findings into our 'USE framework for resistance to IT change', where we should reckon that the main focus of these shifts from (inter)organizational, to group, to individual. In line with the USE IT model,[21] this subdivision is made into macro- and micro-resistance (*see* Figure 7.1, p. 136).

Attitude (will) to change (micro-resistance)

People who are expected to participate in the change project must have personal motivation and a sincere will to engage themselves in the development. Comprehension and acceptance of the basic idea in the project is an important condition. Will does not occur unless real effort at developing the organization can be perceived.

Ability to change (macro-resistance)

The level of knowledge and skills of those who are involved in a 'change' project needs to be high enough to be able to contribute to the project. Job-specific skills enabling people to use new tools and technology and to act according to new procedures and tasks must be adequate. But ability also means comprehension of project vision and understanding one's own role in implementing the new technology. The user experience also adds up to the ability to change.

Opportunity to change (macro-resistance)

There is a need for organizational systems (surrounding people and structures) to support the development process and implementation of the new technology. Sufficient resources, top management support and commitment are essential to give everybody the feeling that change and development can be achieved.

These subdimensions of resistance fit underneath the user satisfaction research model of Mahmood et al.[69] as they call it user background and organizational support. The perceived benefits that complete the user satisfaction are in the USE IT model situated under the relevance determinant[70] and described in the next section.

Relevance

Saracevic defines relevance as a measure of the effectiveness of a contact between a source and a destination in a communication process.[17] This is a somewhat abstract wording of what we would call the degree to which the user expects that the IT system will solve their problems or help to realize their actually relevant goals. There are three dimensions that are kept implicit in Saracevic's definition that we wish to stress. We use the word 'expects', since we want to make more explicit that relevance is a factor that is important in the course of the adoption process, not only in evaluation. Second, instead of effectiveness we use 'solve problems and goals'. By doing so, we imply that effectiveness has two dimensions: to take away existing negative consequences (problems) and to reward with positive consequences (reach goals). Third, the word 'actual' is crucial in our view of relevance. Relevance is not to be confused with the degree to which the user considers outcomes as being positive. The set of outcome dimensions that someone considers 'positive' is larger than the set of outcome dimensions that are relevant. Imagine a physician who basically considers IT outcomes of a computer decision support system, such as, assistance in diagnosis, disease prevention or more appropriate dosing of drugs,[8] as 'positive'. This does not automatically imply that the IT adoption is relevant to him. It is only relevant if these outcomes are high on his goal agenda. That is why we use the word 'actual'.

Again, this is a more explicit wording of a dimension that is implicitly included where Saracevic uses the word 'effectiveness' in his definition. The actually relevant goals may be a mix of short-term goals and long-term goals. If, for example, smooth communication with hospitals or pharmacy is his prime actual problem or goal, he will only consider the IT innovation as relevant when it actually helps to improve that communication, notwithstanding the fact that he might have a positive attitude towards that innovation as long as the innovation helps to solve other problems or other goals that are on the lower positions in his agenda ranking. We discovered in our case studies that it is not sufficient for an innovation to effectuate a positive attitude among users. The IT innovation should be relevant.[29]

Micro-relevance is a related concept that can be used to describe a similar phenomenon once the new IT is installed. Micro-relevance is defined as 'the degree to which IT use helps to solve the here-and-now problem of the user in his working process'. The use of new equipment or new IT procedures is a conscious activity. In every conscious activity that is goal-oriented to a specific goal, there is a reason why that course of action is being chosen. Similar to what was discussed above on 'relevance', not every course of action that a user basically considers as 'positive' is 'micro-relevant'. Again, let's illustrate this with an example. Imagine that a patient with a viral infection visits a physician. The physician might notice the similarity to a number of other patients he has met that week and decide on diagnosis and treatment fairly quickly. To this doctor, the use of a decision support system to determine diagnosis is not micro-relevant. However, a colleague of his may not feel so confident and thus use the system. We discovered that micro-relevance is a key factor in explaining IT use in our case studies. Figure 7.1 (*see* p. 136) gives an overview of relevance as we propose to use it.

Relevance and micro-relevance are notable refinements of the way the role of the user is being discussed in the existing literature. Thornett[8] implicitly refers to relevance and micro-relevance when he discusses limited adoption and use of decision support systems (DSS) by primary physicians where 'consultation time is lengthened by their use and there is no appreciable impact on patient satisfaction'.[8] It is an example where other outcomes that are basically considered as positive (as mentioned above: better diagnosis, more appropriate dosing of drugs, and other) are overruled by limited relevance and micro-relevance.

Saracevic provides a historic positioning of relevance.[17] The roots lay in the 1930s and 1940s when the distinction between information and relevant information was made by Bradford.[17] In order to make the distinction between relevant and non-relevant information, he discusses the nature of communication. By doing so, he recognizes that relevance to a subject depends on specific dimensions, such as for example, the subject's knowledge, representation and values. He discusses a number of (philosophical) approaches to relevance. The elaboration we propose above builds on the radical pragmatism perspective or, more specifically, Cooper's utility function: 'Relevance is simply a cover term of whatever the user finds to be of value about the system output, whatever its usefulness, its entertainment, or aesthetic value, or anything else'.[71] Wilson adds to this that relevance is situational.[72] Ballantine *et al.* put it in the following way: 'Depending on the type of task, the information generated by the system may be more or less appropriate, which will affect its success or failure'.[73] Saracevic distinguishes various other approaches to relevance, of which a number focus on the basic source of relevance, like, logical relevance, the nature of interference and the pertinent view of relevance.[17] We are very much aware of the fact that our elaboration of relevance does not in full retain the differences between those points of view. It is merely a practical elaboration that we use to predict user adoption.

The pragmatic perspective[74] of relevance that we choose resembles the notion of 'relative advantage' as discussed in the innovation diffusion literature by Rogers. Rogers[14,75] reserves a central role for 'relative advantage', which is the user's view of 'the degree to which an innovation is better than the idea it supersedes'. Relative advantage can be economic or social. Rogers states: 'The nature of the innovation largely determines what specific type of relative advantage is important to adopters, although the characteristics of the potential adopter also affect which dimensions of relative advantage are most important'. Based on a review of hundreds of empirical studies, Rogers concludes that relative advantage explains 49% of the rate of adoption of innovations.

It is most notable that the organizational factors are not explicitly included in our user relevance framework. It should be kept in mind that the user's agenda of problems and goals depend on his role in society.[76] The influence of the organization on this agenda depends on many aspects, including the involvement with other organizations, time and place. As a consequence, our framework reflects the actual impact that organizational goals and preferences have on the user, and thus, on organizational behavior.

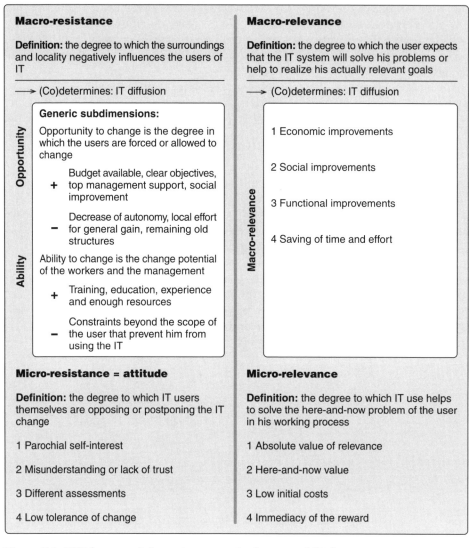

Figure 7.1 USE framework for resistance and relevance of IT change.

Requirements

At the semantic level[12,15,16] we are concerned with how pattern types relate to what happens in the world. On this level we deal with the meaning of the system, but this term brings a lot of different meanings about its definition.[77] The meaning of a sign relates to the response the sign elicits in a given social setting.[78] It is situational of nature since we have a range of pattern types that signify a certain meaning and a user (group) that interprets the expression.[79] Therefore it is necessary to establish requirements as thoroughly as possible. Wieringa defines requirements as desired properties needed to achieve the desired composite system properties.[80] Pressman makes a distinction between normal requirements, expected requirements and exiting requirements.[81] Before defining requirements ourselves we want to study the problem at a deeper level.

'Many system designers do not appear to realize that with their present approach they are designing only partial systems'.[25] Pressman argues that all needs of the end users should be identified. The notion of variance emerged from some early sociotechnical work design experiments in Norway.[82] A variance is defined as 'a tendency for a system or subsystem to deviate from some desired or expected norm or standard'. Key variances are the deviations on goals and functions; operational variances stem from the organizational problems. Together they get close to the main problem that we are addressing, the information gap between designer and user.

Iivari and Koskela[74] include three quality constructs on the semantic level, which they call the input/output requirements: informativeness, accessibility and adaptability. Informativeness describes the potentiality of the information systems, accessibility the quality of the user–IS interaction and adaptability points to the ability of the systems to change.

DeLone and McLean enumerate the criteria for IS success from nine earlier studies.[12] They declare themselves that there is not 'one' measure of IS success but there are many dependent variables. They call their taxonomy Semantic Level Information Quality. Usefulness or relevance is mentioned eight times in the nine studies. Schuring and Spil have studied the importance of relevance and made it a separate determinant on the pragmatic level.[29] Timeliness is empirically used five times and adopted in our model. We keep using the term 'accessibility' as a broader term, including convenience of access. Accuracy is studied four times and adopted under informativeness. We do not understand why there is no notion of adaptibility or ability to integrate in the DeLone and McLean study. We adopt ability to integrate as the degree that the new system is imbedded in the organization.

Brender and McNair use the ISO 900x structure and use the strategic, tactical and operational level to perform their user requirements specification.[83] Larsen also makes this distinction.[20] The strategic level is concerned with the problem definition, including objectives and global task description. The tactical level is interpreted as a preferred approach and the operational level includes a set of functional, performance and capacity criteria.

The requirements determinant is defined as 'the degree to which the user needs are satisfied with the product quality of the innovation'. We divide the requirements into macro- and micro-requirements (*see* Figure 7.2, overleaf).

- Strategic general requirements and tactical approach is the degree to which the users agree with the objectives and methods used.
- Functional requirements and performance requirements specify what the content of the innovation should be. In this study we chose timeliness (accessibility), accurateness (informativeness), ability to integrate and content as main quality criteria but we acknowledge that this is specific for this study and not a complete list.

Resources

Under the semantic level most researchers situate the syntactical level.[74] They give efficiency criteria to measure the quality of the information system on this level (design costs, operations costs and maintenance costs). Shannon and Weaver call it level A, the technical problem,[16] and Stamper divides it into three levels (syntactic, empirical and physical).[15] Main quality criteria on these levels are formal specification, reliability and costs.

The resources determinant is defined as 'the degree to which material and immaterial goods are available to design, operate and maintain the information system'.

The design costs can mainly be seen as time and capability of users and designers,[84] but also the size of the project and the complexity of the problem could be measured to assess the risk of the innovation design. Also hardware and software costs fall under this header. Formal specification on the syntactic level can be checked on the semantic level with the quality criterion accurateness (data, system and information).

The operations costs are mainly human resources but the abnormal costs can be derived from the reliability of the system.[74]

The maintenance costs can be shown with the quality criteria adaptability and portability that also link to the ability to integrate on a higher level.

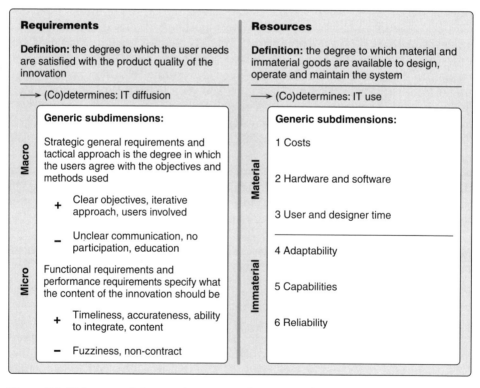

Figure 7.2 IT framework for requirements and resources determinants.

Multiple case studies results

Case study method

Nykänen distinguishes four major evaluation perspectives: goal-oriented, stand-ardized, effectiveness-based and stakeholder-based perspective.[85] In the goal-oriented evaluation the emphasis is on rationality: measurement criteria and the means to achieve the goal can be derived from the goal itself. This is possible if the criteria are clear and there are no conflicts of interest among the stakeholders. The downside of the goal-oriented perspective is the inability to see other than the anticipated consequences of actions. In the standardized (or normative) evaluation, causes and consequences are not in the scope of interest, but compliance with rules, agreements, budgets and principles is monitored (e.g. quality systems). In the effectiveness-based view the input/output ratio of actions is economically evaluated. The problem with this perspective is in expressing intangibles (e.g. health) in monetary terms. According to the stakeholder-based perspective, all actions are not always rational, aiming at one mutual goal, and therefore the criteria should be collected from several stakeholders' views. The perspective has a lot of qualitative characteristics and it can be a quite laborious framework for a study design.[86]

This study used the stakeholder-based perspective and was set up to both assess the situation regarding the electronic prescription system 'EVS' (elektronisch voorschriftsysteem) in the Netherlands and the theory that is described above that was set up to provide an instrument that could be used to analyze the diffusion situation of the prescription system. This resulted in a case study protocol that covers all the topics that are mentioned in the framework in open-ended questions. In line with the case study approach by Yin,[87] we discerned different case situations on the basis of our theoretical framework. Particularly, the network situation (individual, group practice, healthcare center) of GPs and the degree of adoption of previous ideas (laggard (no computer) to innovator (using ICPC codes and electronic patient record)) served as a basis to make categories of GPs. A total of 56 case studies were conducted. Each GP was visited in their own working situation and interviewed for over an hour. We agree with Brender that the kernel point of assessment is that of understanding the business processes.[88]

Electronic prescription in The Netherlands: an introduction

The Electronic Prescription System (EPS) that we studied is an IT system that gives GPs recommendations on the therapy that can be given to patients on the basis of the diagnosis of the practitioner.[89] This diagnosis is coded by use of the International Code for Primary Care (ICPC). The value of the system, as compared to the traditional situation, lies in the fact that the system takes patient characteristics into account. The recommended therapy is customized on the basis of the age and gender of the patient, and existing pharmaceutical therapy for other diseases, and is based on the formulary, which is a list of drug preferences that is set up by professional associations. Figure 7.3 shows the working principle of the EVS.

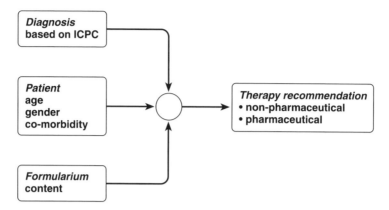

Figure 7.3 Working principle of the EVS electronic prescription system.

The EVS is available as an add-on to practically all information systems that exist for GPs in this country (GP-IS).

Empirical results of GP electronic prescription system

Empirical resistance of GP

The main problem formulation for this study was to find the obstacles of implementation of the EPS system. Under the header 'resistance of the GP', questions were asked about problems or wishes that the GP experienced as important at the moment of asking, during implementation of the EPS. Figure 7.1 gives an overview of all the situational resistance factors mentioned. Here we will summarize the results of the main five:

- time (55%)
- user interface 33%
- free choice 30%
- ICPC 27%
- unwilling 20%.

Fifty-five percent of the GPs said they were under immense time pressure. We think that this made the EPS less relevant to the GPs,[70] but it also levered the resistance because the GPs thought they would need more time for a consult using the EPS instead of less time. These statements are confirmed by British research.[90]

Thirty-three percent of the GPs had problems with the quality of the software. The main problems were not related to the new EPS but more to the old GP IS that was not able to give a good user interface. The EPS we described as 'spoilers on a T-Ford'.[91]

Thirty percent of the GPs say they do not want to be written the law by a new system and want to remain free to choose in prescribing drugs to their patients. Some say the recommendations are too conservative, others say they want to be able to try out new ideas. All of them say they want the freedom of choice.

Twenty seven percent of the GPs think that the ICPC is a problem when using the EPS system. Some state that it is rather difficult to find a related ICPC to the diagnosed disease. Others state that it is not necessary to use ICPC for general diseases like flu because it costs time and it does not help the process.

Twenty percent of the GPs are unwilling to use the EPS. That means that they have not looked at it and will not look at it just because they do not like the change. Here we see clearly a low tolerance of change.

Empirical relevance to the GP

Under the header 'relevance for the GP', questions were asked about problems or wishes that the GP experienced as important at the moment of asking, during implementation of the EPS. Figure 7.4 gives an overview of all the situational relevance factors mentioned. Here we will summarize the results of the main seven:

1 communication
2 time
3 money
4 software
5 free choice
6 International Code Primary Care (ICPC)
7 formulary.

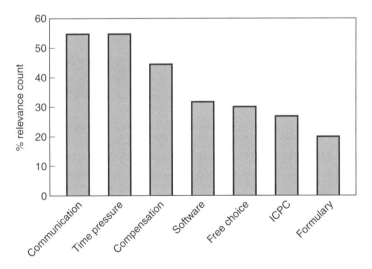

Figure 7.4 Multiple case study results on relevance.

In more than half of the case studies, the GPs said that improvements have to be made to communication with colleagues, pharmacists and hospitals. They state that a standard way of working is very important to reach such a communication. The EPS system does not deliver these features. Saarinen and Saaksjarvi measured the improved internal communication and improved inter-organizational communication under the header 'impact of the IS on the organization'.[19] None of these success factors was satisfied in our cases.

In 55% of the case studies, and independently of each other (the term was not mentioned by the interviewee), the GPs stated that there should be a diminishing of the time pressure. Both in the description of the EPS, as found in the international literature, EPS will not diminish the time of the consult.[8,90]

Forty-five percent of the case studies reported that the GP expected a fee in return for going to the trouble of implementing and using EPS. At the moment of interviewing it was not clear what financial profit the new system would deliver for the GP. What was known was that it would save the government and insurance companies a large amount of money on costs of medicine.

In about 20 case studies, lack of trust in the existing software and in the software supplier were mentioned as a barrier for (wanting to) use the new EPS. They said that first things had to change in the GP-IS market and in the GP-IS itself before EPS could be a success.

About the same number of GPs want to retain freedom of choice in prescribing medication for their patients. Although this seems to be a resistance matter it is also a relevance matter, because the EPS does not comprehend new ideas and new treatments that are already known in the general practice.

Although the use of ICPC seems useful to many GPs (in structuring and communicating), the time it will need to find the right code and the omissions of some codes form a barrier for EPS use.

Twenty percent of the GPs make use of a personal or regional formulary. The EPS makes use of a formulary from the Dutch Council for GPs and GPs are often unable to keep their own formulary when an update of the software is installed.

Finally, once the computer system was installed, use of the system was mostly sparse. The way of working was relatively complicated and added relatively little value in most patient–doctor contacts.

Empirical requirements to the GP

General requirements

The objectives for this innovation were mainly money driven. The system should decrease prescription costs by €150 million per annum. To the GPs we interviewed, the goals were not clear.

Functional and performance requirements

Content

The functionality of the GP information system can be divided into administrative functionality and medical functionality. We observed that the administrative use of the system has the upperhand. Only 15 GPs (27.3%) made use of the SOAP (subjective, objective, assessment, plan) module in the systems, which is a prerequisite for the use of the EPS.

Communication with other GPs, hospitals and pharmacists is a requirement that is high on the agenda of the GP (55%). However, the new EPS does not support this communication at all.

Timeliness

Time pressure is one of the most important problems facing today's GPs. Timeliness of the system is therefore an important performance criterion. Due to a bad user interface, the GPs are not able to work several records in parallel and therefore lose time in opening and closing the patient's record.

Accurateness

The accurateness of the system is good and might be too good. The system was rigidly designed to avoid failures and therefore has many signal functions. For instance, when prescribing medicines for influenza, the GP is given a lot of alternatives and warnings where he or she already knows exactly what to prescribe.

Also the accurateness of input is a problem because 30% of the GPs think it is unnecessary and sometimes difficult to generate a code for all 'vague' diseases like stomach ache, headache and so forth.

Ability to integrate

The EPS is delivered on CD-ROM as a stand-alone system. This means that it is not integrated in the GP information system and also not in the communication configuration of the GP. The GP therefore has to start the program for each patient and cannot work in parallel, the more so because the system is not window-based.

Empirical resources to the GP

Costs

For the GPs there are no costs involved in getting the system but they need time to install and operate the system. In general €30 million was spent in designing and implementing the system. Strangely, all system suppliers said they did not get money to change their GP information system. The operating and maintenance costs are not seen as a problem by the GP. The reward for using the system is seen as a problem. Extra office support was promised by the government, but in practice was not given and was not clear.

Hardware and software

The GPs have no faith in the suppliers of GP information systems. Mergers and take-overs mean the suppliers and GPs are in a deadlock situation where maintenance seems to be the only thing that happens. Thirty percent of the GPs regard the quality of the GP information system as an obstacle to using the new EPS. We described it as 'spoilers on a T-Ford'.

User and designer time

From our questions to the GPs it is very difficult to analyze the time spent in designing the system. In operating the system the GPs lose time because they have to put more information in the computer and use some time in consulting the system. With an average time of six minutes per consult this is a big problem.

Adaptability

From a maintenance point of view, the system is very adaptable, since a new version simply has to be distributed without having to change the rest of the GP system. Nevertheless, we advised that the entire GP system had to be updated with the EPS as an integrative communicative subsystem.

Capabilities

One of our final conclusions in the main report[91] is that we think it is crucial for the continuance of the project that the average GP is addressed rather than the innovative GP. In designing the system, GPs were involved, but only voluntary GPs who were bound to consist of the innovative GPs.

We also found big differences in IT capabilities. Some GPs still used the paper record and no computer and some GPs did all their activities on the computer. Due to these differing IT capabilities, various introduction programs will be necessary to diffuse the system into all GP practices.

Reliability

According to the GPs, the system is reliable. Breakdown of the system seldom occurs. The maintenance is reasonable, although one GP states: 'We have to be at a patient's house in ten minutes and they can stay away for ten days.'

Conclusions

Resistance of GPs is not *the* determinant of the use of the EPS (only 27%). Resistance is the cumulative consequence of effects of the other determinants and therefore it looks as if resistance is the most important determinant. This means that many studies work on the effect and not on the cause of the lack of IT use.

Relevance has long since been a central notion to IT theory. The elaborated approach that we proposed in this chapter was used in 56 case studies. These cases provided us with enough evidence that for this particular (electronic prescription) system in this particular (healthcare) branch, relevance was the most important determinant for failure of diffusion and use of the system.

Although in many studies the social criteria of success are mentioned as more important than the technical criteria, we cannot confirm this for these 56 cases. In most cases, the resources were not sufficient to use the new EPS. On top of that the requirements of the users were not sufficiently met by the system. We would like to draw the following conclusion for the healthcare organizations. Before starting a new project to build or buy a new information system in healthcare organizations it is necessary to explicitly measure the resources available. The next step is to make a contract containing functional and performance requirements, both agreed upon by a broad group (laggards and innovators alike) of end users and the designers responsible for the system.

Finally, we can conclude that assessing the IT diffusion and IT use of the EPS with the USE IT model was a multiple case study balancing sociotechnical determinants. The model has been used in two other healthcare situations and is now been used in a telecare project for stroke patients and a diffusion project of an electronic patient record in a hospital. We would encourage other researchers to work with the model in other environments (including outside healthcare) and we would also encourage the use of the interview schedule.

References

1   Ammenwerth E *et al.* (2003) Evaluation of health information systems-problems and challenges. *International Journal of Medical Informatics.* **71**(2–3): 125–35.
2   Berg M (2001) Implementing information systems in healthcare organizations: myths and challenges. *International Journal of Medical Informatics.* **64**: 143–56.
3   Pare G and Elam J (1999) Physicians' acceptance of clinical information systems: an empirical look at attitudes expectations and skills. *International Journal of Healthcare Technology and Management.* **1**(1): 46–61.
4   Southon G (1999) IT, change and evaluation: an overview of the role of evaluation in health services. *International Journal of Medical Informatics.* **56**: 125–33.
5   Walley P and Davies C (2001) Implementing IT in NHS hospitals – internal barriers to technological advancement. In *Proceedings of the First Hospital of the Future Conference.* Enschede, The Netherlands.
6   Schuring RW and Spil TAM (2004) HCADO: IS implementation, adoption and diffusion in healthcare. In: Call for proposals for the 38th HICSS conference, Hawaii (www.HICSS.org).
7   Kimberley JR and Evanisko MJ (1981) Organizational innovation: the influence of individual, organizational, and contextual factors on hospital adoption of technological and administrative innovations. *Academy of Management Journal.* **24**(4): 400–17.
8   Thornett AM (2001) Computer decision support systems in general practice. *International Journal of Information Management.* **21**: 39–47.
9   Beuscart-Zéphir MC (1997) Cognitive evaluation: how to assess the usability of information technology in healthcare. *Computer Methods and Programs in Biomedicine.* **54**: 19–28.
10 Beuscart-Zéphir MC *et al.* (2001) Integrating users' activity modeling in the design and assessment of hospital electronic patient records: the example of anesthesia. *International Journal of Medical Informatics.* **64**: 157–71.
11 Fleisner P and Hofkircher W (1998) The making of the information society: driving forces, 'Leibilder' and the imperative of survival. *Biosystems.* **46**: 201–7.
12 DeLone WH and McLean ER (1992) Information systems success: the quest for the dependent variable. *Information Systems Research.* **3**(1): 60–95.
13 Davis FD (1989) Perceived usefulness, perceived ease of use, and user acceptance of information technology. *MIS Quarterly.* **September**: 319–40.
14 Rogers EM (1995) *Diffusions of Innovations.* The Free Press, New York.
15 Stamper R (1973) *Information in Business and Administrative Systems.* John Wiley & Sons, New York.
16 Shannon CE and Weaver W (1949) *The Mathematical Theory of Communication.* University of Illinois Press, Chicago.
17 Saracevic T (1975) Relevance: a review of and framework for the thinking on the notion in information science. *Journal of the American Society for Information Science.* **26**(6): 321–43.
18 Michel-Verkerke MB, Schuring RW and Spil TAM (2003) Use IT or leave IT: a model to reveal user satisfaction of ICT-support in healthcare processes ex ante and ex post. In: *Proceedings of the 3rd International Conference The Hospital of the Future,* Association for Healthcare Technology and Management, Warwick.

19 Saarinen T and Sääksjärvi M (1992) Process and product success in information systems development. *Journal of Strategic Information Systems.* **1**(5): 266–77.

20 Larsen TJ (1998) Information systems innovation: a framework for research and practice. In: *Information Systems Innovation and Diffusion: issues and directions,* pp. 511–34. Idea Group Publishing, Hershey, PA, US.

21 Spil TAM (2002) Assessing resistance of professional users as a determinant of IT-diffusion and IT-use in healthcare. In: *Proceedings of ECITE 2002,* Paris.

22 Garrity EJ and Sanders GL (1998) Dimensions of information success. In: Garrity EJ and Sanders GL (eds) *Information Systems Success Measurement,* pp. 13–45. Idea Group Publishing, Hershey, PA, US.

23 Leavitt HJ (1965) Applied organisational change in industry: structural techno-logical and humanistic approaches. In: March JG (ed.) *Handbook of Organizations,* pp. 1144–70. Rand-McNally, Chicago, IL.

24 Offenbeek Mv and Koopman P (1996) Interaction and decision making in project teams. In: West MA (ed.) *Handbook of Work Group Psychology.* John Wiley & Sons, Chichester.

25 Mumford E (1995) *Effective Systems Design and Requirements Analysis.* MacMillan, London.

26 Thong JYL and Yap CS (1995) CEO characteristics, organizational characteristics and IT-adoption in small businesses. *Omega.* **23**(4): 429–42.

27 Venkatesh V *et al.* (2003) User acceptance of information technology: toward a unified view. *MIS Quarterly.* **27**(3): 425–78.

28 Schuring RW and Spil TAM (2001) Relevance as a major driver of innovation diffusion of ICT in healthcare organisations. In: *Proceedings of the Hospital of the Future: 1st International Conference on Management of Healthcare and Medical Technology.* University of Twente, Enschede.

29 Schuring RW and Spil TAM (2003) Relevance and micro-relevance for the professionals as determinants of IT diffusion and IT-use in healthcare. In: Grant G (ed.) *ERP and Datawarehousing in Organizations: issues and challenges.* IRM Press, Hershey.

30 DeLone WH and McLean ER (2002) Information systems success revisited. In: *35th Hawaii International Conference on System Sciences,* Hawaii.

31 Chismar WG and Wiley-Patton S (2003) Does the extended technology acceptance model apply to physicians. In: *36th Hawaii International Conference on System Sciences,* Hawaii.

32 Henry JW and Stone RW (1999) End user perception of the impacts of computer self-efficacy and outcome expectancy on job performance and patient care when using a medical information system. *International Journal of Healthcare Technology and Management.* **1**(1/2): 103–24.

33 Spil TAM and Schuring RW (2003) Assessing requirements and resources of information systems as determinants of IT-diffusion and IT-use in healthcare. In: *Proceedings of IFIP 8.6/03.*

34 Pijl GJvd (1994) Measuring the strategic dimensions of the quality of information. *Journal of Strategic Information Systems.* **3**(3): 179–90.

35 Sperber D and Wilson D (1986) *RELEVANCE, Communication and Cognition.* Basil Blackwell, Oxford.

36 Spil TAM and Schuring RW (2004) Requirements determine why professionals USE IT in healthcare. In: *Proceedings of the 15th IRMA conference,* New Orleans.

37 Ansoff I (1965) *Corporate Strategy.* McGraw-Hill, New York.

38 Goodstein LD and Burke WW (1991) Creating successful organizational change. *Organizational Dynamics.* **20**(4): 5.

39 Lanning H (2001) *Planning and Implementing Change in Organisations – a construct for managing change projects.* Helsinki University of Technology, Espoo, Finland.

40 Raghaven SA and Chand DR (1989) Diffusing software engineering methods. *IEEE Software*. **July**: 81–90.

41 Carey JM (ed.) (1988) *Human Factors in Management Information Systems*. ABLEX Publishing Corporation, New Jersey.

42 Coch L and French JRPJ (1947) Overcoming resistance to change. *Human Relations; Studies Towards the Integration of Social Sciences*. **1**(2): 512–32.

43 Lewin K (ed.) (1952) *Field Theory in Social Science, Selected Theoretical Papers*. Dorwin Cartwright, London.

44 Lawrence PR (1954) How to deal with resistance to change. *Harvard Business Review*. **32**(2): 49.

45 Zuboff S (1982) New worlds of computer-mediated work. *Harvard Business Review*. **March–April**: 142–53.

46 Malinconico SM (1983) Hearing the resistance. *Library Journal*. **108**(2): 111–13.

47 Folger R, Skarlicki DP and Teslu P (1999) Research notes – personality as a moderator in the relationship between fairness and retaliation. *Academy of Management Journal*. **42**(1): 100–10.

48 Piderit SK (2000) Rethinking resistance and recognizable ambivalence: a multi-dimensional view of attitudes toward an organizational change. *The Academy of Management Review*. **25**(4): 783–94.

49 Binney G and Williams C (1995) *Leaning into the Future: changing the way people change organizations*. N Brealy Publishing, London.

50 Kotter JP and Schlesinger LA (1979) Choosing strategies for change. *Harvard Business Review*. **March–April**: 106–13.

51 Wissema JG (1987) *Angst om te veranderen? Een mythe!* Van Gorcum, Assen.

52 Fuller FF (1969) Concerns of Teachers. *American Educational Research Journal*. **6**: 207–26.

53 Schmidt R *et al.* (2001) Identifying software project risks: an international Delphi study. *Journal of Management Information Systems*. **17**(4): 5–36.

54 Zmud RW (1979) Individual differences and MIS success: a review of empirical literature. *Management Science*. **25**(10): 966–79.

55 Lapointe L, Lamothe L and Fortin JP (2002) The dynamics of IT adoption in a major change process in healthcare delivery. In: *Proceedings of the 35th HICSS conference*, Hawaii.

56 Scott J (1985) *Weapons of the Weak: everyday forms of peasant resistance*. Yale University Press, New Haven, CT.

57 Prasad P and Prasa A (2000) Stretching the iron cage: the constitution and implications of routine workplace resistance. *Organizational Science*. **11**(4): 387–403.

58 Strebel P (1996) Why do employees resist change? *Harvard Business Review*. **May–June**: 86–92.

59 Duck JD (1993) Managing change: the art of balancing. *Harvard Business Review*. **November–December**: 109–18.

60 Mittelstaedt RA *et al.* (1976) Optimal stimulation level and the adoption decision process. *Journal of Consumer Research*. **3**: 84–94.

61 Gatignon H and Robertson TS (1989) Technology diffusion: an empirical test of competitive effects. *Journal of Marketing*. **53**: 35–49.

62 Szmigin I and Foxal G (1998) Three forms of innovation resistance: the case of retail payment methods. *Technovation*. **18**(6/7): 459–68.

63 Ram S and Sheth JN (1987) *Bringing Innovation to Market, How to Break Corporate and Customer Barriers*. Wiley, New York.

64 Markus ML (1983) Power, politics and MIS implementation. *Communications of the ACM*. **26**(6): 430–44.

65 Dent EB and Goldberg SG (1999) Challenging 'Resistance to Change'. *Journal of Applied Behavioral Science*. **35**(1): 25–41.

66 Zaltman G and Duncan R (1977) *Strategies for Planned Change*. Wiley, New York.

67 Metselaar EE, Kolk JMvd and Wortelboer FQC (1996) Werken aan veranderings-bereidheid (in Dutch). In: *Handboek effectief opleiden*, pp. 135–58. Delwel, The Hague.

68 Ajzen I and Madden TJ (1986) The prediction of goal directed behavior: attitudes, intentions and perceived behavioral control. *Journal of Experimental Psychology*. **22**: 453–74.

69 Mahmood MA *et al.* (2000) Variables affecting IT end-user satisfaction: a meta-analysis of the empirical literature. *International Journal of Human-Computer-Studies*, **52**: 751–71.

70 Schuring RW and Spil TAM (2002) Explaining plateaued diffusion by combining the user-IT-success factors (USIT) and adopter categories: the case of electronic prescription systems for general practitioners. *International Journal of Healthcare Technology and Management*. **4**: 303–18.

71 Cooper WS (1971) A definition of relevance for information retrieval. *Information Storage and Retrieval*. **7**(1): 19–37.

72 Wilson P (1973) Situational relevance. *Information Storage and Retrieval*. **9**(8): 457–71.

73 Ballantine J *et al.* (1998) Developing a 3-D model of information systems success. In: Garrity EJ and Sanders GL (eds) *Information Systems Success Measurement*, pp. 46–59. Idea Group Publishing, Hershey, PA, US.

74 Iivari J and Koskela E (1987) The PIOCO model for IS design. *MIS Quarterly*. September: 400–17.

75 Rogers EM and Scott KL (1997) The Diffusion of Innovations Model and Outreach from the National Network of Libraries of Medicine to Native American Communities. Paper prepared for the National Network of Libraries of Medicine. Pacific Northwest Region, Seattle, WA.

76 Barnard CI (1938) *The Functions of the Executive*. Harvard University Press, Cambridge, MA.

77 Cohen LJ (1962) *The Diversity of Meaning*. Methuen, London.

78 Liu K (1993) Semiotics applied to information systems development. PhD thesis. University of Twente, Enschede.

79 Spil TAM (1993) The evaluation of SISP: From a quality undergrowth to a semiotic clearing. In: *Proceedings of the first ECITE Conference*, Henley on Thames.

80 Wieringa RJ (2001) *Requirements Engineering: frameworks for understanding*. Wiley, Chichester.

81 Pressman RS (1982) *Software Engineering: a practitioner's approach*. McGraw-Hill, New York.

82 Mumford E (1983) *Designing Human Systems for New Technology*. Manchester Business School, Manchester, UK.

83 Brender J and McNair P (2001) User requirements specifications: a hierarchical structure covering strategical, tactical and operational requirements. *International Journal of Medical Informatics*. **64**: 83–98.

84 Salmela H (1997) From information systems quality to sustainable business quality. *Information and Software Technology*. **39**: 819–25.

85 Nykänen P (2000) Decision support systems from a health informatics perspective. In: *Department of Computer and Information Sciences*. University of Tampere, Tampere, Finland.

86 Hakkinen H, Turunen P and Spil TAM (2003) Information in healthcare process – evaluation toolkit development. In: *Proceedings of the 36th Hawaii International Conference on System Sciences*, Kona, HI.

87 Yin RK (2003) *Case Study Research: design and methods*. Applied Social Research Series, Volume 5. Sage Publications, London.

88 Brender J (1999) Methodology for constructive assessment of IT-based systems in an organisational context. *International Journal of Medical Informatics*. **56**: 67–86.

89 Althuis TR and Rikken SAJJ (2000) Electronic support for general practitioners in prescribing drugs. *Health information developments in the Netherlands.* **April**: 62–6.

90 Mitchell E and Sullivan F (2001) A descriptive feast but an evaluative famine: systematic review of published articles on primary care computing during 1980–97. *British Medical Journal.* **322**: 279–82.

91 Lagendijk PJB, Schuring RW and Spil TAM (2001) *Elektronisch voorschrijf systeem.* Enschede, Universiteit Twente.

Appendix: Interview-protocol care provider USE IT version 14.0

Date interview:

Name interviewer:

Name interviewee:

Job interviewee:

Organization:

P   **Primary process**

P1   What care do you provide?
Most care providers contribute to different care processes.
In our research we make the following distinction:

- Diagnosis   %
- Investigations outside the consulting room   %
- Treatment   %
- Nursing   %
- Acute incidents occur: the whole day through/several times a day/several times a week
- Acute incidents dominate my work very much/somehow/a little/not

The categorization may be adjusted to the investigated care process as long as it is clear to what % of patients or tasks the innovations applies (*see* REL 7)

How do you act at each of the above-mentioned tasks?

- Do you follow a fixed pattern?
- How long does a patient contact take?
- Do you use equipment?
- Do you use (human) support? If so, for whom else does this supporter work?
- Where do you perform your tasks? Could they be performed elsewhere?
- Do you always sit or stand in the same position towards the patient? (Make a sketch)
- Do you have to look up or ask after things?
- Do you have to prepare anything?

P 2   What other tasks do you have apart from providing care?

How much time or energy do these tasks take from you?

- Time   %
- Energy   %

P 3   What exceptions or disturbances make this kind of care or the coordination of this care fail?

P 4   Do you use a care protocol or medical guideline for the care you provide?

- Do you comply with this protocol entirely or partially?
- What parts do you use, what parts don't you use?
- Does using the protocol fit with your way of working?

P 5   Who refers patients to you?

P 6   To whom do you refer patients?

P 7   What other care providers or institutions are simultaneously involved with the care for your patients?

- Do you work together?
- Or do you work 'in parallel'?

P 8   How do you experience the cooperation with other care providers in respect to the providing of the care?

P 9   With what care providers should you cooperate (more)?

- Why?
- With whom should you exchange more information?
- What information?

P 10   What do you find important in the contact with other care providers?

REQ   Requirements

I 1   What information about the patient do you need to perform your job properly? (Distinguish according to the separate tasks, mentioned in P 1 and P 2)

What information do you receive from

- The patient?
- The patient's surrounding?
- Other care providers?
- With what purpose?
- In what frequency?

What form does this information have?

- Letter (sent by post or handed over personally)
- Fax
- Email
- In paper record
- In electronic record

I 2   Does this information suffice?

- Do you experience problems?
- Do you miss information?

I 3   What information do you generate yourself when providing care?

What information do you give to:
- The patient?
- The patient's surrounding?
- Other care providers?

- Managers?
- External parties (e.g. insurance company, government)?

What form does this information have?

- Letter (sent by post or handed over personally)
- Fax
- Email
- In paper record
- In electronic record
- Record only used for this patient group or this type of care
- Record only used by your own discipline
- Record only used in your institution

I 4 How do you appreciate the quality of the proposed (or implemented) innovation? Regarding the:

- Content
- Objectives
- Method
- Possibility to integrate it in the present situation
- Timeliness
- Correctness

I 5 Were the right end users involved with making or selecting this innovation?

REL **Relevance**

R 1 What do you experience, **for you personally**, as important in your daily work when you look at the care you provide?

R 2 What aspects in the ability to provide care, do you experience as a bottleneck or problem?

- Concerning the providing of care
- Other aspects

Are there any specific actions in the previously discussed processes that cause bottlenecks or problems?

R 3 Do you know proposals for improvement, concerning these patients, for which you would do your utmost?

R 4 How important are these proposed improvements in the chain of care in relation to other possibilities to improve aspects of your job?

- Can you name other proposals for improvement, which are more important?
- Can you name other proposals for improvement, which are less important?

R 5 In what way could the use of ICT matter to you?

- What application are you thinking of?
- For what purpose or for what situation?

R 6 What aspect of your job would you miss, if it was removed?

R 7 How important are your tasks for these patients, **for you**, in comparison with your tasks for other patients?

- Why are these patients so important or of so little importance for you?

Res	**Resistance**

A 1   To what extent are you convinced that the use of ICT is necessary to improve the provision of care?

- What experience do you have with ICT?
- How much time are you prepared to spend?
- Do you use ICT to communicate?
- How often do you use the Internet?
- How often do you use specific systems yourself?

A 2   Do you experience obstacles when implementing innovations?

- Workload
- Management support
- ICT support
- Money
- Your skills

A 3   How much time and energy do you think you can find to implement the changes that will occur when introducing innovations and ICT in this kind of care?

A 4   Do your colleagues or managers stimulate you to participate in changes?

A 5   Can you name other innovation projects this organization is working on? Are these projects equally important (or more or less important)?

Res	**Resources**

M 1   What ICT facilities do you have at your disposal at your workplace?

- Hardware
- Software
- For communication
- Data

M 2   Which of these ICT facilities do you use when providing care?

- Hardware
- Software
- For communication
- Data

M 3   Is the technical support sufficient to guarantee the quality of the system?

- Reliability
- Availability
- Security
- Privacy

M 4   Do you think you will have support to implement changes?

- Time
- Money
- Training
- Management support

C	**Concluding questions**

C 1   Is there anything you would like to add?

C 2   May we contact you to think with us in the development of a ICT application?

Chapter 8

Implementation of a telerehabilitation system using change management principles

Pamela G Forducey, Lori Smith, Kawaljeet Kaur and
Cynthia Scheideman-Miller

The need for alternative healthcare delivery models is real and critical. Innovative telecommunications technology has developed as a cost-effective strategy to meet the challenge of improving medical services to individuals.[1] One example of this type of technology is telemedicine, which is the use of electronic communication and information technologies to provide or support clinical care at a distance. A new term, 'telehealth', is often used to reflect the inclusion of preventative services in addition to diagnostic and medical treatment applications, and is one method that can reduce the limitations of our current healthcare system. As with any alternative delivery model, telehealth must satisfy the criteria of improving quality of life and achieving meaningful functional outcomes for individuals with chronic health conditions and resulting acquired disabilities.[2]

Rehabilitation is the process of restoring a person to a state of health or useful activity through training, therapy and guidance. It is the observation of these authors that rehabilitation patients often receive intensive acute inpatient rehabilitation but frequently have access to only variable and limited post-acute outpatient rehabilitation services, especially in rural communities. Integration of long-term care and other needed non-medical social services is often lacking, which is a significant concern to rehabilitation professionals since individuals with acquired disabilities, such as brain injury or spinal cord injury, often continue to improve throughout their lifetime. Given this reality, the efficacy of community-based, non-medical services/perspectives should be evaluated. These services include, but are not limited to, supported living programs, centers for independent living, case management services, supported employment programs and telerehabilitation.

Telerehabilitation is defined as the remote delivery through telecommunication technology of a variety of rehabilitative services for persons with disabilities. It is a versatile interdisciplinary medium that is used by health professionals to facilitate post-acute rehabilitation in the home and community settings.[3,4] Telerehabilitation interventions primarily occur in real time via two-way interactive audio-visual linkage, as opposed to a 'store and forward' method. Nineteen different programs surveyed by the Office for the Advancement of Telehealth (OAT) in

2001 included some kind of telerehabilitation activity at their site. Services included occupational therapy, physical therapy, speech–language pathology, physiatry, psychology, audio-verbal therapy and vocational rehabilitation. The majority of these programs are currently funded by federal, state or private grants. Long-term feasibility of these telehealth programs is dependent on the economic and organizational sustainability of the program.

Over the past three to four decades, multiple and diverse researchers have speculated why one organization is more likely to adopt innovation than another organization. A variety of factors have emerged from economic, political, psychological, sociological and managerial perspectives.[5] The seminal study conducted by Kimberly and Evanisko (1981) focused on the health sector and identified factors to explain variability in the adoption of both technological and administrative innovations by hospitals. Data were collected from both hospital administrators and chief medical officers in each hospital surveyed as well as from the American Hospital Association Annual Survey of Hospitals. Individual (characteristics of hospital leaders), organizational (structural characteristics such as level of specialization and size) and contextual (competition in community and size of city) variables were found to be better predictors of hospital adoption of technological innovations than of administrative innovations. Comparative analyses also revealed that the education level of the hospital administrator, the size of organization and the presence of competition in the local environment were significant predictors of both technological and administrative innovation. Organizational-level variables, size in particular, were better predictors of both types of innovation than either individual or contextual level variables.

As we considered our own organizational initiative in launching a telerehabilitation program, several variables noted in this research contributed to our strategy and implementation approach. The most positive influences for technological adoption were the variables of organizational size, hospital administrative support and functional success in the service line of rehabilitation. Despite our confidence in the administrative decision for advancing our mission through increased technological innovations, we also had to rely on our own experiences of prior change initiatives and lessons learned. The value of considering these lessons within the context of our organizational culture was critical. Prior experiences have taught us to plan early for barriers to success. As a result of these experiences, a teaching model emerged within our system in an attempt to become more efficient and effective in system change initiatives. This model assists our organization in both planning for barriers and providing hope for the endurance of the initiative.

Banner and Gagne[6] emphasize that there are common characteristics to all organizations:

- goal direction
- identifiable boundaries
- social interaction
- structured activity
- culture.

Our organizational system captured these characteristics and created components that we believed should be addressed throughout the life span of the telerehabilitation project to promote success. A visual model was developed that would serve as a pictorial guide to maintain our focus and balance. This model was instrumental to the implementation of our telerehabilitation program in Oklahoma. These authors describe the implementation of the telerehabilitation program through focused effort on the five components outlined in Banner and Gagne's model. The five components of integrated organizational design, all of which should be addressed for a balanced approach to change, are *strategy* (goal direction), *structure* (identifiable boundaries), *people* (social interaction), *process* (structured activity) and *customer (*end user).

The culture of an organization is the product of the interaction between these components. The customer is the hub around which these components interact and evolve. The interrelationship of these components is shown in Figure 8.1. All of these components can be traced to the different layers of the onion model described earlier in this book. Lessons learned during the process are included in the corresponding sections. Although this chapter focuses on 'change management', the third layer of the onion model, a successful change initiative is a multidisciplinary task, and cannot be dealt with in isolation.

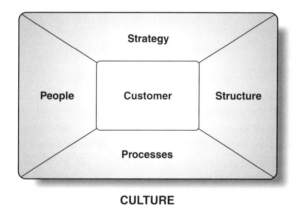

CULTURE

Figure 8.1 Interrelationship between components of change and culture.

Facility background

INTEGRIS Health Inc. is an Oklahoma-based not-for-profit healthcare organization with hospitals, a rehabilitation hospital, physician clinics, mental health facilities, independent living centers and home-health agencies throughout urban and rural Oklahoma. In 1993, Baptist Medical Center (BMC) created Oklahoma's first telemedicine network by connecting six rural INTEGRIS Health hospitals for voice, video and data connectivity. In 1994, BMC went from a single hospital located in an urban area to several hospitals located throughout Oklahoma and became known as INTEGRIS Health. The INTEGRIS Telehealth Network (ITN) was built for two primary reasons, CEO commitment and potential external competition. Since there was no provision for telemedicine reimbursement in 1993, the ITN primarily was used for continuing medical education (CME) and administrative and community-based services, and was self-supportive with staff to cover it 24 hours, seven days a week.

INTEGRIS Rural Health received a rural telemedicine grant (1997–2000 and 2000–03) from the Health Resources and Services Administration (HRSA), OAT to improve access to healthcare for rural individuals across the life span, reduce isolation of rural practitioners, and to collect and disseminate this data. The grant was used to expand the ITN sites and provide medical primary care and specialist consultation. INTEGRIS Health expanded telehealth services to include analog-based technology. They are currently partnering with a software company in a Rural Utilities Services grant in 2003 with a focus on disease management for patients in rural residences. The system recently converted to H323 (a multimedia teleconferencing standard) capable bridge, which expands its quality and capability. Today, evolving services are providing access to clinical information services (through Cerner applications), financial information and services (through PeopleSoft systems), and decision support (real-time Cerner decision support action). Teleradiology is active at four sites and will be expanded. INTEGRIS Health provides for ownership and maintenance of telemedicine equipment. From 1999 to 2003, INTEGRIS Health Information Technology[IT] received the Hospital and Health Networks Most Wired Award.

Needs assessment for telerehabilitation in Oklahoma

It is the supposition of these authors that telehealth is most likely to succeed if the healthcare needs of the community are not adequately met by conventional or traditional healthcare treatment modalities. Needs assessment should be a reflection of the organizational strategy, mission and vision, and is guided by the specific cultural and institutional context, which constitutes the first layer of the onion model. Executive buy-in is easier if the change complements the long-term strategic objectives of the organization. It should be noted that an innovative program such as telerehabilitation should be built on 'demand' and not on 'need'. The need may be present, but it takes a demand for the service to generate business. Frequently, it is the healthcare consumers, individuals with disabilities and their caregivers, who are making the demands of their healthcare providers and insurance companies. The advent of the Internet has led to greater consumer empowerment and many individuals with chronic health conditions are assuming a more proactive role in the maintenance of their healthcare.

Oklahoma is a predominantly rural state with 63 of the 77 counties federally designated as rural. Rural patients receive fewer home health services and attain less favorable discharge outcomes as compared to the urban patients; a factor primarily attributed to resource constraints and a lower availability of skilled care disciplines.[7] Twenty-four of these counties are designated as medically underserved areas (MUAs), three counties are designated as health professional shortage areas (HPSAs), and 28 counties are designated as both MUA and HPSA. Telemedicine can be used in HPSA, MUA, prison inmates, school systems, long-term care facilities, Indian health centers, worker's compensation or self-insured industries, general population and specialist consultation with other facilities. Seven of the 77 counties are designated as frontier counties with fewer than six people residing per square mile. Besides the distance barriers, there are sociological and economic factors that play a part. The eastern part of the state primarily has agriculture and lumber industries. These lifestyle components expose people to a high risk of injuries with few local specialized services available for rehabilitation and recuperation. Since 1981, 15 Oklahoma hospitals, usually the sole hospital in their communities, closed secondary to low patient census and closure of physician practices. Twenty-three more rural hospitals are in danger of closing in the next three years.[8]

A comprehensive, coordinated rehabilitation program can reduce mortality and improve functional outcomes following an acquired disability. While such findings suggest longer periods of rehabilitation benefit the patient, pressures from third-party payers to reduce lengths of stay appear to be the stronger influence. Financial constraints imposed by the Prospective Payment System (PPS) mandate inpatient rehabilitation facilities to re-examine resource utilization and organizational effectiveness. According to one study, charges at rehabilitation facilities are increasing by an average of 7% each year, but the length of stay is decreasing by approximately 8% annually.[9] This translates to the fact that patients with chronic medical conditions may be leaving acute inpatient rehabilitation facilities before they are functionally ready, which results in increased reliance on community-based rather than hospital-based resources. Liss et al.[2] suggest that telecommunication-based interventions may be used efficiently and effectively for populations with chronic disability, including those who do not have previous experience with the technologies. Rosen[10] points out that the individual can stay in their community without losing the expertise available in the larger hospitals, which would result in reduced travel expenses for the physician/therapist and patient; possible delivery of a greater proportion of therapy by less expensive community providers with occasional teleconsultation by specialists; as well as a shift of the overhead of housing a patient from the service provider to the family.

Identification of stakeholders and champions

Stakeholders may be internal or external to the organization and are individuals, groups or organizations with an interest in a given focus area. For the telerehabilitation program, the internal stakeholders included hospital administrators, clinicians/therapists, clinical support staff and information technology specialists. External stakeholders were third-party payers, case managers, referring physicians, patients and their caregivers. Stakeholders were identified and their diverse interests defined, understood and updated as the situation evolved. Recognizing and working with the underlying concerns, desires and fears that motivate an individual are critical for their participation in the change process. Each stakeholder is unique and will have a different set of concerns and questions, which all need to be addressed. One frequently overlooked group of stakeholders is the knowledge holders who possess critical skills to contribute to the problem-solving process. This group generally includes the researchers, rehabilitation engineers, clinical development specialists and policy makers. Knowledge holders can play a key role of educating and facilitating discussion between stakeholders. Change acceptance starts with the stakeholders; and education of the stakeholders is vital. Change champions are stakeholders who buy into the new concept or idea and play a pivotal role of championing the project.

The INTEGRIS telerehabilitation program was trademarked INTEGRIS Tele-Rehab for name-branding and focused on gaining support from the top, but building the program from the ground up. The program had both an administrative and a clinical champion. The director of the telemedicine program was the administrative champion, educating the key administrative people about the telemedicine program and services, thus creating administrative and executive buy-in. The administrative champion also communicated with the rural sites and the system support staff. The director of clinical development served as the clinical champion, focusing on educating and gaining support of therapists, clinicians, and rehabilitation patients and their caregivers. Both champions had the ability to think outside the box, and adopt alternate methodologies to accomplish their goals. A technical champion is also crucial to the success of a telerehabilitation program and should not be overlooked at any stage of program development.

Strategy

Strategy is a pattern in a stream of decisions, positioning an organization within its environment and resulting in the 'behavior' of the organization. It is future-oriented and sets direction for the organization. Strategy ties the organization together with a common sense of purpose of shared values, enabling the organization to develop a clear concept, specific goals, and consistency in decision making. Setting clear strategy goals is the most crucial component of any change. Strategies should align with the mission, vision and values of the organization. Strategy should be *simple*, as it is a template for decision making; *competitive*, as it defines the product and services at which the organization will excel; *innovative*, as it requires new perspectives from both outside and inside the organization; *responsive*, as it defines the organization in terms of stakeholders and the competition; *evolving*, as it requires room for improvising; and *involving*, as it should not be isolated to the top levels of the organization.

The vision of INTEGRIS Health is *to be the healthcare delivery system of choice, committed to caring service, quality outcomes and cost competitiveness*. Specific INTEGRIS Health goals for the next five years that directly relate to the INTEGRIS Rural Telemedicine Project include patient goals, physician goals and community goals.

Patient goals include providing geographic accessibility, creating demonstrably better outcomes and providing cost-effective care. Physician goals include providing technology and sophisticated tools for care management. Community goals include providing care that exceeds stakeholder expectations and improving the health status of the community.

INTEGRIS Rural Telemedicine Project concentrated on four areas in order to achieve these goals (*see* Table 8.1).

Table 8.1 Rural telemedicine project goals and objectives

---

1 Solidify the growing reputation of INTEGRIS in the telerehabilitation field
   • by the formation of a Telerehabilitation Planning Group including a patient advocate
   • through collaborations with other rehabilitation and academic centers in clinical applications and research
   • with publications and presentations at the state and national levels to government departments, healthcare associations and providers, and at related conferences.
2 Establish a market presence by
   • proving efficacy, cost savings and improved accessibility through the pilot study
   • marketing indirectly through articles in national publications and local newspaper as well as news reports on television
   • direct marketing through brochures distributed to healthcare providers by the Oklahoma Healthcare Authority and contact with school districts
   • marketing directly to the patients and caregivers by working through special interest groups, such as the Brain Injury Association, and Rural Health Association.
3 Develop services based on the needs of the rural facilities
   • need assessments based on Joint Commission for Accreditation of Healthcare Organizations (JCAHO) deficiencies
   • needs indicated by rural primary care physicians and other healthcare professionals
   • shortages as indicated by state statistics
   • needs indicated by government and community members.
4 Promote telemedicine on a state level
   • work with the Governor's Telemedicine Advisory Council to promote telemedicine to third-party payers, legislators, and general public
   • help build the Oklahoma State Website and INTEGRIS website, which includes projects and services available through INTEGRIS
   • work with the Department of Health and other state departments to promote a state-wide network of telemedicine providers.

The primary reasons for misalignment of mission, vision and values are unclear strategic direction, lack of cohesion and open communication channels in the senior management team, leadership that is too top-down or lenient, ineffective vertical communication between management levels in the same department, lack of institution-wide coordination and integration, and lack of down-the-line leadership development and training. To prevent misalignment, most of the system goals are echoed by the individual hospital goals. The INTEGRIS tele-rehabilitation strategy is revisited annually and modified according to the current needs and circumstances.

Development of the TeleRehab program at INTEGRIS Health

The foundation of the TeleRehab was established in 1999 when a speech teletherapy pilot study was initiated in an elementary public school in Hugo, Oklahoma. The administrator of the telemedicine program approached administrators at the Hugo Hospital to determine if there was a 'need' for telemedicine and learned that the local school was unable to recruit a speech–language pathologist for students with disability. Schools are federally mandated to provide speech therapy services to the students; however, hiring a speech therapist is not only economically challenging for the schools but is often not feasible due to lack of therapist availability in the rural areas. This rural school was already using audio-visual equipment for distance learning, so school personnel were familiar and comfortable with the equipment.

Permission for a pre-pilot study was obtained from the school board, and eight students were provided with speech therapy in the local rural hospital, which was already using telemedicine for emergency room visits. Speech teletherapy was conducted for four weeks, and the results, including complete cost analysis, were presented to the Hugo school board. Based on these results, the school board approved therapy services via TeleRehab for one year.

Expansion of services to other schools followed the same pattern of demonstration of efficacy resulting in approval by the school board. Currently, our organization has contracts with four different rural school systems throughout Oklahoma and employs two full-time equivalent speech teletherapists who conduct approximately 168 hours of direct service per month to students with both acquired and congenital disabilities.

Clinical and administrative champions should do their homework before venturing into an uncharted territory. Learning from the experience of other organizations is beneficial. This information can be obtained from websites, trade journals, focus groups, phone calls and site-visits. It is also helpful to find a mentoring organization of a similar nature providing telemedicine services. However, when INTEGRIS Health started its telerehabilitation program, there was very little telerehabilitation activity in the country. Since INTEGRIS was treading new terrains, it was decided to focus on one discreet area that would be less controversial and more likely to succeed. This area proved to be school-based speech therapy services. Once these services were successfully in place, the program proceeded to build on its success by adding other allied health disciplines and expanding the market base. The TeleRehab program has subsequently expanded to include physical therapy, occupational therapy, physiatry, vocational rehabilitation and psychology. The tool used for process development by INTEGRIS Health was PDCA (Plan, Do, Collect, Analyze), which follows an iterative cycle of planning the process improvement, doing process improvement, collecting data and analyzing data (Figure 8.2). The PDCA model also forms the anchor for organizational learning and success, which is the innermost layer of the onion model and the desired end-point of all effort.

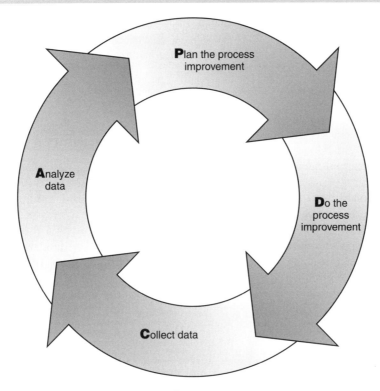

Figure 8.2 PDCA model for process development.

Services are currently offered to schools and third-party payers (such as workman compensation and self-insured industries) as well as to the general public. The current TeleRehab network covers north-central, northeastern, southeastern, south-central and western Oklahoma (Figure 8.3). Services fall under one of the three categories.

- Direct patient intervention where the therapist either works directly with the patient or guides the remote therapist or caregiver.
- Mentoring with the patient present, which includes teaching manage-ment strategies, activity selection with grading, and handling training and development.
- Consultation where the patient is not present, which includes concepts and practice discussion, session analysis and feedback, and planning.

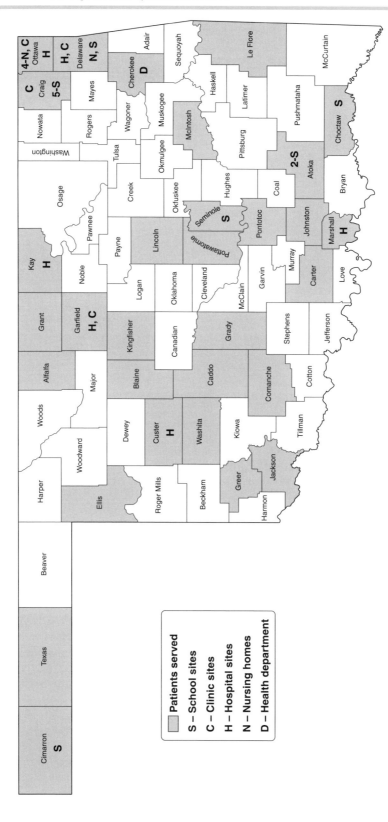

Figure 8.3 Coverage of INTEGRIS TeleRehab Network as of October 2003.

Structure

Structure provides the building blocks for the program. Structure considerations center on such questions as:

- Do all layers of the organization have the adequate information, resources and tools to support the innovative program?
- Does the organization have the structure in place to monitor quality, service, cost-effectiveness and team work?

In order to have these questions answered, general structure components deal with:

- information access and dissemination
- physical plant layout
- outline of functional departments and their integration and fit to other departments
- centralization versus decentralization
- equipment (automation/specialization)
- human resource development such as recruitment and retention of staff, job role and function
- financial structures including payment and distribution, cost containment and maintenance
- policy development
- competency development of staff.

Business model

The INTEGRIS TeleRehab business model is not static, but keeps on evolving as technology, consumer and clinician acceptance, and reimbursement components change. The business model defines the scope, goals, competitive advantage, value constellation and value chain of the business unit. At INTEGRIS, there is a separate cost center for telemedicine with a dedicated director and a telemedicine coordinator. Establishing TeleRehab as a separate cost center facilitates management of the program. However, this should be done once the program is well planned and implemented. Making the program autonomous allows easier financial tracking. Having TeleRehab as a separate business unit also addresses the ambiguity of program ownership secondary to diverse stakeholders.

Both the grant-based telehealth projects and the start-up telehealth companies should have a clear and focused business plan. The content of the plan varies based on the specific program. However, it generally incorporates information about the company profile; principal services being offered; target customers; projected sales or consultations; partnerships with other organizations, if any; overview of needs assessment; cost profiles; contractual agreements, if any; quality measures; risk management; competition; sales and marketing techniques; company management; financial management; and research and development (R&D).[13]

Organizational commitment

Telehealth implementation and sustainability require interdepartmental support and resources. Organizational commitment is required at all stages of conception, implementation and management of the program. Education of the executives and the stakeholders is paramount for continued organizational commitment. The telehealth program at INTEGRIS Health has mixed executive buy-in. The program was accepted at its inception largely because of the funds coming from the HRSA grant. However, the program is increasingly gaining support. After five years of initiation of the program, telehealth has been included as part of INTEGRIS Health strategic plan at the organizational level. TeleRehab has also transitioned from being a project to a program, and is now considered part of the normal INTEGRIS Health business, instead of being an experimental R&D model.

Economic model

Sustainability does not always equate to profitability in the initial phase of telehealth implementation; however, a stream of revenue and profit are essential for long-term sustenance of the program. Grant funding is helpful as seed money to help with one-time costs associated with the initial set-up. A significant number of telehealth interventions are not reimbursed. Currently, the Center for Medicare and Medicaid Services (CMS), the primary federal funding agency for healthcare, requires face-to-face evaluation for reimbursement, except for image applications such as radiology. A number of demonstration grants are currently underway to establish the efficacy of telehealth as an alternative healthcare delivery model, and make a case for reimbursement initiatives and legislature. Long-term viability depends on contracts and third-party reimbursements. Diversifying sources of revenue, with a combination of stable but marginal revenue sources with an intermittent but high return on investment, is a safe strategy.

Contracts

Contracts are often associated with agencies or organizations that require interventions for a number of people over an extended period of time, such as schools or prisons. Contracts can be based on a flat-fee model or an hourly rate. The contracts for school therapy program at INTEGRIS Health underwent four stages of evolution. The first stage comprised of a flat fee, regardless of the number of hours used or the number of students seen. At one point, when extensive technology problems precluded service delivery for six weeks, billing adjustments had to be made. The next year, the contract was modified to bill based on the number of hours used. However, this model had the negative effect of school teachers canceling speech teletherapy session at will, which resulted in unproductive time for the speech teletherapist that could have been spent with other patients. A hybrid contract model was introduced in the third year. This required reimbursement of half of the anticipated sessions, whether they were used or not. The hybrid contract reduced the number of cancellations, thus increasing compliance and benefiting both the students and the teletherapy program. The final modification to the contract was a slight increase in charge to help pay for the extra time for paperwork required for schools to receive Medicaid reimbursement for some students. This has been a popular feature of the INTEGRIS speech teletherapy program as it helps the schools receive funds for special education that would otherwise be unavailable to them. Clear outline for the service care delivery, agreements on quality standards and regulatory requirements should be addressed in the contract. Table 8.2 (*see* p. 166) provides a template for cost analysis of telehealth as a substitute for face-to-face visits, along with estimated value for each variable.[14]

Fee for service

Reimbursement through the third-party payers is the largest source of revenue for telehealth programs. Rules governing reimbursement for telehealth services vary from state to state and the type of service provided. Under current Medicare regulations, only physician and psychology telehealth services are reimbursed. Beginning in 1999, Congress mandated CMS to pay for telehealth services to patients in HPSA. Efforts have also been underway at the state level pushing reimbursements for telehealth consultations. California, Oklahoma and Texas have now eliminated face-to-face evaluation as a requisite for reimbursement. Reimbursements are limited to the interventions at the remote clinic settings and do not include therapy provided at the patient's residence. Third-party payers are now reimbursing telehealth services in several states, and about 12 states have partial Medicaid reimbursements.[15] At INTEGRIS, therapists work with the administrative sections of the organization for billing and compliance purposes. Current Procedural Terminology (CPT) codes, documented therapy procedures, service units and costs for TeleRehab sessions have been developed and are documented for reimbursement purposes. TeleRehab therapists have given numerous presentations for state legislature and CMS to educate and build a case for reimbursement for telerehabilitation-based interventions.

Infrastructure and equipment

Infrastructure and equipment fall under the 'technical innovation' layer of the onion model. However, it is imperative to base the decisions regarding the infrastructure in the context of other layers such as 'cultural and institutional context', 'actors, network and alliance' and 'mental models and clinical perspective'. Irrespective of how advanced the technology is, it is ineffective if not adequately utilized.

Set-up costs include the costs of the infrastructure including audio-visual equipment, lease lines, phone bills, hiring of new personnel if needed, marketing and training costs. Infrastructure cost associated with the implementation of a telehealth program can be significant. Infrastructure should be adapted to the technological needs of the application, cost, comfort level of the users and availability of resources in the remote areas. If targeting rural populations, it is advisable not to invest in the computer-or Internet-based platform since the majority of the rural population is limited in their access and knowledge of computers. Simplicity of installation is preferred. Universal Access Fund provision of the 1996 Telecommunications Deregulation Bill provides funds to subsidize certain telecommunication services to rural, non-profit healthcare providers.[16] INTEGRIS telehealth system interfaces with OneNet, the Oklahoma

Table 8.2 Template for cost analysis of telehealth and face-to-face visits with estimated values

No.	Questions concerning variable costs	Estimated value
1	How often is the telehealth system a successful substitute for a face-to-face visit?	90%
2	What % of patients would drive to a specialist if TM was not available?	70%
3	How many miles will patients drive (round trip) to the telehealth facility?	16
4	What is the cost of transportation per mile?	$0.31
5	How many hours of a patient's time will a telehealth consultation take?	1.14
6	What value do the employers and patients place on their time?	$13.44
7	What is the average payment to physicians per telehealth consultation?	$65
8	What is the hourly cost of telehealth broadcasts?	$35
9	How many hours of technical support are needed for each hour of consultation?	1
10	What is the average number of consultations per hour?	4
11	What is the hourly cost of technical personnel who operate the system?	$30
12	What is the hourly cost of having a nurse at the spoke site?	$20
13	How many minutes of nurses' time will be used for each consult?	20
14	What is the cost of the spoke's supplies used for each consult?	$8
15	How much additional hub overhead is generated for each consult due to billing, etc.?	$2
16	How much spoke overhead is generated for each consult for record keeping, etc.?	$5
17	What is the average total fee paid to a physician's clinic for a face-to-face consultation?	$65
18	How many hours will a visit for a face-to-face consultation take?	7.63
19	How many miles (round trip) will patients drive to see a specialist?	304
	Questions concerning fixed costs	*Example*
20	What is the cost of equipment and improvements?	$144 128
21	What is the average life of the equipment and improvements?	8
22	What is the organization's cost of capital?	5%
	Therefore:	$21 238
23	What is the annual cost of the hub's administrator?	$27 000
24	How many fixed hours of technical support per week are needed to maintain the system?	16
25	How many square feet of hub office space are needed?	500
26	What is the value of the hub's office space per foot?	$11
27	How many square feet of office space are needed at the spoke?	350
28	What is the spoke's cost of office space per square foot?	$11
29	What is the annual cost of the spoke's administrator?	$4000
30	How many hours of administrative assistant time will be needed per week?	10
31	What is the hourly cost of administrative assistant time?	$11.70
32	How much will be spent on training and travel?	$2000
33	What is the amount of hub overhead for phones, system overhead etc.?	$5000
34	What is the amount of spoke overhead for phones, system overhead etc.?	$2500
35	What are the hub site's annual fixed telecommunications costs?	$5724
36	What are the spoke site's annual fixed telecommunications costs?	$4728
37	How many hours of line time will be needed for telehealth administration?	24
38	What % of the overhead will be allocated to consults?	50%
		Estimated cost
	Comparable face-to-face visit cost	$183.34
	Telehealth visit cost	$144.34
	Savings per TM visit	$39.01
	Total fixed costs	$113046
	Break even point (telehealth consults)	1449

Telecommunications backbone, which also links Oklahoma public schools and several hospitals. Connections have also been made to various educational and hospital networks in other states for conferencing and research training.

Bandwidth consideration is an important aspect of designing the infrastructure. When using videophones, there is a great disparity in the quality of video. This is important when looking at fine motor movements, as in speech therapy. There is also an individual tolerance level among therapists as to the level of clarity and smoothness of motion that will be acceptable. The therapists are therefore involved in equipment selection. Bandwidth is directly proportional to the data-carrying capacity and the cost. INTEGRIS Health Rural Telehealth project began with a focus on high-end technology. H.320 video conferencing systems with T1 lines were used. While the first pilot study was successful, it identified challenges associated with the use of this technology. Patients had to travel to the nearest site where this equipment was available, although this was still considerably less than the distance to a specialty rehabilitation outpatient site. This was a highly reliable technology utilizing a transfer rate of 384 kbps at 30 frames per second. The cost of equipment and the line lease were the major limiting factors. Travel by patients was not always feasible, so the focus shifted to exploration of technology options that could be utilized at home.

Low-technology equipment was experimented with in 2000, and rapidly gained favor from metro and rural healthcare providers because of increased convenience, ease of scheduling and increased application potentials. 'Plain Old Telephone System' (POTS) was used for the telerehabilitation connections. H.324 desktop videophones were utilized for these interventions. Desktop videophones are easy to install and require the user to just plug the videophone into any ordinary phone jack. Operation involves dialing a telephone to establish an audio connection and then pushing a button for video. The unit provides real-time video communication with adequate quality video and audio connection. The maximum transfer rate is 33.6 kbps with video streaming at 18–22 frames per second and costs $1600 to $2500 depending on the model and capabilities. Home-use equipment should be compatible with the phone systems in the area. A complete list of different camera equipment, including the recommended specifications, benefits, drawbacks and approximate cost for each, is available at http://telehealth.hrsa.gov.

Purchase and implementation of the system does not alone constitute the infrastructure. Factors such as network management responsibility, equipment insurance and room design should be taken into consideration. Room design, including lighting, sound and video placement, is important. Light should be on the patient, and not behind them. Half of the teletherapy sessions conducted by INTEGRIS have been in the residential settings. The camera should face away from the windows and ceiling lights. Background movements such as fans, and any fish tanks in the room, should be avoided as they result in excessive disconnects. Backgrounds and paints should be flat, and preferably monochromic.

Processes

Processes complement and frequently overlap the program structures. Processes for establishing a telehealth program should focus on protocols and service delivery, training, outcome measures, and regular evaluation and feedback.

Protocols

INTEGRIS TeleRehab program has developed protocols for referrals, screening, admission, evaluation, recertification, discharge, billing, coding, documentation and use of data for research purposes. This has been a constant learning process, which has been developed over time from experiences with the program. The protocols have followed refinement and written documentation of the workflow. A team of managers, therapists and other support staff meet bi-weekly to refine strategy and discuss cases, coding and billing issues.

Training

The majority of implementation and operational problems associated with telehealth can be traced to inadequate training. Training modules should be prepared for telehealth coordinators, clinicians and support staff. The primary focus of training is on therapist comfort and familiarization with the new technology, including operation, installation and troubleshooting of the equipment. New verbal skills, including unambiguous description and instruction, are necessary to compensate for the lack of hands-on demonstration or examination. Training also covers cognitive knowledge, physical examination skills, ability to communicate with the patients through audio-visual means and suitable documentation of a telehealth encounter. Education of target healthcare providers and consumers is accomplished via direct demonstrations, continuing medical education (CME) or continuing education unit (CEU) courses, and brochures. Training can be imparted through a combination of direct demonstration, instructional tapes or written materials. It is advisable to develop a formal training program over time that includes skills assessment and trainee evaluation.

Documentation and outcomes measures

Anecdotal evidence is not sufficient to scientifically establish the efficacy of a program. Collection and analysis of outcomes measures help in establishing the efficacy of the program and aid legislators in reimbursement issues. Outcomes measures also highlight any inherent deficiencies in the program and provide a framework for further program improvement and refinement. Outcomes measures collected for TeleRehab focus on clinical outcomes, subjective and objective quality of life, customer satisfaction and research opportunities. Cost analysis outcomes include revenue dollars, frequency of hospitalizations, number of consultations, travel costs saved and value added to the institution's mix of services. Technical outcomes include mean time between failures, connection and display problems, and rate of usage. INTEGRIS Health is also investing in developing a database for outcomes measures for telerehabilitation. A prototype is currently being developed in Microsoft Access that will be later upgraded to Structured Query Language (SQL) with a Java front end.

People

Effective management of people during a change process is often the key to a successful change initiative. People can be categorized as innovators, early adopters or late adopters. Innovators are the risk takers who can cope with a high degree of uncertainty during adoption of a new innovation and are highly suitable as champions for a new project. Early adopters are the target population for education and conversion during a change process. The late adopters wait for the change to be a proven concept before adopting it.[11] People involved in the TeleRehab program are the administrators, therapists/clinicians, information technology specialists, researchers, patients and their caregivers. These correspond to the 'actors' of the fourth layer of the onion model. Education and user involvement at all levels of the change process are critical. Individuals have difficulty sustaining new behaviors in an old environment, so the goal should be to change the environment as well. The environment should expect, encourage and support personal accountability, diversity, open expression, conflict as a source of creative tension and growth, participation at all levels, and caring and respect for all members of the organization.

Therapists

Therapist acceptance and utilization are the cornerstones of a successful telerehabilitation program. Experienced interdisciplinary teletherapists identified attributes important for a productive and meaningful teletherapy intervention or encounter. Attributes of successful teletherapists include flexibility, professional maturity, creativity, motivation, clinical competence, sense of humor, good interpersonal skills, person-first philosophy, intuition, tenacity, excellent problem solving, empathy and good communication skills. Unfamiliarity with technology and an inability to touch the patient for examination are potential sources of therapist dissatisfaction. Therapist resistance can be overcome by proper education and training. Proper orientation of the new teletherapist is paramount. A TeleRehab staff member is usually present during the first session to assist with any questions or problems with the equipment. Motivation in healthcare goes beyond monetary incentives. Quality of care and patient satisfaction reinforce clinician satisfaction. Technology is only a 'tool' to provide service; the people involved determine the success of the program.

Customers/consumers

Patients and their caregivers are an important and often overlooked component of a telerehabilitation program. Certain inclusion criteria have been identified for patients who participate in teletherapy. TeleRehab patients have generally participated in successful inpatient hospitalization or outpatient service. Patients should be medically stable, and a support person is generally required if the patient requires supervision for physical and/or cognitive impairments. The patient's support person is trained about the operation and basic troubleshooting of the audio-visual equipment being used. In addition, this support person must be able to comprehend audio-visual instructions, should be physically able to help with therapy and should be compassionate towards the patient. Whenever possible, the initial evaluation of the patient is done face to face in the presence of their caregiver, which facilitates the subsequent teletherapy sessions. Involvement of distant healthcare providers in the initial patient encounter via Tele-Rehab is beneficial.

Remote therapists

Development of collaborative efforts with the rural therapists is of significant importance. Despite generalization, each rural area has a unique culture and unspoken rules. Having a local person as a guide or mediator often facilitates gaining trust and overcoming resistance or hesitancy on the part of the users to try an alternative healthcare delivery model. Territorial issues sometimes arise when partnering with rural therapists. Rural therapists are generally independent due to lack of peer support. Cultivation of a symbiotic relationship requires patience and education on the part of teletherapists.

Dealing with resistance

Resistance to change is a common phenomenon that accompanies a change initiative. Resistance can be deliberate or subconscious, and it typically interferes with the successful implementation of a change initiative. Resistance can be encountered at all levels of the organization. The reasons for resistance can be economical, psychological, social, intellectual, prior unfavorable experiences, organizational or operational.[12] Resistance and other human factors constitute the 'mental models with clinical perspective' layer of the onion model. User involvement and education facilitates the change process. Honest and open communication is key to dealing with the user's concerns.

Results

As of October 2003, a total of 3397 TeleRehab sessions were conducted by INTEGRIS in a variety of settings.

Table 8.3 Patient interventions by discipline

Discipline	No. of consults	Hours
Audio/verbal therapy	82	77
Neuropsych	23	19
Occupational therapy	39	21
Physiatry	126	32
Physical therapy	473	397
Speech language pathology	2651	1619
Vocational rehabilitation	3	3
Total	3397	2165

User satisfaction

Satisfaction surveys are routinely given to providers, patients and caregivers. Patient satisfaction ratings have generally been positive. Nine out of ten negative comments were related to technology issues. Analog lines are affected by weather conditions, especially wind, which can be a considerable problem in Oklahoma. For the school-based speech teletherapy program, students were slightly less satisfied than the patients (Figure 8.4), which can be attributed to the fact that they were not given an option to choose between TeleRehab and face-to-face interventions. The relationship between the student and the therapist also influenced the satisfaction rating. The satisfaction of patients was also affected by increased accessibility and travel costs saving.

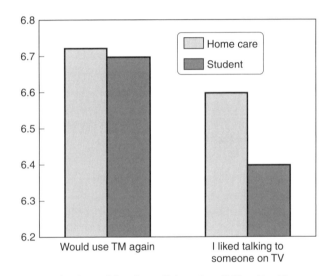

Figure 8.4 Patient satisfaction with telemedicine. 1 = dislike, 7 = like very much.

Among the therapists, speech therapists rated telerehabilitation lower than other allied health disciplines (Figure 8.5). These lower ratings have been traced to technology problems during the early phases of the school teletherapy program. The technology issues have subsequently been addressed resulting in higher speech therapy ratings. TeleRehab forces therapists to interact with patients verbally rather than through tactile means, which can be less satisfactory for some therapists during the initial period.

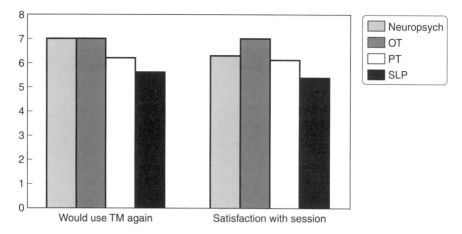

Figure 8.5 Provider satisfaction with telemedicine by discipline. 1 = unsatisfied 7 = very satisfied.

Constant user feedback and evaluation are important for reassessing, rethinking, redesigning or reengineering the program. The TeleRehab program implementation is a constant change process. Feedback and evaluation are crucial during the initial phases. The business plan and the workflow processes should be reassessed periodically based on the feedback.

Cost savings

Cost savings can be direct (reduced provider travel) or indirect (reduced length of stay or adverted emergency department admissions because of early intervention). If the program is considered a cost of doing business because of the value it adds to the institution, this should be documented. TeleRehab is a resource to other departments to help increase their revenue or decrease costs. Revenue is a combination of grant funds, reimbursements and educational programs. Value of telehealth should also be assessed in terms of the visibility and stability it provides to the organization. Savings during a six-month period included:

- Home care miles saved: 13 874   ($49 946 saved at 0.36/mile)
- Home care productivity saved: 231 hours   ($4158 saved at $18/h)
- Hospital readmissions reported as averted: ($10 000 saved: 2 at $5000/admit)
- Provider (not home health) miles saved: 36 912
                                                              ($13 288 saved at 0.36/mile)
- Provider productivity saved: 615.2 hours   ($14 760 saved at $24/h)

Total savings in travel, productivity and adverted non-pay hospital admissions: $92 152.

The cost savings to other departments were:

- Clinical services (home health/hospice/wound care/averted no-pay) $266 500
- Telecommunications (Network line lease reimbursement) $200 000
- Administrative travel $361 527
- Total $828 027

For patients, savings in terms of travel costs were $64 366 (178 794 miles at the rate of $0.36/mile). Average mileage to provider was 36 miles; 71% of the patients did not have their own transportation and 25% would not have received help without TeleRehab.

Conclusion

Adequate change management is a necessity in today's dynamic healthcare environment. Change efforts fail by trying to shortcut the steps in the organizational change process. Strategy, people, structure, and customers are the five critical components of change.

Strategy should always be finalized first as it lays the groundwork and outline for the rest of the change process. Lessons learned:

1   When implementing a new initiative, people frequently make the mistake of changing the structure first as it is the most visible of the change elements. However, without adequate groundwork, purely structural change is not successful or sustainable.
2   Having frequent milestones with short timelines keeps the people focused; however, the timelines should be realistic and practical. TeleRehab should be viewed as a support service with rehabilitation as the primary or actual service, and TeleRehab an extension of the traditional rehabilitation services.

Structure and *processes* are the building blocks of the long-term change process, and they frequently overlap. A sustainable change is a function of attention to the global picture, stakeholder buy-in, skills, managed risks and continued action. Lessons learned:

1   Program strategy, personnel, structure and processes should be revisited regularly, with changes made as needed.
2   While contracting for services, it is important to promise only what can be delivered. The program should preferably start with a targeted niche area, and then build on that success. Diversifying the services offered is an important component.
3   Continuous feedback and evaluation resulting in continuous process improvement is essential. The new change effort must be anchored in the culture and process of the organization, only then will it result in a long-term successful change implementation.

People are critical to the adoption of a change management process. The change management process is deeply inter-related to the other components or layers of the organizational design as outlined in the onion model. A new change initiative should always start with the need assessment for change. Lessons learned:

1   Identification and involvement of stakeholders are important at all points of the change process and during the maintenance phase.
2   Change advocates are the keystones of successful change initiatives and the majority of change failures can be traced to human factors such as lack of risk-taking ability or perseverance.

3 Education and user training are essential for the users to be comfortable with the change process.

The *customer* (consumer) is the core of traditional or innovative healthcare business. So it is only fitting to conclude our chapter with the customer component. Consumers are assuming a much more proactive role in the maintenance of their healthcare and have become equal stakeholders with healthcare professionals. Lesson learned:

1 It is the belief of these authors that the end-users of innovative telehealth programs such as TeleRehab are the individuals with chronic health problems and resulting disabilities. Decisions about their healthcare are made mutually, rather than by the more traditional medical model in which the physician dominated these interactions. This trend will continue to advance as consumers educate themselves further and assume more active roles, acting in collaboration with their healthcare providers to receive alternative services beyond the traditional medical model.

References

1 Forducey PG, Ruwe WD, Dawson SJ, Scheideman-Miller, C, McDonald NB and Hantla MR (2003) Using telerehabilitation to promote TBI recovery and transfer of knowledge. *NeuroRehabilitation.* **18**: 103–11.
2 Liss SJ, Glueckauf RL and Ecklund-Johnson EP (2002) Research on telehealth and chronic medical conditions: critical review, key issues, and future directions. *Rehabilitation Psychology.* **47**(1): 8–30.
3 Burns RB, Crislip D, Daviou P, Temkin A, Vesmarovich S, Anshutz J *et al.* (1998) Using telerehabilitation to support assistive technology. *Assistive Technology.* **10**(2): 126–33.
4 Glueckauf RL, Nickelson DW, Whitton JD and Loomis JS (2002) Telehealth and healthcare psychology: current developments in telecommunications, regulatory practices, and research. In: Boll T, Baum J, Frank R (eds) *Handbook of Clinical Health Psychology: models and perspectives in health psychology.* American Psychological Association, Washington, DC.
5 Kimberly JR and Evanisko MJ (1981) Organizaational innovation: the influence of individual, organizational, and contextual factors on hospital adoption of technological and administrative innovations. *Academy of Management Journal* 1981; **24**(4): 689–713.
6 Banner DK and Gagne TE (1995) *Designing Effective Organizations: traditional and transformational views.* Sage Publications, California.
7 Schlenker RE, Powell MC and Goodrich GK (2002) Rural urban home health care differences before the Balance Budget Act of 1997. *The Journal of Rural Health.* **18**(2): 359–72.
8 Carter R (2000) *Republicans' Outline: 2000 rural agenda.* Oklahoma City, Oklahoma.
9 Schopp L, Johnstone B and Merveille OC (2000) Multidimensional telecare strategies for rural residents with brain injury. *Journal of Telemedicine & Telecare.* **6**(S1): 146–9.
10 Rosen MJ (1999) Telerehabilitation. *Neurorehabilitation.* **12**(1): 11–26.
11 Rogers E (1995) *Diffusion of Innovations* (5e). Free Press, New York.
12 Worthley JA (2000) *Managing User Resistance. Managing Information in Healthcare: concepts and cases.* Health Administration Press, Chicago, pp. 165–203.
13 Darkins AW and Cary MA (2000) *The Business of Telehealth. Telemedicine and Telehealth: principles, policies, performance, and pitfalls.* Springer Publishing Company, New York, pp. 204–15.

14 Stensland J, Speedie SM, Ideker M, House J and Thompson T (1999) The relative cost of outpatient telemedicine services. *Telemedicine Journal.* **5**(3): 245–56.

15 Kane J, Marken J, Boulger J *et al.* (1995) Rural Minnesota family physicians' attitudes towards telemedicine. *Minnesota Medicine.* **78**: 19–22.

16 Brecht RM and Barrett JE (1998) Telemedicine in the United States. In: Viegas SF and Dunn K (eds) *Telemedicine: practicing in the information age.* Lippincott Raven, Philadelphia, PA, pp. 25–30.

Section 5

Actors, networks and alliance in e-health

Chapter 9

The Three Rivers Telehealth Network: creation of a distributed network

Deborah K Justis, Charles R Doarn and Ronald C Merrell

Introduction

Although the concepts of telemedicine and e-health have been around for many years, it has only been in the past several decades that it has become an option for rural health. Each year the capability increases and the costs continue to decline. In rural communities throughout the US, equipment and telecommunication links are increasingly affordable. However, along with the decreasing cost, the funding for new programs is also decreasing. State budgets have never been tighter, and Federal grant programs are more and more competitive, one reason why growth in rural areas has been slow. Nevertheless, grant funding and federal assistance that is available helps communities afford to initiate telemedicine programs (http://telehealth.hrsa.gov/grants/funds.htm). In addition, with changes in Medicare reimbursement structures, telemedicine is being reimbursed more today than perhaps only five years ago, making it worth the investment in time and effort to attempt to obtain funding.

Using the layers of an onion model, as described in the introduction to this book, when the Virginia Commonwealth University Health System (VCUHS) set out to establish a network, the culture of the community was assessed, the available technology was considered (including connectivity), leaders and champions were sought in the VCUHS as well as in Three Rivers Health District, and alliances were developed to create strong relationships to form the network. The network members learned about telemedicine and explored its uses in education, and as a useful significant adjunct to healthcare where distance is a challenge. As access issues continue to be a challenge, the role of a strong network becomes even more important to provide high-quality healthcare to this rural community.

Creation of the network

Sustaining telemedicine programs is another challenge altogether. Studying healthcare in rural communities is paramount in creating successful networking strategies for a telemedicine project to be sustainable. The role of the people in the network in a rural community is much more important than the connections created through telecommunications. The dynamics of the healthcare providers, patients and others within the community can be of benefit to the entity of the network, or tear it apart. Much like Seale *et al.* state in Chapter 11 of this book, Three Rivers Telehealth Network was created with emphasis on strategic partnerships, identifying local champions, working with a dedicated team, securing buy-in from management as well as local government representatives and obtaining community support. These efforts were necessary to raise chances for long-term success. The emphasis in creating this network has to be on the people and relationships rather than the technology. The strength of these relationships was tested when the grant proposal was not accepted, delaying funding for the initial phase. The alternate plan went into effect right away. The relationships and the increased access to healthcare offered through the creation of the network proved to be more important than receiving the initial funding.

Setting

In the Commonwealth of Virginia, the challenges of rural medicine are evident in the Three Rivers Health District in Eastern Virginia. This area consists of ten rural counties surrounded on three sides by rivers (Potomac River on the north, North Anna, Pamunkey and York River chain on the south) and the Chesapeake Bay on the east. The population is diverse within the ten counties. A few of the counties serve as retirement communities, one is considered a 'bedroom community' for the greater Richmond area. However, these counties have a lower income than the state average and all are medically underserved. The community of Three Rivers Health District has a saying about people who live in their community. If you reside in Three Rivers, you are a 'from here', if you have moved into the area you are a 'come here'. As is typical of many rural areas, it is much more difficult to find acceptance as a 'come here.'

When the VCUHS began to investigate the idea of creating a Telemedicine Network in Three Rivers, it knew that being a 'come here' was not going to help establish a successful, sustainable network. In order to gain acceptance, from the beginning the VCUHS, an academic, urban hospital, took on the role of coordinator but did not assume the exclusive role of provider. The VCUHS studied the health statistics and the number of health-related visits to the VCUHS clinics from Three Rivers. This study indicated that 16 000 visits were made in 2001 from the ten counties included in the Three Rivers Health District. Moreover, this region's health statistics were alarming. The death rate of the citizens in Three Rivers was much higher than in the Commonwealth of Virginia for cardiovascular disease (22% more deaths in 1996–2000), pulmonary disease (16% more deaths in 1996–2000) and many types of cancer (26% more deaths in 1996–2000).[1] These health disparities and the high number of clinic visits prompted the VCUHS and several healthcare providers in Three Rivers to begin to formulate a plan for implementing a telemedicine program to link providers and patients in a distributed telemedicine network in the area.

Plan

A distributed network was chosen as a more effective model than a hub-and-spoke model. In this model, members can connect to each other, providing education and/or consultations *to* and *from* any network site. In the hub-and-spoke model, all peripheral sites (spokes) connect to a central site (hub) to receive care/education. Three Rivers has several specialist groups and three hospitals serving the area. Since it is well documented that rural physician recruitment and retention is a problem,[2,3] it was made clear from the beginning that the VCUHS did not want to take patients from the rural physicians, but rather to enhance their ability to provide care and supplement specialty care where it was not locally available. Hicks *et al.* describe the importance of rural community pride to the rural population, as 'Members of the community often view their local hospital with civic pride and recognize that the hospital is a key factor in efforts to attract and retain physicians and other healthcare personnel and resources'.[4] Recognizing this, the VCUHS sought and received the support of the Three Rivers Health District Health Director during the early planning stages, and worked closely with hospital administrators, community physicians, patients and regional health departments determining the area healthcare needs and possible solutions. It was determined early that some healthcare needs (such as cardiology, where there are sufficient cardiologists in the area) could be met by local physicians and practitioners, and some needs would require the VCUHS staff support (such as neurology, where there are significant shortages in the area). The year after the network was initiated the community lost all inpatient obstetrical services. This crisis has made the network even more important. As leaders of the network, it becomes even more important and more valuable to obtain full funding to link all participants.

Another need identified through requests from the healthcare professionals was the lack of available continuing education opportunities. According to the State and Federal Bureau of Primary Care, Three Rivers consists of several physician shortage counties. Therefore, travel for required continuing medical education further reduces the number of available physicians at any one time, thus impacting healthcare responsiveness. In order to meet the needs of the physicians and other health providers in the area, the network could be used for providing education. The network members hope that the experience with receiving education via video-teleconferencing might increase the number of telemedicine referrals by the same groups of practitioners. The use of the network for education can also provide a potential source of revenue for the network, as well as a recruitment and retention tool for the area. Grigsby *et al.* point out, 'Expanded continuing education is often seen as a pre-requisite for attracting and retaining professional staff'.[5] This goal of retention and recruitment through enhanced educational opportunities fits well with the overall goals of the Rappahannock Area Health Education Center (RAHEC) (www.rahec.net/RAHEC%20Site.htm), the newest member of the network.

Network formation

When the original plan did not receive the expected funding, leadership of the network changed. By changing the organization of the network group to include the RAHEC as the organizing agency, the network becomes a 'from here'. RAHEC is a known support agency in the area. Their staff are from the community, and they have a history of working to improve the healthcare of the Three Rivers area.

Under the leadership of the RAHEC, and based on the assessed needs, Three Rivers Telehealth Network continues to have two purposes: to provide consultative specialty care via telemedicine to the residents of Three Rivers Health District; and to provide educational opportunities to the health practitioners in the area as well as community members. Two community hospitals, both under 100 beds, a community health center and public health clinic (combined), an Area Health Education Center (AHEC) along with an urban academic medical center have all joined together to form this network. During the year spent preparing to initiate the Three Rivers Telehealth Network, the VCUHS telemedicine coordinator met with several groups, including physicians, to listen to their specific needs for both inpatient and outpatient specialty consultations, such as dermatology, neurology, infectious disease, endocrinology and rheumatology.

Since most medical schools do not include telemedicine in their curriculum, many of the physicians in the rural community were not aware of the numerous opportunities offered through a telehealth network. The telemedicine coordinator was also able to share with the rural physicians the subspecialties available from VCUHS, which are especially amenable to care provided over telemedicine. New reimbursement opportunities were explained, which was well received by the physician groups.

Each rural healthcare facility has identified a medical champion and an administrative champion for telemedicine. As the time has passed, these champions have become even more important in sustaining enthusiasm for the project. Dr Puskin stresses the importance of the clinical champion, 'Minimally, there must be clinical leadership or these systems are doomed to failure, since it is practitioners who drive telemedicine use'.[6] Mascovice agrees, 'If the major purpose of the network activity is service integration, the rural physician group practice, rather than the hospital, may be the main coordinating element'.[7] An administrative champion is also needed to help with resource management at the rural sites during the operationalization phase of the project. These champions have a vested interest in the success of the network, as they have invested time and promised in-kind donations to ensure its long-term success. The administrative champion at one facility has found funding to replace worn-out equipment when the grant did not receive funding.

Keeping the goal of improving the health of the community in mind, the Three Rivers Telehealth Network was especially sensitive to the issues of keeping a safety net in place for the members of the Three River Community. In the rural community, where recruitment and retention is especially difficult, it is vital to comprehend the importance of forming a network, when pursuing a telemedicine project *without* forming a network would result in competition with local providers for patients, especially those who have insurance. If the network takes the paying patients from the local safety-net providers, but does not provide care for the uninsured, the safety net collapses. It follows that the network will not thrive in the area, as long as there is a choice of provider by the local insurer.[8]

It is just as vital to promote the perception of the local hospitals. According to Hicks, when a patient is transferred to a larger urban facility, especially if tests are repeated, the confidence in the rural hospital is decreased, which can result in the patient bypassing the local hospital and going straight to the urban medical center.[4] With telemedicine, the local hospital can provide a more advanced assessment, which increases confidence from the local patients, potentially avoiding loss of patient revenue to the academic medical center. For example, currently the hospitalist from the rural facility calls a VCUHS physician on the phone for consultations. With telemedicine the consult is billable, and the patient is actually seen by a VCUHS specialist. Patients and families can be reassured that even if the patient stays in the community hospital they are receiving the same care as if they had been transferred to the VCUHS. Hicks goes on to point out that network development is one way to redefine the rural hospital for survival in the managed care environment, by providing more services through telemedicine links.[4]

Understanding the motivation of a rural healthcare provider to join a network and identifying the benefits they are expecting are important steps in forming network relationships. Retention of network members will be easier if expectations are made clear from the beginning of the relationship. Moscovice *et al.* list three motivations for forming networks in rural areas.[7] A 'resource dependence model' assumes that during a time of financial uncertainty, it is beneficial to reduce dependence on one source outside the organization. Control of the environment, then, is one motivation to join a network. A second model assumes a reduction in transaction costs, or 'the costs of running the economic system'. The third model holds that the belief that networks improve access to and quality of healthcare is widespread, therefore communities expect healthcare providers to collaborate.

The Three Rivers Telehealth Network formed for many of the reasons stated in the literature. By enabling the physicians to link to sources of education and clinical care outside their immediate geographic area, they reduce dependence on an already short supply of physicians. By joining the network together in a distributed model, we utilize economies of scale, increasing the numbers of visits, decreasing the per unit cost of each visit. The network will also potentially increase income to physicians and facilities within the connected areas by increasing the number of patients seen who would not have been able to be transported but can be seen on telemedicine. The network formation will also increase expectations of healthcare providers to collaborate as individuals and physicians to see successful consultation outcomes. The standard of care becomes utilization of the network. Each of the members will contribute to and receive benefits from the network. Each member has clearly stated that the goal of the network is to see an improvement in the health of the population it serves.

Referring back to the model of the onion layers, the third layer, change management, was considered in the plans. Forming a successful rural health network also involves acceptance of change, a difficult concept for some rural communities. In order for this change to be accepted by the rural community members, they must 'feel ownership for the project'.[6] Mueller *et al.* list three main ingredients to mold change in a rural community: resources, leadership and community capacity.[8] When the Three Rivers Telehealth Network was created, the planning team took into account that resources to provide care via telemedicine would have to be provided, and applied for a Federal grant to purchase needed equipment, pay for consultations for the uninsured, help with telecommunications cost, and support salaries to create and sustain the infrastructure of the network. Now, without funding, the network is still successful. With funding the network will be even more useful, so RAHEC and others are seeking funding from several sources.

Local leadership is the second ingredient mentioned by Mueller. When requesting feedback from the community about the network idea, one county administrator was present; additionally, the Three Rivers Health District Health Director has been a key player in the planning of the network. The third ingredient is community capacity. Mueller suggests looking to Medicare and Medicaid for incentives to increase capacity. Since reimbursement is always a question when the idea is presented, the network members are well versed in Medicare and Medicaid policy regarding reimbursement for telemedicine from the rural areas. This will provide incentive for the involved urban and rural physicians alike. Capacity in the realm of available inpatient bed space has also been an issue. The VCUHS is frequently full and 'on diversion'. With the telemedicine network, and trusting relationships built between providers, the patients who would have been transferred can be cared for in the community hospital. This benefits the community by increasing local revenue, the payer by avoiding transportation and the family, who can remain close to the patient.

Results

Success of the Three Rivers Telehealth Network can be measured by the enthusiastic support for the network from the members and their parent organizations. Support was sought and received from each of the network sites in the area. One of the local hospitals has decided to purchase new equipment for the telemedicine project. Seeking the expertise of the network members has proven helpful to this hospital's information department. The testing of current equipment has begun, with donated time and effort from involved sites. Presentations to community members, including potential users in three counties, as well as local physicians were well received. Overcoming the barriers of working in a rural community has begun by gaining the acceptance of the physicians and patients, both potential users of the network.

Future

The Three Rivers Telehealth Network is just beginning to scratch the surface of the wealth of opportunities for improving the health of the Three Rivers population. For example, the network will be able to take advantage of economies of scale as it grows to include other providers in the area. Defining the relationships between the network members is an important first step in creating the network as its own entity. The options for defining relationships in a network vary from ownership to informal ties between care providers. Moscovice defines an integrated rural health network as 'a formal organizational arrangement among rural healthcare providers (and possibly insurers and social service providers) that uses the resources of more than one existing organization and specifies the objectives and methods by which various collaborative functions will be achieved.'[7]

In order to clarify the relationship between network members in the Three Rivers Telehealth Network, every member has signed a Memorandum of Understanding (MOU). This helps each member to solidify his or her commitment to seeing the network succeed. The healthcare providers in the area include two hospitals owned by a corporation, one privately owned hospital, several private physician offices and county health departments. The members have no interest in establishing relationships which involve vertical or horizontal integration, but will continue in this symbiotic relationship, 'supporting each other in the provision of their services and helping each other to achieve joint competitive advantage.'[7] The strategic advantage for each network member, enhanced by the telehealth links, include an increase in the referral base for each facility, revenue incentives including facility fees for providing consultation presentation, and enhanced recruitment and retention for healthcare providers through increased educational opportunities.

The organizational structure of this network does not fit into the description by Luke *et al.* of a quasi-firm. The survival of each member is not dependent on the survival of the network. The importance of the network to the strategic plans of each participant does not qualify this as a quasi-firm, as defined by Luke *et al.* The intended permanence of the network, however, is important. This network has a potential plan for growth and permanence. In the future the network may move from the network classification to a tighter coupling and higher degree of strategic importance to its members.[9]

As a network matures, the relationships between the members will change. The goal of the members is for the Three Rivers Telehealth Network to become its own entity. At a recent gathering, the group decided to form a charter. The members agree it will be necessary to support the infrastructure by contributing financially to sustain the network's infrastructure. Moscovice and Hicks remind us that the operation of a rural health network takes time and dedication to succeed. Human nature looks to each idea for 'what's in it for me?' Since members of a distributed network will financially benefit both directly and indirectly, the incentive to participate in care via telemedicine, and thus reap the financial rewards, is greater.

The goals of the Three Rivers Telehealth Network include continuous assessment. The initial plan was developed based on needs assessed from the potential network users. 'Ongoing assessment of rural practitioner needs by the specialty centers and their rural partners must be built into the management of telemedicine systems for them to be successful'.[6] There are more people who are already expressing a desire to be part of the network. As needs are assessed, the network members will continue to look for ways to incorporate others into the network. As Dr Puskin so aptly summarizes, 'Telemedicine is a tool to break down barriers to patient care and professional education. It is the highway of the 21st century by which we are moving information, not patients. Community needs and healthcare requirements – not technology – should drive telemedicine system development'.[6]

References

1 Virginia Department of Health, available at www.vdh.state.va.us/stats
2 Felix H, Shepherd J and Stewart MK (2003) Recruitment of rural health care providers: a regional recruiter strategy. *J Rural Health.* **19**(Suppl): 340–6.
3 Scammon DL, Williams SD and Li LB (1994) Understanding physicians' decisions to practice in rural areas as a basis for developing recruitment and retention strategies. *J Ambul Care.* **5**(2): 85–100.

4 Hicks L and Bopp K (1996) Integrated pathways for managing rural health services. *Health Care Manage Review.* **21**(1): 65–72.
5 Grigsby W (2002) Telehealth: an assessment of growth and distribution. *Journal of Rural Health.* **18**(2): 348–58.
6 Puskin D (1995) Opportunities and challenges to telemedicine in rural America. *Journal of Medical Systems.* **19**(1): 59–67.
7 Moscovice I, Wellever A and Christianson J (1997) Understanding integrated rural health networks. *Milbank Quarterly.* **75**(4): 563–86.
8 Mueller K, Coburn A, Cordes S *et al.* (1999) The changing landscape of health care financing and delivery: how are rural communities and providers responding? *Milbank Quarterly.* **77**(4): 485–510.
9 Luke R, Begun J and Pointer D (1999) Quasi firms: strategic interorganizational forms in the health care industry. *Academy of Management Review.* **14**(1): 9–19.

Chapter 10

A comparative study of the diffusion of computerized health records among general practitioners in Australia and Sweden

David Bomba

What are health, health informatics and e-health, and how do they all fit together?

Health is a complex social phenomenon. Health is not just about medicine or the practice of medical methods by doctors. Health is much broader than just medicine, inextricably related to political, economic, legal, environmental and social issues through time. Evidence of this argument is provided by the World Health Organization's (WHO) definition of health:

> . . . a state of complete physical, mental and social well-being, and not merely the absence of disease or infirmity, is a fundamental human right and that the attainment of the highest possible level of health is a most important world-wide social goal whose realisation requires action of many social and economic sectors in addition to the health sector.[1]

From the outset, this implies a broader approach to the study of health which goes beyond traditional disciplinary boundaries. Health is not the exclusive domain of medical practitioners. Thus, it is argued that health informatics, which is defined as ' . . . an umbrella term used to encompass the rapidly evolving discipline of using computers, networking and communications – methodology and techno-logy – to support health related fields . . .'[2] rather than medical informatics. Health informatics is more reflective of an approach that tries to embrace a multidisciplinary approach to the study of healthcare provision. This is not to deny the importance of medical clinicians; however, health needs to be viewed as a partnership made up of network alliances involving many actors. The following definition of primary healthcare has been adopted:

> primary care is the provision of integrated, accessible healthcare services by clinicians who are accountable for addressing a large majority of personal

healthcare needs, developing sustained partnership with patients, and practicing in the context of family and community.[3]

The term e-health has also emerged more recently as another umbrella descriptor which attempts to portray the convergence, collaboration and alliance building between numerous actors and disciplines; this book being an example of this idea. Telemedicine is seen to play a significant role in future e-health activities, despite its poor utilization to date.[4] The WHO, in its 1993 report, indicated the importance of telemedicine at a global level.[5] However, research into the utilization of computerized medical records (CMRs) among general practitioners (GPs) is seen as a critical area of study in an emerging e-health vision. The term 'GP' as used hereafter can be used interchangeably with the terms 'family practitioner/ physician' as is the practice of the World Organisation of Family Doctors.[6]

Dickinson indicates that in Australia, 80 to 85% of the population will visit their GP within any given year.[7] GPs can be considered as the main point of entry to primary healthcare in most health systems around the world and therefore GPs can be seen as the gatekeepers of health information, both locally and nationally.[8] This health information is presently an under-utilized information resource in Australia and is generally buried away in hand-written files stored in various isolated paper card file systems at disparate GP sites. General practice in Australia has been described as a black hole, 'so big and impenetrable is this black hole that those charged with the job of analyzing the nation's health needs at a grassroots level are practically working in the dark'.[9] The cost of healthcare in Australia (GP visits, prescriptions, pathology tests, radiology and specialist visits) was estimated at approximately $7.5 billion (Australian dollars) and the problem of trying to collect some structured information about these events is further exacerbated by the low levels of computer use by GPs.[9]

The use of CMRs in general practice could lead to new processes and ways of looking at healthcare. For example:

- epidemiological research
- analysis and tracking of disease trends by database queries and data mining
- prescription pattern monitoring
- calculation of patient and health treatment costs
- providing greater scope for teleconsultations and telemedicine.

The central argument is that CMR systems are seen as a fundamental building block for primary healthcare globally. In order for grander visions of global telemedicine, virtual hospitals and e-health to take place, CMR adoption and use among GPs is therefore seen as a key linking element and needs to be explored. This work explores the discrepancies in the utilization of CMRs; specifically, how can high and low rates of CMR adoption among GPs in different countries be explained? All too often in the medical informatics literature, there is a preponderance of technical or black box studies of CMRs, technics. This is not to say that technical approaches are not informative, but they need to be balanced with approaches that give CMRs a wider social and political context of understanding as to why some technologies may or may not be adopted. The process of technology design, i.e. why has a technology been designed in a particular way as opposed to another design, is inextricably linked to the alliances and actors involved in technology construction.

The meaning of health is to a large extent a reflection on the (de)constructions made by GPs through patient healthcare records over time, for example identification of novel types of diseases, classification of diseases, disease trends, etc. It can be argued that what happens at the micro level within GP practices is the basis for shaping macro-level national health policy developments, allocation of resources and identification of priority care needs. Macro-level health policy in turn shapes micro-level GP activities, for example availability of funds and grants for priority research areas. Information technology (IT) can be designed and used to aid this policy process, for it is the information and how it is captured and made available to others that is the central element in the technology design debate. Privacy concerns can be seen as a manifestation of technology design debates.[10–12]

Historically, the patient record has been the documentational building block for healthcare and medical practice as is often traditionally attributed to Hippocrates 5BC. The patient health record as such can be considered as a minimum documentational practice. This minimum standard is set by governments through legislation such as Health and Health Services Acts, thus making the record a legal document created by healthcare workers during the provision of healthcare to a patient. Traditionally, these have been centered on a paper-based paradigm of healthcare, despite patchwork revisions to legislations designed to be more reflective of contemporary technological changes. Computerization of the patient record is an attempt to move from a paper-based paradigm of healthcare provision to a computerized or electronic-based paradigm. This fundamental change is not without problems and consequences. Linnarsson indicates that the computerization of the patient record needs to be seen as much more than just the simple automation of a manual process.[13] The process of change has many legal, political, health, economic, organizational, technical and social implications and barriers. This is demonstrated in the work of Berg, who examined the rationalization of medical work practices.[14] This is a major change in the organization of how healthcare is practiced, divisions of labor, funding mechanisms and the way organizations operate; hospitals and GP practices being examples of such organizational structures. CMRs are representative of information systems that allow greater control over patient and practice information and respectively greater accountability and evaluation.[15]

What is a computerized health records (CMRs) system?

Various authors have looked at the potential role of computers in medical practice over the decades.[16–21] The actual meaning of CMRs is, however, reflective of a social and political process through time, (de)constructed by actors who have an interest or stakehold in CMRs. Hence, conceptually, the patient record should be considered as a socially constructed technology which exists within a larger system of health technologies, networks and actors. For this reason various individuals and organizations have attempted to define and shape the debate over CMRs. A key organizational actor has been the Institute of Medicine (IOM) in the US.[22,23] The IOM defines the computer-based patient record in the following way:

> *an electronic patient record that resides in a system specifically designed to*
> *support users by providing accessibility to complete and accurate data, alerts,*
> *reminders, clinical decision support systems, links to medical knowledge, and*
> *other aids.*[22]

This definition is a rather ambitious, broadly ranging ideal. It does not necessarily exist in practice, despite systems which may try to approximate this ideal. There is also a tendency to focus on clinical systems rather than on a more holistic organizational or practice management system which also includes non-clinical components such as accounting and budget management. This will come under the spotlight more so in coming years, especially in healthcare systems where GPs operate, or may be encouraged to operate, as private business entities rather than government-funded employees.

The significance of information and telecommunications systems within healthcare cannot be denied. In the US, Schneider *et al.* argue that telemedicine could save billions of dollars by using the telecommunications system to exchange health information between providers.[24] In Australia, the telemedicine vision can be characterized by a growing number of pilot and experimental projects.[25–28] Pradhan provides a useful account of the area and some of the issues.[29]

Theoretical background for understanding actors, networks and alliances in e-health

Market competition can be interpreted as organizational politics and the battle over the control of economic modes of production and information markets, with the health sector being one such market.[30,31] Hence, CMRs can also be explained as a development within a more competitive market framework; information as a commodity which gives competitive economic advantage and reduces uncertainty.[32–38] Therefore, (information) technology studies are reflective of theories for understanding the organization and control of market and social structure.[39–43] E-health is therefore an extension of competitive thinking in healthcare.

Rigby indicates:

> *Healthcare organizational structures are frequently seen as a hierarchy of*
> *networks and alliances. The individual healthcare organization has a network*
> *relationship to other healthcare organizations. Additionally, there will be*
> *alliances with related organizations. Internally, the health organization can be*
> *viewed as a network of departments or clinicians liaising directly with one*
> *another . . .*[44]

E-health organizations in the future may be defined more by their telecommunications networks rather than just their physical presence. The idea of 'frames of meaning' is essentially derived from Collins and Pinch[45] and Bijker *et al.*,[40] who use the term 'technological frame' to represent ' . . . the *interaction* of various actors . . .'. Hence, as used here, this frame is representative of the negotiation space or (de)construction space, of meaning between actors and actor networks in different discipline frames. This builds on the idea of actor networks within different meaning frames.[40,46] For example, GPs are essentially actors in organizational, professional and social networks, formal and informal, e.g. the general practice setting; or professional bodies like the Australian Medical Association (AMA), the Royal Australian College of General Practitioners (RACGP), the Australian College of Health Informatics (ACHI) and the Health Informatics Society of Australia (HISA). All attempt to shape the meaning and artefactual form of patient records with other actors both within meaning frames and between actors within other professional networks, e.g. government administrators, policy planners, strategists, third-party insurers, patients, nurses, pathologists, pharmacists, radiologists, CMR vendors, software standards bodies and others. Conflict is therefore inherent in this negotiation of meanings and artefact translation process. This creative disruption is perceived as benefiting some professional groups of actors more than others, and as a possible destabilization of the status quo. Some perceive a possible gain in power over other actors while some perceive a loss in power, restructuring, hence the utility of a socio-political paradigm of understanding CMR diffusion and non-diffusion. Technical black box design, translation and diffusion are socio-political processes among various actors and need to be understood as such.

CMRs need to be viewed as an organizational construct. At a theoretical level, the question then arises as to whether actors can also be inanimate objects such as software programs like computerized health records systems. CMRs should be considered as actors as they embody inherent political and social ideals about how GPs should organize their health/medical thinking and work behavior, directly and indirectly by way of the design. A software standard (e.g. HL7) may be embodied by a CMR program and therefore reflects a set of particular values as espoused by other actors in professional networks (for example standards organizations such as the European Standards Organisation (CEN), ANSI, IEEE, ISO, ITU). Along similar lines, decisions about the type of organizational schema to be used to structure a patient record, for example Weed's problem-oriented record[47] and the medical nomenclature to be used for diagnosis (e.g. SNOMED, ICD-10, Read). These all reflect attempts to structure not only the GP–patient consultation but also promote a particular way of thinking. Hence, the technology is symbolic of the embodiment of these ideals and not just a neutral tool to be used; CMRs are actors themselves since they influence work behavior in a particular direction. It must be acknowledged that CMRs may be put to uses never envisioned by actors at the design stage, and this should be seen as the creativity or novelty process of reinvention and change over time. Thus, the deconstruction of what CMRs mean also occurs in order to reflect changes in thinking about healthcare systems and to reposition the value of CMRs accordingly in a global e-health environment. It may well be argued that CMRs are both a threat and an opportunity for GPs to either increase or decrease their personal and professional self-interest both individually and as a profession. This will be a reflection on how GPs, individually or collectively, shape the debate over CMRs. The outcome of this is still hard to predict as some actors are more vigilant and powerful than others in looking after their own self-interest. More interesting is the interaction that takes place among actors, especially when those actors cross disciplinary and market boundaries as a result of converging interests and motivations. From an actor network point of view the crossing of market boundaries represents a communication interaction and information exchange between actors from different networks, and a gradual convergence or closer integration of various actor networks in a global e-health system.

The classic work of Luke *et al.* provides a useful framework of thinking about quasi firms and how a wide variety of loosely coupled inter-organizational arrangements can be designed to achieve strategic objectives in healthcare.[48] The authors attempted to classify quasi-firms, how they can be created and mechanisms for strategic decision making. Table 10.1 below extends the research agenda offered by Luke *et al.* and provides a perspective on how network alliances may further develop and the types of impacts they may have.

Table 10.1 Quasi-firms' strategic decision making

Organisation identity	Information enablement	Effects
Internal departmental unit	Expert knowledge bases; telecommunications	Departments work to external standards; can 'trade' widely
Local alliances	Local area networks, etc.	'Virtual' organization, but no overall control
Global and national trading	Telemedicine and Internet	Bigger business, but unresolved control and accountability issues

Source: Rigby, 1999.[44]

The International Medical Informatics Association (IMIA) can be seen as an international alliance of actors pursuing various health informatics agendas. IMIA was initially established in 1978 as a special interest group of The International Federation for Information Processing, until 1989, when it gained status in its own right. It has many national and corresponding institutional members and links to the WHO. Figure 10.1 is a simple overview of the linkages between various organizational actors and their relationship to each other.

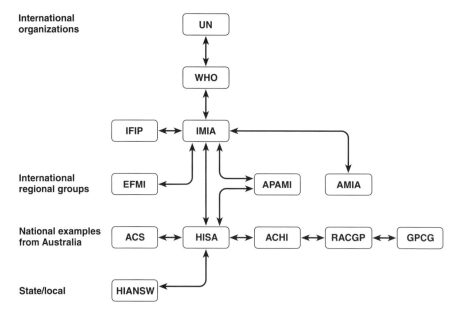

Figure 10.1 Overview of some organizational actors and alliances constructed to promote health/medical informatics utilization.

New networks (or the realignment of existing networks) and organizational alliances are forming all the time in e-health as governments and patients have greater expectations over how computer technology and telecommunications can be utilized, for example, use of the World Wide Web. Consumer health informatics is reflective of this thinking.[49–52]

CMRs in a diffusion context

Through the work of Rogers we can begin to think about *what* happens, the rate of diffusion (as depicted by the S-shaped curve) and *why* the rate of diffusion may vary in different settings, but not always *how* the process of diffusion actually happens.[53] Rogers provides a useful framework of analysis such as the perceived attributes of innovations (relative advantage, compatibility, complexity, observability and trialability); type of innovation decision (optional, collective, authority); communication channels (e.g. mass media or interpersonal); nature of the social system (e.g. its norms, degree of network interconnectedness, etc.); and the extent of change agents' promotion efforts.[53]

It would be somewhat optimistic, given current knowledge about information systems failure,[54] to think that there exists a general unifying pattern of diffusion which serves to explain *what* happens, *how* it happens and *why* for all cases. There will be varying rates of diffusion between individuals, within organizations and national systems. For example, in studies of military e-health systems, well-designed formal bureaucratic structures were not sufficient to ensure acceptable utilization rates of e-health technologies; research yielded that organizational and cultural dimensions related to uncertainty avoidance and may explain some variance in utilization rates.[4] Therefore, cross-national studies are useful for helping to identify the reasons for utilization variance. Straub also looked at the effect culture has on diffusion by examining the diffusion of email and fax in Japan and the US.[55] Furthermore, Geffen and Straub looked at gender differences in the utilization of email using a cross-sectional survey instrument.[56] They argued that gender needs to be added to an IT diffusion model, since gender differences may be related to beliefs and use of computer-based media. The findings indicated that men and women differ in their perceptions but not in their use of e-mail.

This work adds to the Technology Acceptance Model (TAM) proposed by Davis (1989),[106] which is essentially a causal model trying to correlate system use with perceived ease of use and perceived usefulness. The origins of this model can further be traced back to the Theory of Reasoned Action by Ajzen and Fishbein.[57] Another approach is offered by Heikkilä who argues that '. . . the willingness to adopt is more dependent on the adopter-technology fit, and the sustained use is more dependent on the task-technology fit', possibly with peers serving as a moderating reference group.[58] This also points to learning processes as being vital to sustained utilization as advocated by several authors.[59,60] Kidd *et al.* also argue that the learning process is incremental and full utilization of CMRs takes time.[61] Rogers argues that information exposure is the most important explanation for diffusion.[53] Valente takes this one step further and argues that exposure (contagion) is not enough, but rather that the focus needs to be on the frequency of exposure.[62] The more a person is exposed to an idea or technology the greater likelihood there is that utilization at some level may take place. But this is not to deny that it may also serve to reinforce an individual's decision to reject the idea.

Past studies of electronic data interchange (EDI) are also informative; Emmelhainz argued that organizations with low utilization and knowledge of EDI tended to postpone EDI adoption until there was only one type of standard in the industry.[63] This may also be the case with CMRs and needs to be investigated further. A Swedish survey conducted in 1994 identified 27 different suppliers of CMRs, of which only a few were deemed able to meet reasonable user require-ments.[64,65] Finally, in a market environment, competition between GPs may lead to greater utilization rates of CMRs as those GPs who adopt and learn to use CMRs strategically may squeeze non-users out of the market place. This interpretation is more reflective of a competitive advantage way of thinking.[32,33,66,67]

GP computer utilization

A great number of discussion papers, reports and studies have been published since 1991 in Australia. The main impetus for this sudden movement would appear to be a series of overseas events, primarily the work of the IOM and its landmark study into the computer-based patient record. The only publication work of any significance in this context before this time in Australia were the RACGP study (1985) and the CAPP (1986–90) project.[68,69] These spawned the work of O'Toole, Crampton and Lord, and the Crampton RACGP Survey.[70–72] It must be noted that, despite chronological appearances, some of the work may have been stimulated by events in the US prior to publication of the IOM's report in 1991. This also needs to be seen in the broader context of initiatives which took place in the UK and Europe, such as the work of the International Federation of Information Processing (IFIP) and IMIA and, prior to the work of the IOM, the work of Greisser *et al.* on data protection in health information systems.[73] Another significant initiative was the UK government's 'Micros for GPs' scheme, estab-lished in 1972, which, after a long gestation period, received an injection from the government of £24 million in 1989, to allow GPs to purchase computers and software.[70,74] Tied into this initiative was the government-supported develop-ment of Read Codes,[75] to try and structure the clinical input of medical terms used by GPs in their computer systems to allow analysis of clinical data, (un)aggre-gated, so as to help in health service planning, epidemiological research and auditing.

The RACGP (1985) study revealed that 54% of the RACGP respondents viewed computers as having some potential to improve practice management but not clinical records.[68] Only 19% agreed that computerizing patient records would improve the quality of patient care and only 14% supported the sharing of information among other healthcare actors. Also of interest was that only 20% of RACGP respondents agreed that patients had a right to see their entire record.

O'Toole provides an initial attempt to document the field of medical record computing in Australia from a GP's point of view.[70] O'Toole argues that the generalist practitioner of the 1980s faces a situation of growing information overload relative to practitioners in previous periods. This tension is characterized as the generalist-specialist dichotomy with ever-increasing levels of specialization and the fragmentation of knowledge. One attempt to try and deal with this information-processing dilemma is through the use of computer technology. O'Toole optimistically argues that the computer is the answer to these problems.

The Computer Assisted Practice Project (CAPP) represents one of the largest attempts to explore computer implementation and use issues in general practice Australia.[69] It is from this study that a number of spin-offs continue to have relevance even to the present day, e.g. computerized prescribing, computer age/sex/disease registers, computerized drug databases, attitude surveys, coding and standards issues. Conducted over a five-year period (1986–90) the CAPP study primarily consisted of a number of subprojects. In essence, 22 general practices across Australia were evaluated for their use of a practice computer system (*Medrecord*), and their opinions and experiences were analyzed using both qualitative and quantitative methods. The project showed that computerized accounting and medical records achieved a high level of acceptance among doctors, staff and patients. This was followed up by a report in 1994 by the RACGP which extended the project timeline (1986–93) and focused somewhat more on the usage and problems surrounding computer records. The main problems identified centered around data entry, accidental data loss and presentation.

Also of significance was the national survey of computer use among RACGP members by Crampton.[71] The basic finding was that 41% of GPs used a computer in their general practices for such activities as accounts, billing and word processing, but only 2% used computers for clinical purposes. Younger GPs and those in group practices were more likely to use computers. Also, cost had a bearing on the attitudes of GPs towards the use of computers.

Other relevant surveys that have looked at various aspects of computerization in general practice in Australia include the work of Douglas and Saltman, Liaw, Fry, Cacek, and Bolton and Gay.[76–80] In the Douglas and Saltman study of 1900 GPs, respondents indicated they used computers mainly for front-desk-type applications such as accounts (34%) or word processing (33%), while only 5% used the computer for recording clinical information.[76] Furthermore, many GPs were found to be using traditional, paper based 8″ × 5″ cards and less than half were using any accredited medical records system at all.

Based on previous studies, it has generally been claimed that the adoption rate of CMRs by GPs in Australia has been low, ranging from 2% to around 8%, with computerization levels around 40%.[68,71,80] This is in contrast to the UK, where 50% of primary practitioners use the computer for clinical notes and 90% of primary care practitioners work in computerized practices.[81] As a further comparison, in Singapore, the adoption rate is said to be somewhere between 30 and 50%[82] and less than 30% in Hong Kong.[83]

A brief background to the Australian and Swedish health systems

It must never be forgotten that the critical longer-term questions facing e-health researchers are not just how technologies can be designed to help patients, but whether the use of technology leads to actual improved patient health outcomes and how this is measured?

Generally, governments are involved in the management of healthcare resources, costs, outcomes and equity issues. Nevertheless, these may all be interpreted differently, for example equity may be seen as the redistribution of healthcare costs as opposed to accessibility to healthcare services. Health systems and health policy are often reflective of a complex historical and political mix of changes to the organization of funding arrangements and responsibilities between various levels of government (e.g. national, state and local), for example the Australian healthcare system. The Australian healthcare system can be described as reflective of a philosophical position located somewhere between the UK National Health Service (NHS) and the US health system, with a gradual movement away from government funding and public health insurance to a more privatized system based on individual private health insurance.[84,85]

It would appear that the UK, the Swedish and the Australian health systems share some common features but also have some distinct variations. It becomes evident that the more health systems devolve from a centralized system to a more decentralized regional/local system, the more variation and experimentation in budget devolution and patient needs-assessment planning is evident across counties in Sweden, the UK or across states and GP divisions in Australia.

The healthcare system in the UK is based on a system of care provided by GPs who can be seen as private contractors paid by the NHS, just as GPs in Australia are paid by the Australian health insurance system (Medicare). Experimentation with the idea of purchasers and providers is evident in both the UK and Swedish healthcare systems, where local councils purchase healthcare services from their regional and national organizing bodies in order to tailor provisions to the specific healthcare needs of their respective communities. GPs are essentially given a budget to work with in order to try and buy the health services required for their patients. This can be problematic since patient needs will vary, for example between rural and urban areas. However, problems of definition and classification over what constitutes rural areas serves to add more complexity to the problem, especially since government funding formulas are tied into such definitions.[86] Case-mix and DRGs can be seen as a manifestation of this attempted tailoring process at the hospital level.

The Swedish healthcare system, makes use of a patient registration list system by which a list of patients (about 2000 per GP, but variations do occur) is assigned to each district GP. The Swedish system has experimented (1994/95) with the house doctor system (a patient can choose which GP they wished to belong to) but with only mixed success, in that some GPs had excessive lists while others had diminishing list numbers. Some counties have adopted the system (e.g. Uppsala) while others have reverted back to the old district doctor list system.

The UK and Swedish systems can be characterized as systems in a state of continuing flux;[87,88] similarly the Australian system is one facing mounting economic pressure to change. The cost of the publicly funded Medicare system in Australia is rapidly escalating to well over $7.5 billion.[9] This can be seen as a problem arising from an over-supply of GPs leading to over-servicing and outright rorting of the system by some GPs. As indicated, this problem is escalating as more medical doctors are pumped out of educational institutions every year leading to a mismatch between supply and demand. This over-supply of GPs places more of an economic burden on the national Medicare health bill that taxpayers eventually have to help fund (through a levy on taxable income), since more medical doctors equates to greater consumption of various medical services. Hence, both GP over-servicing behavior and supply need to be constantly monitored.[89] This would suggest some form of direct regulatory strategy from the government. There is predominantly an imbalance between rural and city areas in that there is an over-supply of GPs in large city areas and an under-supply in smaller rural regions.[90]

Historically, rural areas in Australia have been disadvantaged in terms of access to health services.[91,92] This stems in part from the fact that political, legislative and economic power in Australia is generally located in the national and state capitals rather than at the local government level. Thus, health budget devolution to local government can be viewed as an attempt to try and redress part of this power imbalance. Financial responsibility is shifted to local government, but this does not necessarily address the need for more revenue to fund increasing demand for healthcare services.

Good health and equal access to health services for everyone are the goals of both the Australian and Swedish healthcare systems as articulated through national policy and a range of legislations including the National Health Act, the Health Insurance Act and the Medicare Levy Act in Australia, and the Health and Medical Services Act in Sweden. A fundamental principle of both systems is public sector responsibility to provide and finance health services for the entire population. In Sweden, health is organized in a decentralized way through bodies called Landstinget, which are situated in each of the 25 counties. The respons-ibility and operational management for healthcare services rests primarily with the local county councils who have the power to levy taxes to raise the finances required to run these services. This is a reflection of the Swedish welfare state ideology and also a reason for the generally high tax regime used to fund social services. The Australian healthcare system is administered by the federal govern-ment in conjunction with the respective state governments and area health services (who are responsible for public hospitals) through funding grants and the Medicare Levy. The history of Australian welfare programs has been one of targeted welfare rather than universal social programs as in Sweden. Hence, GPs in Sweden operate mainly under a public umbrella healthcare system funded by the county councils while GPs in Australia mainly operate as private businesses within a public system. They thus receive minimal direct financial assistance with CMRs, however the Practice Incentives Program is an attempt to readdress this issue.

Questionnaire design

Field visits and interviews were conducted with GPs both in Australia and Sweden in order to help with the identification of the issues to be investigated. The questionnaire itself went through several drafts and pilot testing for face validity before distribution. Responses were sought for questions relating to demographic data, educational background and training, computer use/non-use, adoption barriers, computer security awareness, software/hardware plat-forms as well as present and possible future trends in the use of CMRs. The questionnaire comprised of a common section for all respondents and then two nested sections, one for GPs who were CMR users and another for those who were non-computerized. Both open-ended and closed questions were included where appropriate. The design of the questionnaire included a coding schema for easier transcription into a spreadsheet and imported subsequently into SPSS for data analysis. All mail-out questionnaires were accompanied by covering letters and prepaid return address envelopes. The questionnaire was developed in English and Swedish.

Sample selection

Sample selection can take various forms, random, non-random or some quasi combination of the two. A random sample of GPs was chosen as being an appropriate approach based on the experience of other researchers in the area.[21,71,79,80]

The Swedish GP sample and mailing list was made available courtesy of the Department of Family Medicine, Uppsala University. The survey was sent to a random computer-generated sample of GPs in Sweden ($n = 600$). The first and only mailing was conducted in November 1994 for return before mid-December. A 50% ($n = 298$) response rate was gained and there were no follow-up or reminder notices to increase the response rate.

The Australian mailing list was made available courtesy of the Commonwealth Department of Human Services and Health. A random computer-generated sample was provided and the state of New South Wales was also randomly chosen for sampling ($n = 600$). The first and only mailing was carried out in November 1995 for return before mid-December. A 49% ($n = 293$) response rate was gained and there were no follow-up or reminder notices to increase this rate. The respective samples were deemed to be representative of their respective GP populations based on national data.

Survey findings

The main findings of the survey indicate that there has been a high rate (72%) of diffusion of computers and CMRs among GPs in Sweden and a low rate (14%) of diffusion among GPs in Australia. Moreover, use of computers by Australian GPs is still predominantly confined to front-desk-type applications (e.g. accounts/ billing, word processing) as opposed to clinical CMR use (e.g. patient notes, script writing, recall and referral, test ordering). On further analysis, only 16% of the Australian computer user respondents (14% overall) indicated that their main computer use was for patient records, as opposed to 93% of the 72% of Swedish respondents. This means that of the 14% of Australian respondents who do use computers, only 2% use them specifically for clinical purposes while the other 12% make some use of CMRs but do not consider it to be their main use. This supports the more general findings of the survey work conducted by Cacek, who found that of the 35% of Australian GPs using a computer, 78% were using computers for word processing and 63% for financial management.[79]

Findings further indicate that the high rate of diffusion in Sweden has mainly been achieved by direct financial funding schemes from the Swedish government and county councils. Furthermore, 80% of the Swedish respondents indicated a strong belief that CMRs will be an essential technology for healthcare in the future, as compared to only 55% of Australian respondents.

Among GPs who are CMR users, results from both samples support the claim that CMRs are helping to improve the way GPs work (Australia 82% and Sweden 69%), but the consensus is less than overwhelming. Both samples indicated improvements in the following areas: having increased quality control over patient information (as opposed to hand-written notes); faster access to patient records; and easier access to patient information when dealing with telephone enquiries. These can be considered as relative advantage attributes of CMRs,[53] or even long-term economic advantages, due to savings in time, effort and organization (whether of information or staff). Overall, 92% of Australian respondents still process patient records manually, while 95% of the Swedish respondents process records electronically using a computer. Only one respondent in Sweden indicated keeping hand-written patient records. Table 10.2 provides a comparative view of beliefs and adoption rates.

Table 10.2 Beliefs and CMR adoption rates

	Australia (NSW) (n = 293)			Sweden (n = 298)		
	Total	Males	Females	Total	Males	Females
GPs who believe CMRs are an essential technology for healthcare in the future	55% (n = 158)	73% (n = 115)	27% (n = 43)	80% (n = 236)	61% (n = 144)	39% (n = 92)
Total responses	286			294		
Missing	7			4		
GPs who use CMRs	14% (n = 42)	90.5% (n = 38)	9.5% (n = 43)	72% (n = 215)	57% (n = 123)	43% (n = 42)
Total responses	292			298		
Missing	1			0		
GP CMR users who believe CMRs have improved work practices	82% (n = 36)	94% (n = 34)	6% (n = 2)	69% (n = 140)	59% (n = 83)	41% (n = 57)
Total responses	44			204		
Missing	249			94		

Statistical testing indicated significance at the 0.05 level for cross-tabulation of GPs who use CMRs and gender in the Australian sample, as can be seen in Table 10.3. This is the only response that supports the hypothesis that a relation exists between gender and CMR use. Nevertheless, no such relation was found in the Swedish sample. Furthermore, no other correlations between belief about CMRs and gender were found to be significant in either sample.

Table 10.3 Tests of significance for GP CMR use and gender

	Value	Degrees of freedom	Asymptotic significance test (2-sided)	Exact significance test (2-sided)	Exact significance test (1-sided)
Pearson	8.366[b]	1	0.004		
Chi-square continuity correction	7.327	1	0.007		
Likelihood ratio	9.974	1	0.002		
Fisher's exact test				0.003	0.002
Linear-by-linear association	8.337	1	0.004		
No. of valid cases	292				

[a] Computed only for a 2 × 2 table.
[b] 0 cells (0.0%) have expected count less than 5. The minimum expected count is 11.79.

There are also similarities between the make-up of GPs in both the Swedish and Australian samples, especially in relation to employment status; 77% of respondents in both samples regard themselves as being employed full time and 23% of respondents regard themselves as being employed part time. The male to female ratio in Australia was 72:28, while the Swedish ratio was 60:40. Hence, GPs tend to be male, employed full time and are aged in their mid-forties (Australia: mean = 45 years, standard deviation = 5.6 years; Sweden: mean = 46 years, standard deviation = 10.5 years). In Sweden, GPs tend to cluster to form group practices more than in Australia (Sweden, mean = 5, s.d. = 2; Australia, mean = 3, s.d. = 2), where GPs predominantly operate more in solo or partnership practice. In fact, 50% of the respondents in Australia operated in practices with three or fewer members. The most obvious difference between the two samples is in the types of practice. In Sweden, 92% of GP respondents are predominantly in public practice, while 95% of GP respondents in Australia are in private practice. Furthermore, the numbers of staff employed per practice was significantly higher in Sweden (mean = 18, s.d. = 13) than in Australia (mean = 5, s.d. = 5), which is reflective of the larger public service and pro-government employment policies in Sweden versus cost-controlled and profit-oriented operations in Australia.

The claim that in both Australia and Sweden the trend is towards the clustering of GPs with other allied practitioners (for example, dentists) in one center or practice[93,94] is also supported by the survey. In Sweden, this is seen to aid cooperation and the sharing of medical resources among primary care practitioners, while in Australia this move is not merely for cooperation but more importantly to create super clinics which achieve greater economies of scale, throughput and returns. Australian respondents also indicated seeing a lot more patients per week (mean = 132, s.d. = 73) than GPs in Sweden (mean = 63, s.d. = 19).

The non-computerized samples offer some distinct differences in GP attitudes. In the Australian sample, of the overall non-computerized respondents (86%), 63% believe CMRs will improve the way GPs work but 67% do not plan to implement CMRs within the next three years. Follow-up questions indicated that 65% did not feel that they had a problem managing patient health records, which may, if answered truthfully, account for why non-computerized GPs felt that they did not need to computerize. A significant number of the Australian GPs are obviously not convinced of the benefits of CMRs over paper records, and 77% indicated that they have taken no planning steps towards implementing CMRs whatsoever. Respondents indicated that they were concerned over lack of software standards and data portability between software systems. There was also some concern over the problem of converting from paper to computer and the time, cost and effort involved in such an endeavor, especially if there was no support involved.

In contrast, 68% of the Swedish non-computerized respondents indicated they were having problems managing patient records and that CMRs were perceived as helping to resolve these problems. Within the Swedish non-computerized sample (28%), 72% believe that CMRs will improve the way GPs work and 90% plan to introduce CMRs within the next three years. Table 10.4 provides a comparative view of non-computerized attitudes of GPs towards CMRs.

Table 10.4 Attitudes of GPs (non-computerized) towards CMRs

	Australia (NSW) (n = 293)			Sweden (n = 298)		
	Total	*Males*	*Females*	*Total*	*Males*	*Females*
Non-computerized respondents	86% (n = 250)	69% (n = 172)	31% (n = 78)	28% (n = 83)	68% (n = 56)	32% (n = 27)
Total responses	292			298		
Missing	1			0		
Non-computerized respondents who have problems managing patient records	35% (n = 93)	73% (n = 68)	27% (n = 25)	68% (n = 56)	68% (n = 38)	32% (n = 18)
Total responses	268			82		
Missing	25			216		
Non-computerized respondents who believe CMRs will improve the way GPs work	63% (n = 164)	73% (n = 119)	27% (n = 45)	72% (n = 55)	71% (n = 39)	29% (n = 16)
Total responses	259			76		
Missing	34			222		
Non-computerized respondents who plan to implement CMRs within the next 3 years	33% (n = 82)	72% (n = 59)	28% (n = 23)	90% (n = 71)	66% (n = 47)	34% (n = 24)
Total responses	246			79		
Missing	47			219		

In both samples, there were some respondents who indicated that they kept no back-up records or had no disaster recovery plan for patient records. In the case of keeping back-ups, Australian respondents (81%) were found to be guiltier of this than Swedish GPs (19%). This is attributable to the fact that Australian GPs are predominantly non-CMR users and do not keep paper-based back-up records. Nevertheless, both samples overwhelmingly consider themselves as responsible for the accuracy of patient information contained in patient records. Again, ideological differences become apparent, in that of the Australian sample, 95% believe that it is the GP who owns the patient record, while 44% of the Swedish respondents believe that the government owns the patient record. Clearly, GPs feel that they are responsible in some way for the patient information, but interestingly Australian GPs, much more than their Swedish counterparts, do not seem responsible enough in protecting this valuable resource. A legal precedent may yet be set in this area, along with the testing of the validity of CMRs in the courts. Legislation is traditionally based around a paper-based paradigm rather than an electronic one. Only 3% of Australian respondents indicated that they thought the patient owned the information and no respondents thought that the government owned the information. Swedish responses more strongly favored a model of joint ownership of patient information between government, GPs and patients than did the Australian sample. This may be linked to the funding mechanisms for CMRs, since 88% of the Australian respondents indicated receiving no government help with computerization as opposed to 77% of Swedish respondents who did receive financial help to computerize from central and local governments. Table 10.5 provides a comparative view of general security, responsibility, ownership and support issues among all GPs surveyed.

Table 10.5 General security, responsibility, ownership and support issues among all GPs

	Australia (NSW) (n = 293)			Sweden (n = 298)		
	Total	Males	Females	Total	Males	Females
All GPs who keep no back-up records	81% (n = 226)	71% (n = 161)	29% (n = 65)	19% (n = 54)	65% (n = 35)	35% (n = 19)
Total responses	279			284		
Missing	14			14		
All GPs who have no disaster recovery plan	90% (n = 158)	75% (n = 119)	25% (n = 39)	91% (n = 32)	72% (n = 23)	28% (n = 9)
Total responses	176			35		
Missing	117			263		
All GPs who consider themselves responsible for the accuracy of patient information	98% (n = 286)	71% (n = 204)	29% (n = 82)	99% (n = 287)	60% (n = 173)	40% (n = 114)
Total responses	292			291		
Missing	1			7		
All GPs who believe they own the patient records	95% (n = 275)	72% (n = 198)	28% (n = 77)	14% (n = 37)	62% (n = 23)	38% (n = 14)
Total responses	289			264		
Missing	4			34		
All GPs who have received government help with computerization	12% (n = 34)	71% (n = 24)	29% (n = 10)	77% (n = 216)	60% (n = 130)	40% (n = 86)
Total responses	276			280		
Missing	17			18		

Computer-using respondents indicated having had a wide range of computer experience. Despite the low use of CMRs among respondents in Australia, experience with CMRs was longer (mean = 44 months, s.d. = 41 months) as compared to Sweden (mean = 25 months, s.d. = 23 months).

The general software/hardware trend is towards PC Windows-based platforms with software that integrates CMRs with other functions, e.g. accounts/billing, appointments scheduling, word processing, e-mail, etc. The potential for a *GP Office*-like software is apparent. In the Australian sample, computers being used solely as stand-alone workstations were as common as those in a multi-user network configuration. In Sweden, however, 97% of respondents had their computers set up in a multi-user network configuration. This is a reflection of the larger staff and GP numbers needing to share computers in a practice. The password remains the most common form of security protection in both samples. Table 10.6 provides a comparative overview of computerized GPs.

Table 10.6 Computerized GPs

	Australia (NSW) (n = 293)			Sweden (n = 298)		
	Total	Males	Females	Total	Males	Females
Computerised GPs who use a coding scheme to classify patient morbidity (e.g. ICD-10, etc.)	19% (n = 9)	100% (n = 9)	0% (n = 0)	89% (n = 185)	55% (n = 101)	45% (n = 84)
Total responses	48			209		
Missing	245			89		
Computerised GPs who follow some type of patient information management guidelines or practice	25% (n = 11	100% (n = 11)	0% (n = 0)	75% (n = 147)	58% (n = 85)	42% (n = 62)
Total responses	44			195		
Missing	249			103		
Computerised respondents indicating that passwords are their main form of computer security	98% (n = 34)	91% (n = 31)	9% (n = 3)	94% (n = 186)	56.5% (n = 105)	43.5% (n = 81)
Total responses	38			198		
Missing	255			100		
Computerised GPs who encrypt their patient database	27% (n = 11)	82% (n = 9)	18% (n = 2)	33% (n = 51)	61% (n = 31)	39% (n = 20)
Total responses	41			156		
Missing	252			142		
Computerised GPs who have outside dial-in access to their patient database	24% (n = 10)	90% (n = 9)	10% (n = 1)	13% (n = 216)	69% (n = 130)	31% (n = 86)
Total responses	42			196		
Missing	251			102		

Within both samples, very few had to undertake any computer-related subjects as part of their medical education. This may well be attributable to the fact that desktop computers were not around nor as accessible when the majority of respondents were undergoing their medical education (the mean year of medical education completion in the Australian sample was 1974, s.d. = 10 years; and in Sweden 1977, s.d. = 6 years). Nevertheless, this would indicate that there is no predisposition to adopt CMRs by having undertaken computer-related subjects at university and subsequent CMR adoption. The Swedish results would indicate that high CMR adoption is possible without there necessarily being an association between computer use at university and CMR adoption. In the Swedish case, the decision to adopt CMRs is more a result of direct funding availability (a type of authority decision) from the government, while in Australia the decision to adopt CMRs is more of an individual optional or collective group practice business decision.

The most common sources of information about keeping up to date with computers were through colleagues, journals and conferences. It is interesting to note that journals preceded colleagues in the Australian sample (51%:18%), while in the Swedish sample it was the reverse (26%:48%).

GP respondents in Sweden indicated that the lack of a CMR software standard among GPs was their main barrier to adoption, while Australian respondents indicated that cost was the major inhibiting factor. Another barrier to adoption that arises from the qualitative responses is finding the time to transfer from a paper-based patient records system to a CMR system, especially the laborious task of having to enter patient information into the system.

Discussion

'It is perhaps easiest to begin by stating what statistics is not. Statistics first of all is not a method by which one can prove almost anything one wants to prove'.[95] Statistical testing and presentation of the data only provides for one level of analysis and reporting. It was important to present the response breakdown by gender, since it was hypothesized that men and women perceive CMRs differently, which influences their decision to adopt or not to adopt the technology. The results on this are inconclusive; gender may be an element not just in CMR utilization among GPs but also an attribute that may need to be added to the diffusion model proposed by Rogers.[53] However, as with any analysis, 'The best data analysis comes not from keystrokes and printouts, but from spending time thinking'.[96]

The high rate of diffusion in Sweden supports the idea that perceived belief about a technology could be an important characteristic in the adoption process, hence a possible extension of the five-characteristic model of adoption as proposed by Rogers. Nevertheless, Rogers does capture this thinking in the idea of homophily and heterophily used to describe actors in similar or different social network groupings based on belief, education, social status, etc. Therefore, the relationship between belief and adoption/non-adoption needs to be investigated further. It may well be that belief, above all else, influences an actor to want to adopt. Nevertheless, it may also be the case that there is no generalizable association between belief and actual adoption, since availability of funding may, in fact, be the key adoption factor, therefore funding availability may need to be added to the adoption model proposed by Rogers.

The clustering of GPs with allied practitioners in Australia could cause over-servicing by GPs, especially under the publicly funded Medicare system. The fact that Australian respondents indicated seeing many more patients per week can be seen as a further reflection of the attitude that primary healthcare is more of a business. Throughput becomes a measure of financial return, which stands in opposition to that of sharing among public sector GPs in Sweden, who have a set list of patients for their area and for each of whom they are paid a set amount from the public purse. Nevertheless, patients, more so in Sweden than in Australia, also have to make a co-payment when visiting the GP, which may act as a deterrent for patients from seeing a GP. Greater application of compulsory co-payments in the Australian GP scene could be worth investigating but not as another revenue stream for the GP on top of the existing Medicare payment. Instead, the patient co-payment could be used to help pay for the Medicare payment, which in turn would be a contribution to helping to reduce the Australian Medicare bill.

The relatively high level of favorable attitudes but relatively low rate of adoption in Australia is somewhat similar to the 'KAP-gap' (Knowledge, Attitudes, Practice) problems of family planning diffusion surveys carried out in Third World countries during the 1960s.[53] This may be due to a combination of a low degree of observability of the long-term benefits and socio-political drawbacks such as gradual loss of ownership, power and control over patient data access. GPs are also reluctant to computerize because of the fear of choosing software that may become obsolete or may be incompatible with other systems.

In terms of the most common source of information for GPs, in Australia, journals preceded colleagues, while the reverse was the case in the Swedish sample. This is significant, since according to the innovation decision process model presented by Rogers,[53] mass media awareness is considered to be the main communication channel for creating knowledge awareness. In this model, persuasion to adopt occurs at a more interpersonal level usually after mass media knowledge awareness has taken place. The Australian sample responses would appear to support this model, but the results from the Swedish sample, suggest that mass media channels do not play such a key role in knowledge awareness and that from the outset, interpersonal communications with colleagues are more significant in the formulation of attitudes. This would also indicate a more collective based decision-making process among the Swedish sample, as opposed to a more individualized process in Australia. This is possibly a significant point worthy of follow-up, since more respondents in the Swedish sample have adopted CMRs; hence, the innovation-decision process model proposed by Rogers may need to be modified or rejected. Future studies may wish to follow up on this aspect by including another, more specific follow-up question about how respondents found out about CMRs in the first place, rather than just about computer developments (e.g. mass media, interpersonal or other).

In the context of spatial diffusion, another question worth pursuing may be to see if proximity to colleagues plays a role in persuasion to adopt or reject; for example, do the colleagues from whom information was received work within the same practice, live in the same city, or elsewhere? Furthermore, this implies that word of mouth can be seen as an important form of communication among GPs, possibly more so than mass media communication channels when considering making a decision to adopt or to reject. In Australia, this could be attributable to internalizing something a GP may have read in a journal and then testing that information with colleagues prior to either accepting or rejecting information and ideas. It could also point to a mistrust of mass media sources and preference for reliance on the opinions and experiences of colleagues. Thus, face-to-face communication, conferences and workshops must be considered an important part of the process of communicating information to others. The slow rate of CMR adoption in the Australian sample could further be interpreted as a possible mismatch between perceived complexity of the innovation by GPs and the communication channel selected to convey information. CMRs may be perceived by GPs as a highly complex technology. Therefore, interpersonal communication may be more important in communicating information about a technology which may be perceived to be complex, rather than communicating the information through mass media channels.

Results would suggest that financial investment or reimbursement for the purchase of computer equipment would benefit some GPs, but there would still be those who would not know what to do with the technology even if they had a computer on their desk. A computer on a GP's desk needs to be seen as more than just a symbolic ornament. A decision to adopt could, for example, be reflective of a perceived need to keep up with the latest fashion and as a status symbol, giving the appearance of being modern and keeping up with the times, that is, as a form of passive rather than active adoption. This may reflect a lack of computer literacy and knowledge about what computers can do (the second-most important barrier indicated in both surveys). GP respondents in Sweden indicated that the lack of a CMR software standard among GPs was their main barrier to adoption, while Australian respondents indicated that cost was the major inhibiting factor. The results therefore support the conclusions of another Australian study that 'non-computer users do not know enough about the benefits of computerization to make an informed decision about computerizing' and that cost was a 'high priority'.[80] Rogers concurs with these comments, indicating that an individual may not know enough about an innovation for it to be regarded '. . . as relevant to the individual's situation, and as potentially useful . . . the individual's attitudes or beliefs about the innovation have much to say about his or her passage through the innovation-knowledge process'.[53] This further supports the conclusions of Moidu, that 'training is a crucial factor for dispelling fears in the transfer of technology particularly when the end-users have a high interest but a low level of awareness'.[97] Hence, information and knowledge about CMRs is needed so that an environment of persuasion is created in which adoption can take place. More difficult to determine is whether an individual need for a CMR precedes the technology or whether knowledge of CMRs creates a need for the technology. It is also of interest to note patient reactions to GP computer use. Fitter, for example, indicates that '. . . studies suggest that the overall impact on patients is small . . . patients' experiences in computer use have more positive attitudes towards doctors using computers'.[94] This would seem to be reflective of a wider conditioning process occurring in society.

Another barrier to adoption that arises from the qualitative responses is finding the time to transfer over from a paper-based patient records system to a CMR system, especially the laborious task of having to enter patient information into the system. This can be somewhat difficult to overcome, since trying to scan hand-written notes on a card file, which may only be legible to the GP, is not really an option. It implies a longer-term phasing-in process, possibly associated with patients' visits to the GP. As each patient comes to see the GP, their paper records can gradually be transferred to the computer.

Careful consideration needs to be given to the argument that cost is a major barrier to adoption. Certainly, cost is an issue and past research has indicated that adopters underestimate the actual cost of adoption,[58,70] but is it the barrier that we are led to believe? It may well be that the perceived benefits do not outweigh the perceived costs involved, for it would follow that GPs would pay if the advantages were equal to or greater than the cost. A secondary line of thought, therefore, may be that cost is used as a strategy to divert attention from the real issue, and that the perceived cost of having to learn something new outweighs any potential monetary benefit from using CMRs. Time spent on learning to use computers and CMRs cannot necessarily be quantified, but still counts as a perceived cost of adoption. This highlights some of the problems with conducting cost-benefit analyses, since not all benefits or costs can be quantified; there may be qualitative benefits which in subtle ways may influence the overall process of work but are not directly connected with improvement, for example improved appearance and quality of patient records, improved editing capability, time savings and improved data security. Benefits and costs are therefore essentially a matter of perception. The danger in using just a cost-benefits analysis to justify the use or non-use of CMRs on a quantifiable basis is open to serious limitations and critique.

Results from the survey data indicate what can be called an attitude paradox. In the Swedish survey, among the non-users, a positive attitude is associated with an intention to adopt in the near future. In the Australian survey, even when non-users indicate a positive attitude, they have no intention of adopting. Therefore, a positive attitude is not sufficient for adoption but may only be desirable. This finding supports the general belief that new knowledge and attitudes by themselves are not sufficient to bring about a change in behavior. Other socio-political reasons need to be considered rather than just behavioral or technical reasons. The survey work shows a need to clarify legal, social and political debates over CMR ownership, CMR legal status, stakeholder access rights, responsibilities, GP loss of power issues and funding models.

Limitations and suggestions for future research design

Mention needs to be made of the limitations of this study and the limitation of using a survey as a research methodology. Limitations help to understand and locate some of the survey findings in a more meaningful context as well as to help other researchers with the design of future diffusion surveys. The works of Kaplan and Duchon, Leedy, and Neuman are informative in this respect.[98-100]

One key point needs to be made before undertaking a mail-out survey: the investigator(s) need to know that a mailing list sample can be compiled from a comprehensive list of the target population. This is not to say that a sample cannot be composed without a list of the relevant population, but it may have implications for both the design methodology and the feasibility of the project. There may be a cost involved or the actual mailing list may not be available to the public (i.e. it may be seen as a closely held organizational asset).

Respondents may have a vested interest in responding to the survey and hence distort the picture of events. If possible, it would be worthwhile to investigate the non-respondents and the reasons for their non-response. Some GPs may well be reluctant to disclose that they are non-computerized because they perceive the survey to have a positive bias towards computers and CMR usage. Those who are computerized, therefore, may well be more inclined to respond in order to promote CMR adoption. Furthermore, since the focus of this survey was on CMR usage rather than just computer usage, only those using CMRs are likely to have been positively inclined to respond. A different target audience could yield a different perspective, for example instead of GPs who may or may not have a vested interest in CMRs, a survey of practice patients or the general public could be useful in order to ascertain another picture as to the state of computer and CMR usage among GPs, since they could be seen as a more objective third party.

Home computer adoption was not examined, but future research may wish to include questions about home computer usage as this could have some bearing on computer use in the workplace. Also, a question about GP income levels may need to be included to see if there is an association with computer and CMR adoption. However, asking about levels of income can be a sensitive issue. The work of Bolton and Gay (1995) indicates a possible association between income level, practice size and CMR adoption.[80] Larger practices with high incomes tended to adopt CMRs more readily.

Errors can also creep into the survey due to a lack of understanding of the terminology, through definitional problems and differences over what the respondents perceive they use the computer for, especially in cross-cultural studies requiring translations. Respondents may, for example, equate computer usage with CMR usage, hence resulting in an over-representation of CMR usage. This also suggests another limitation in that self-administered questionnaires about computer usage can also be somewhat problematic because users may base their answers on what they think they may do or would like to do rather than on what they actually do in practice. Hence, the need to provide specific definitions of terms as part of the cover letter and also the possible need for further follow-up through observation and interviews. This may only be possible in longitudinal studies and where respondents are willing to identify themselves.

Conclusions and recommendations

As the Australian survey findings showed, a high awareness and favorable attitudes towards CMRs are not necessarily associated with the action to adopt, as can be seen in the case of the Australian non-computerized respondents. This may in part be due to the fact that such individuals do not consider their existing paper record management practices as a problem. The Australian results may further be associated with perceptions of possible undesirable consequences following from the adoption and implementation of computers in the minds of GPs. On the other hand, the Swedish results demonstrate a different situation altogether, as can be seen from the Swedish non-computerized respondents, where a high level of awareness and favorable attitudes are associated with a direct intention to adopt.

The paradoxical findings between the Australian and Swedish studies demonstrate that a positive belief about CMRs does not necessarily correspond to actual adoption. This can further be described as a discrepancy problem between attitude and practice, that is between rhetoric and action. Direct interventionist strategies, such as standards setting, reimbursement schemes, training programs and the offering of grants, can only provide a partial means for controlling the work practice behavior of GPs. Other strategies involve greater information flow through professional networks, journals, conferences, training sessions, etc. This effort involves the mobilization of many organizational networks and disciplines: the (re)creation and merging of journals, courses, degrees and organizations so as to reflect this reorientation or change in thinking about the role of CMRs in an e-health environment.

The results from the Swedish study support the argument that the process of diffusion can be controlled at least to a certain extent. In Sweden, a direct financial incentive has been provided by the governing bodies at the county council level for GPs to adopt CMRs. This can be interpreted as a direct policy initiative to computerize GPs, whether they like it or not, similar to the 'Micros for GPs' scheme in the UK, also a type of forced regulatory obligation.[70] In return, the councils expect standardized monthly aggregated reports from the GPs in order for them to be paid. The Swedish result is even more interesting in that, despite being forced to computerize, GPs still have a positive attitude towards using CMRs. This reflects a deeper belief that the utilization of CMRs is an improvement on past work practices.

Since conducting this study the Australian federal government's Practice Incentives Program, introduced in 2000/2001 is helping to increase the utilization of computers for clinical purposes. Government payments are made to GPs who use computers essentially for prescription writing and electronically sending and receiving clinical information. The government also introduced health privacy legislation as part of its amendments to the Privacy Act (1988), which now covers the collection, storage, use and disclosure of patient information which GPs have to abide by. This came into force in December 2001.[101] At a national level, the most recent study of GP computer utilization was the Western et al. study, which found that 89% of Australian GPs use computers and that computers are more likely to be used for administrative purposes than clinical purposes.[102] This is a substantial increase on the results reported in an earlier national study by AC Neilson, which indicated the computerization level to be at 31%, and that a combination of administrative and clinical use of computers was common; however, less so for clinical purposes.[103] Clinical notes were seen to be the least common.

Suggestions for increased utilization and future research

There is a long-standing need to decide on a national standard for an integrated CMR and practice management software for GPs in Australia and to encourage other health providers to adopt the same standard. The national standard should fit into the general development of a future health communications infrastructure, the Health Connect project between GPs, hospitals, pathology, insurers, government and other healthcare providers.[104] The Australian Coordinated Care Trials were in part an attempt to experiment with CMR use in a more comprehensive and integrated way.[105]

The following are some specific suggestions that resulted from the data collected and, despite being context-specific to the Australian scene, can be more generally extrapolated to other healthcare systems.

- Need for an integrated CMR system must meet GP (and other stakeholder) needs and cater for patient confidentiality/privacy, must have an easy-to-use graphical user interface, screen displays should be easy to read and not cluttered with too much information.
- CMR use should not interfere with the physician–patient encounter; the CMR system should have appropriate security features built into the design (e.g. encryption, passwords, audit logs).
- The system must include a comprehensive query and statistical generation component so that GPs are able to interrogate the practice population database. Graphical and visual tools to display data would also be desirable.
- If a CMR standard cannot be agreed upon, a standard should be encouraged, *de facto*, or at least a minimum data standard should be established for the transmission of health data (e.g. HL7) and security (e.g. public or private key encryption).
- National health policy should specifically address and indicate the importance of CMRs in its vision for a reformed healthcare system. There is a need to develop uniform national legislation for patient information and CMR use; the amendments to the Privacy Act (1988) which came into force in December 2001 are a step in the right direction.
- A national CMR Institute should be set up for greater coordination of resources and research into CMRs. Representatives from the wider community and all interested stakeholders should be involved.
- A comprehensive national health data dictionary would inevitably be a valuable public resource, but this has social implications beyond the mere collection and retrieval of information. Issues of centralization, control, ownership and confidentiality are inevitably associated with such developments. Efforts to develop a standard GP data dictionary can also be considered important and this should be a subset of the greater national health data dictionary. Careful thought will be required to determine what data elements are needed both now and in the future, in order to accommodate all stakeholders involved.
- GP divisions in Australia need to be treated as social diffusion networks. Pilot GP practice success centers within GP divisions can be established and showcased as centers of excellence.
- Target technology champions and opinion leaders as the key information diffusers within GP divisions; these may be the pilot success center GPs. Each success center can act as a regional support site for interested GPs to visit.
- Enlist technology diffusion mediators and facilitators. These individuals should ideally have a broader awareness of health informatics, technology diffusion and an understanding of GP settings and e-health developments nationally and internationally.
- Set up a national GP IT 'help center', which GPs can call toll free when needing help and advice with CMR implementation.
- A wider mass media strategy is desirable (TV, radio, newspapers, WWW) so as to create greater awareness of CMRs, telemedicine, health informatics and e-health within the community.

- Sufficient conference forums presently exist at the national level (e.g. the Australian Health Informatics Conference, the RACGP Computer Conference) for general health informatics information diffusion. What is needed is greater consolidation of the various initiatives, research findings, clinical trials and so on, in order to provide a greater sense of direction. Otherwise, islands of uncoordinated, disparate research will proliferate among private research organizations and universities.
- There is a need for the development of a bibliographic directory of past efforts, as well as existing ongoing research into CMRs and telemedicine, both within Australia and internationally. This could be a home page sitting on the WWW, which would be easier to update than a paper-based publication and could contain hyperlinks to the associated project, the researchers and reports.
- Computer and CMR education, information dissemination, debate, training and support are vital within the GP divisions in Australia. There is a need to develop and integrate computing and statistical competencies into future medical training qualifications and programs. This would allow for more and better epidemiological studies by GPs operating at the practice level.
- Greater involvement of professional bodies in Australia such as ACHI, HISA, RACGP, AMA and interaction with the federal and state health departments.
- Need for more financial incentive schemes for GPs to computerize, for example, Medclaims ($500 rebate from the Australian Health Insurance Commission). This sum could be increased.
- Financial incentives from government, RACGP, AMA, HISA, industry and other possible stakeholders. Financial support (public and private) to encourage CMR development and diffusion is important and cost sharing among stakeholders should be encouraged. As a start, financing issues should be addressed by GP divisions within their IT strategic plans, i.e. how to obtain sources of funding through, for example, collaborative grant applications. Voluntary adoption may be preferable to mandated adoption. The key is to create an environment in which GPs will voluntarily adopt without direct coercion. The alternative is for the federal government to regulate CMRs as a national standard for GPs, which would undoubtedly create some dissent.
- Greater visibility of pilot projects documenting CMR adoption before, during and after implementation. These can be written up as case studies. This allows for verification of the rhetoric about CMR technology against social reality and current practice, for example, e.g. costs, benefits, design problems, unintended consequences, loss of power issues and general practice impact studies.
- Greater collaboration between GPs, researchers, professional bodies, local area health services and government needs to be encouraged, especially in grant applications.
- Research into the use and development of consumer health Web portals, smart tokens/cards, biometric identification and personal digital assistant (PDA) applications by patients and healthcare workers all need to be evaluated carefully as will accompanying workflow process models.

The central argument of this chapter has been that CMR systems need to be seen as a fundamental building block for primary healthcare globally. In order for grander visions of telemedicine and e-health to take place, CMR utilization among GPs is seen as a key linking element. Successful adoption strategies drawn from countries with a high rate of adoption, such as Sweden, can serve as useful learning models for devising national plans. The caveat is that it is still necessary to carefully examine the attitudes of local GPs (the main users) towards CMRs with an eye on international developments in e-health. The development and further diffusion of CMRs, telemedicine and e-health are not only a reflection on the motivations, attitudes and alliances between the actors involved within social and professional networks but also upon government policy, legislation and funding mechanisms.

References

1   World Health Organisation (1978) *Primary Health Care: Report of the International Conference on Primary Health Care*. Alma-Ata. WHO, Geneva.
2   Mandil SH, Moidu K, Korpel M *et al.* (eds) (1993) *Health Informatics in Africa: HELINA 93*. Excerpta Medica, Amsterdam.
3   Van Bemmel J, Musen M and Helder J (eds) (1997) *Handbook of Medical Informatics*. Springer, Heidelberg.
4   Bangert D and Doktor R (2000) Implementing store-and-forward telemedicine: organizational issues. *Telemedicine Journal and e-health*. 6(3): 355–60.
5   World Health Organisation (1993) *Implementation of the Global Strategy for Health for All by the Year 2000, Second Evaluation*. 8th Report on the World Health Situation, Geneva.
6   WONCA (1991) *The Role of the General Practitioner/Family Physician in Health Care Systems*. World Organisation of Family Doctors, Melbourne.
7   Dickinson J (1991) Validity of measurements and research. *Australian Family Physician*. 20(10): 1491–4.
8   Strasser R (1992) The gatekeeper role of general practice. *Medical Journal of Australia*. 156: 108–10.
9   Leech G (1998) Beachhead for data on black hole opening wide for GPs. *The Weekend Australian*. 4–5 April: 42.
10 Westin AF (1976) *Computers, Health Records and Citizen Rights*. National Bureau of Standards, Washington, DC.
11 Donaldson M and Lohr K (eds) (1994) *Health Data in the Information Age: Use, Disclosure, and Privacy. Institute of Medicine*. National Academy Press, Washington, DC.
12 Safran C, Rind D, Citroen M *et al.* (1995) Protection of confidentiality in the computer-based patient record. *MD Computing*. 12: 187–92.
13 Linnarsson R (1993) *Methods, Design and Components for a Computer-Based Patient Record to Promote Quality Care in General Practice*. Doctoral Dissertation.
14 Berg M (1997) *Rationalising medical work: decision support techniques and medical practices*. Doctoral dissertation. Massachusetts Institute of Technology, Cambridge, MA.
15 Feinglass J and Warren-Salmon J (1990) Corporatisation of medicine: the use of medical management information systems to increase the clinical productivity of physicians. *International Journal of Health Services*. 20(2): 233–52.
16 Best WR (1962) The potential role of computers in medical practice. *Journal of the American Medical Association*. 182: 994–1000.
17 Fitter M and Cruickshank P (1982) The computer in the consulting room: a psychological framework. *Behaviour and Information Technology*. 1: 81–92.
18 Fitter M and Cruickshank P (1983) Doctors using computers: a case study. In: Sime ME and Coombs MJ (eds) *Designing for Human–Computer Communication*. Academic Press, London.
19 Brownbridge G, Fitter M and Sime M (1984) The doctor's use of a computer in the consulting room: an analysis. *International Journal of Man-Machine Studies*. 21:65–90.

20 Brownbridge G, Herzmark G and Wall T (1985) Patients' reactions to doctors' computer use in general practice consultations. *Social Science and Medicine*. **20**: 47–52.

21 Crampton M (1995) The computer on your desk: general practice computing in the 1990s. *Australian Family Physician*. **24**(3): 296–7.

22 Institute of Medicine (1991) *The Computer-Based Patient Record – An Essential Technology for Health Care*. National Academy Press, Washington, DC.

23 Institute of Medicine (1997) *The Computer-Based Patient Record – An Essential Technology for Health Care* (revised edn) National Academy Press, Washington, DC.

24 Schnieder M, Mann N and Schiller A (1992) *Can Telecommunications Help Solve America's Health Care Problems?* Arthur D Little, Boston, MA.

25 Watson D (1989) Telemedicine. *Medical Journal of Australia*. **151**(2): 62–6.

26 Brauer G (1992) Telehealth: the delayed revolution in healthcare. *Medical Progress Through Technology*. **18**(3): 151–63.

27 Crowe B (1993) *Telemedicine in Australia*. Australian Institute of Health and Welfare, Canberra.

28 Allen A (1994) Evaluating telemedicine: the cooperative model. *Telemedicine Today*. **2**(1): 8–9.

29 Pradhan M (1996) Telemedicine. In: Hovenga E, Kidd M and Cesnik B (eds) *Health Informatics: an overview*. Churchill Livingston, Australia.

30 Zuboff S (1988) *In the Age of the Smart Machine – The Future of Work and Power*. Basic Books, New York.

31 Milner A (1996) *Literature, Culture and Society*. University College London, Great Britain.

32 Porter ME (1980) *Competitive Strategy, Techniques for Analyzing Industries and Competitors*. The Free Press, New York.

33 Porter ME (1985) *Competitive Advantage. Creating and Sustaining Superior Performance*. The Free Press, New York.

34 Porter ME (1990) *The Competitive Advantage of Nations*. Billing & Sons Ltd, Worcester.

35 Porter ME and Millar V (1985) How information gives you competitive advantage. *Harvard Business Review*. **July/August**: 149–60.

36 Arrow K (1980) The economics of information. In: Dertouzos M and Moses J (eds) *The Computer Age: a twenty-year view*. MIT Press, London.

37 Lamberton DM (1990) *Information Economics: 'threatened wreckage' or new paradigm?* CIRCIT, South Melbourne.

38 Eliasson G (1990) *The Knowledge Based Information Economy*. The Industrial Institute for Economic and Social Research, Sweden.

39 Bijker W (1995) *Of Bicycles, Bakelites, and Bulbs: toward a theory of sociotechnical change*. MIT Press, Cambridge, MA.

40 Bijker WE, Hughes TP and Pinch T (eds) (1987) *The Social Construction of Technological Systems: new directions in the sociology and history of technology*. MIT Press, Cambridge, MA.

41 Winner L (1980) Do artifacts have politics? *Daedalus*. **109**(1): 121–36.

42 Giddens A (1984) *The Constitution of Society: outline of the theory of structuralism*. University of California Press, Berkeley, CA.

43 Callon M and Latour B (1981) Unscrewing the big leviathan, or how do actors macrostructure reality? In: Knorr-Cetina K and Cicourel A (eds) *Advances in Social Theory and Methodology toward an Integration of Micro- and Macro-Sociologies*. Routledge and Kegan Paul, London.

44 Rigby M (1999) The management and policy challenges of the globalisation effect of informatics and telemedicine. *Health Policy*. **46**: 97–103.

45 Collins H and Pinch T (1982) *Frames of Meaning: the social construction of extraordinary science*. Routledge & Kegan Paul, London.

46 Callon M and Law J (1989) On the construction of sociotechnical networks: content and context revisited. *Knowledge and Society: Studies in the Sociology of Science Past and Present.* **8**: 57–83.

47 Weed L (1969) *Medical Records, Medical Education and Patient Care.* Case Western University Press, Cleveland.

48 Luke R, Begun J and Pointer D (1989) Quasi firms: strategic interorganizational forms in the health care industry. *Academy of Management Review.* **14**(1): 9–19.

49 Bomba D and Land T (2003) A survey of patient attitudes towards the use of computerised medical records and unique identifiers in four Australian GP practices. *Journal on Information Technology in Healthcare.* **1**(1): 31–45.

50 Eysenbach G and Kohler C (2002) How do consumers search for and appraise health information on the World Wide Web? Qualitative study using focus groups, usability tests, and in-depth interviews. *British Medical Journal.* **324**: 573–7.

51 Slack W (2001) *Cybermedicine: how computing empowers doctors and patients for better healthcare* (2e). Jossey-Bass Publishers, San Francisco, CA.

52 Jadad AR and Gagliardi A (1998) Rating health information on the Internet: navigating to knowledge or to Babel? *JAMA.* **279**(8): 611–4.

53 Rogers EM (1995) *Diffusion of Innovations* (4e). The Free Press, New York.

54 Sauer C (1993) *Why Information Systems Fail.* Alfred Waller Ltd, Oxfordshire.

55 Straub DW (1994) The effect of culture on IT diffusion: e-mail and fax in Japan and the US. *Information Systems Research.* **5**(1): 23–47.

56 Geffen D and Straub DW (1997) Gender differences in the perception and use of e-mail: an extension to the technology acceptance model. *MIS Quarterly.* **21**(4): 389–400.

57 Ajzen I and Fishbein M (1975) *Belief, Attitude, Intention, and Behavior: an introduction to theory and research.* Addison-Wesley Publisher, Colorado.

58 Heikkilä J (1995) *The Diffusion of a Learning Intensive Technology into Organisations: The Case of Personal Computing.* Helsinki School of Economics and Business Administration, Helsinki.

59 Walker D (1997) Health informatics in Australia. *Informatics in Healthcare Australia.* **6**(4): 135–8.

60 Walker D (1993) To succeed, computers need to become irresistible. *Informatics in Healthcare Australia.* **2**(5): 5–6.

61 Kidd M, Carson N, Crampton R *et al.* (1994) New technology in primary care: benefits, problems and advice. In: Fry J and Yuen N (eds) *Primary Care and Family Medicine.* Radcliffe Medical Press, Oxford.

62 Valente T (1995) *Network Models of the Diffusion of Innovations.* Hampton Press, Creshill. NJ.

63 Emmelhainz MA (1990) *Electronic Data Interchange: a total management guide.* Van Nostrand Reinholm, New York.

64 Spri (1996) *User Requirements on Electronic Health Care Records.* Spri, Stockholm.

65 Spri (1997) *Vad Gör Spri?* Spri, Stockholm.

66 Drucker P (1970) *Technology Management and Society.* Harper and Row, New York.

67 Ansoff HI (1987) Strategic management of technology. *Journal of Business Strategy.* **7**: 28–39.

68 Royal Australian College of General Practitioners (1985) *Vision of General Practice Now and in 1995.* Arthur Anderson and Co, Melbourne.

69 MacIsaac P, Lord T, Crampton M *et al.* (1990) *Computer Assisted Practice Project (CAPP) Report.* Royal Australian College of General Practitioners, Melbourne.

70 O'Toole C (1988) *Computerised medical records.* Masters thesis.

71 Crampton M (1990) Survey of RACGP members' use and attitudes towards medical practice computing. *Proceedings of the RACGP 1990 Computer Conference,* Sydney.

72 Crampton M and Lord T (1988) *Standards for Computerised Medical Records Systems*. Royal Australian College of General Practitioners.

73 Greisser GG, Bakker A, Danielsson J *et al.* (eds) (1980) *Data Protection in Health Information Systems, Considerations and Guidelines*. North-Holland Publishing Company, Amsterdam.

74 Roberts J (1991) General practice: feeling fine, getting better. *British Medical Journal*. **302**.

75 Read JTB (1986) Comprehensive coding. *British Journal of Health Care Computing*. **3**: 22–5.

76 Douglas R and Saltman D (1991) *W(h)ither Australian General Practice?* National Centre for Epidemiology and Population Health, Canberra.

77 Liaw S (1992) *How Is Information Managed in General Practice?* Study for the RACGP (South Australian Faculty).

78 Fry F (1993) IPC Survey Results. *Australian Family Physician*. **22**(2): 87.

79 Cacek J (1994) *A survey of the attitudes of Australian general practitioners to computerisation of medical records*. Masters thesis. Monash University, Melbourne.

80 Bolton P and Gay G (1995) Review of computer usage among RACGP members. *Australian Family Physician*. **24**(10): 1882–5.

81 Hayes G (1993) GP computing – the UK scene, present and future: achievements and incentives. *Proceedings of the RACGP 7th Computer Conference*, Melbourne.

82 Lun K and Goh L (1993) GP computing; the Singapore scene: present and future. *Proceedings of the 7th RACGP Computer Conference*, Australia.

83 Johnston J, Leung G and Wong J (2001) Physicians attitudes towards the computerization of clinical practice in Hong Kong: a population study. *International Journal of Medical Informatics*. **65**: 41–9.

84 Australian Institute of Health and Welfare (1992) *Australia's Health 1992*. Australian Government Publishing Service, Canberra.

85 Bates EM (1983) *Health Systems and Public Scrutiny: Australia, Britain and the United States*. Croom Helm, London.

86 Nichol W (1990) What is rural? Centre for rural welfare research. *Rural Welfare Research Bulletin*. **4**: 4–5.

87 Calltorp J (1989) The 'Swedish model' under pressure – how to maintain equity and develop quality? *Quality Assurance in Health Care*. **1**(1): 13–22.

88 Berleen G, Rehnberg C and Wennström G (1992) *The Reform of Health Care in Sweden*. Spri, Stockholm; Spri Report No. 339.

89 Bridges-Webb C (1992) General practitioners and over-servicing. *Medical Journal of Australia*. **156**: 140–41.

90 Shepherd J (1995) Whither rural practice. *Medical Journal of Australia*. **162**: 232.

91 Humphreys JS (1988) Social provision and service delivery: problems of equity, health and healthcare in Rural Australia. *Geoforum*. **19**(3): 323–38.

92 Humphreys JS and Weinand HC (1991) Healthcare preferences in a country town. *Medical Journal of Australia*. **154**: 733–7.

93 Jeffreys M and Sachs H (1983) *Rethinking General Practice: dilemmas in primary medical care*. Tavistock Publications, London.

94 Fitter M (1986) Evaluation of computers in primary healthcare: the effect on doctor–patient communications. In: Peterson and Schneider W (eds) *Human-Computer Communications in Health Care*. Elsevier Science Publishers, Philadelphia, PA.

95 Blalock H (1979) *Social Statistics*. McGraw-Hill International Editions, Washington, DC.

96 Axford R, Grunwald G and Hyndman R (1996) Information technology in research. In: Hovenga E, Kidd M and Cesnik B (eds) *Health Informatics: an overview*. Churchill Livingston, Australia.

97 Moidu K (1993) Informatics in support of primary healthcare management. In: Mandil SH, Moidu K, Korpel M *et al.* (eds) *Health Informatics in Africa: HELINA 93.* Excerpta Medica, Amsterdam.

98 Kaplan B and Duchon D (1988) Combining qualitative and quantitative methods in information systems research: a case study. *MIS Quarterly.* **12**(4): 571–86.

99 Leedy P (1993) *Practical Research: planning and design* (5e). Macmillan, New York.

100 Neuman W (1997) *Social Research Methods* (3e). Allyn and Bacon, Boston, MA.

101 Bomba D and Hallit G (2002) Will the new Australian Health Privacy Law provide adequate protection? *Australian Health Review.* **25**(3): 141–51.

102 Western M, Dwan K, Makkai T *et al.* (2001) *Measuring IT use in Australian General Practice 2001.* General Practice Branch, Commonwealth Department of Health and Aged Care.

103 AC Nielson (1998) *A Study Into Levels of, and Attitudes Towards Information Technology in General Practice, Vols 1 & 2.* General Practice Branch of the Commonwealth Department of Health and Family Services, Canberra.

104 Commonwealth Department of Health and Aged Care (2000) *The National Electronic Health Records Taskforce. A Health Information Network for Australia.* Canberra.

105 Commonwealth Department of Health and Aged Care (2002) *The Australian Coordinated Care Trials: recollections of an evaluation.* Canberra.

106 Davis FD (1989) Perceived usefulness, perceived ease of use, and user acceptance of information technology. *MIS Quarterly.* **13**(3): 319–40.

Chapter 11

Developing strategic alliances for telemedicine

Deborah E Seale, Sally S Robinson, Alexia Green, Glenda Walker, Christina Esperat, Bobbye Berg and Patty Ellison

Introduction

This chapter focuses on the role of alliances among various actors – individuals, organizations, communities and networks – in an effort to understand the range of human factors that influence telemedicine utilization and sustainability.[1] Actors form alliances to accomplish that which they cannot accomplish alone.[1–9] Healthcare organizations often develop alliances with other organizations to enable the delivery of telemedicine services.[5,9–10] These inter-organizational arrangements are often initiated as a result of grant funding received by one of the participating organizations.[12] All too often these telemedicine alliances are underutilized and end after the grant period.[13]

Luke, Begun and Porter propose that *loosely coupled* inter-organizational arrangements created to achieve short-term objectives tend to dissolve because they are never seen by the participating organizations as strategically important.[14] They argue that *loosely coupled* inter-organizational relationships developed for long-term strategic purposes are more likely to last. A five-step process (FSP) developed to identify organizations appropriate for exploring a telemedicine alliance and guide the development of alliances that assure ongoing telemedicine utilization and assure long-term sustainability is presented. The steps of the process are:

1 build upon existing relationships
2 develop co-champions
3 engage the team
4 secure executive commitment
5 gain community support.

A case study approach is used to describe the real-world application of these steps in building strategic alliances among an academic health science center and health professions programs at three universities. This process was developed over the years from 1992 through 2000 and grew out of the combined experiences of the authors. The first telemedicine alliance is being sustained, but is not growing. The second continues to grow and thrive. Attempts to develop the third alliance were suspended in the second step of the process.

The FSP is not undertaken in isolation of the other *layers* of human factor influences discussed in the editorial commentary.[1] Nor does completion of these steps guarantee a well-utilized and sustainable telemedicine program. However, the process ensures that the telemedicine alliances are strategic in nature, based on shared values and objectives, and aligned with the respective missions and strategic directions of the individuals, organizations, communities and societal sectors involved.

Background

The case study covers the timeframe from 1990 to 2001 and reflects the experience of an academic health science center working with health professions programs in three state universities to establish a telemedicine program. Feature characteristics of these institutions and the development of their inter-organizational relationships over time are described below.

The academic health science center (HSC) is situated in the southwestern region of the US on a barrier island 50 miles south of a major metropolitan area of five million people. The island population is 60000 and the overall county population is 250000. Just over 2000 students and 550 medical residents are enrolled in the academic health science center's schools of medicine, nursing, allied health and graduate biomedical sciences. The HSC employs over 1000 faculty and 10000 staff. The university's state-supported healthcare network includes eight on-campus hospitals and a network of campus- and community-based clinics that offer primary and specialty care throughout a 228-county area.

The three state universities are located 100 to 350 miles from the HSC (*see* Table 11.1). University A is nearest to the HSC and is situated in a city of 110000 amidst a metropolitan statistical area of 250000. The other two universities are located in cities of approximately 30000. University B is in a rural area. University C is in a metropolitan area of over 500000. The enrollments, faculty sizes and ratios of students to faculty of the three universities are similar. However, University B – located in a rural area – offers more undergraduate and graduate degrees with fewer faculty members than its urban counterparts.

Table 11.1 Feature characteristics of alliance universities

Characteristic	University A	University B	University C
Miles from HSC	100	185	350
City population	110000	30000	30000
County population	250000	60000	500000
No. of students enrolled	9800	10000	14000
No. of faculty	490	525	660
Ratio of students to faculty	20	19	22
No. of undergraduate students	76	94	51
No. of graduate degrees	33	60	45
Partner program	Nursing department	Nursing division program	Physician assistant

In 1990, the HSC began offering a joint graduate nursing degree at University A (*see* Table 11.2). HSC faculty used a combination of on-site videotaped classes. The two-hour commute (100 miles), while demanding, was doable. University B also wanted to offer the joint nursing degree. However, the 185-mile (3.5 hour) commute was unrealistic.

In 1991, the HSC received federal funding to initiate an Area Health Education Center (AHEC) charged with developing community–academic partnerships to improve the supply and distribution of health professionals in rural and under-served areas. University A and University B are each within one of the service regions of the AHEC program. Community-based AHEC offices were opened in 1991 and 1992 in both service regions. University representatives serve on the community boards of each AHEC office. University C is not in the AHEC service region.

Table 11.2 Alliance development timeline

1990	Joint graduate nursing program between HSC and University A begins (faculty commuting supplemented with videotapes)
1991	AHEC created by HSC serving University A's region
1992	• HSC opens AHEC serving University B's region • All four institutions/universities conduct video-conference demonstrations
1993	Joint graduate nursing program between HSC and University B initiated (video-conferencing)
1994	Discussion initiated between HSC and University A to develop a telemedicine alliance
1996	HSC and University A form telemedicine alliance: • pediatric telemedicine services offered • joint graduate nursing degree program transitions to video-conferencing Joint physician assistant degree program initiated between HSC and University C (video-conferencing)
1997	HSC and University B form telemedicine alliance: • pediatric telemedicine services offered • joint nursing degree program continues
1998	HSC and University C's attempt to form telemedicine alliance fails
1999	Independent school districts associated with HSC and University A and B join telemedicine alliance
2000	Mental health, maternal child health, asthma programs between HSC and University B begins

All four institutions conducted video-conferencing demonstrations in 1992.[15] As a result of the demonstrations, HSC and University B offered a joint graduate nursing degree via video-conferencing, beginning in January 1993.

HSC and University A began exploring the potential of forming a telemedicine alliance in mid-1994. The steps undertaken to develop this alliance and alliances with University B and University C are the focus of the case study presented later in this chapter.

A telemedicine clinic was opened between HSC and University A in 1996[16,17] and a second telemedicine clinic was opened between HSC and University B in 1997. Both of these telemedicine clinics were implemented without external funding. Once the clinics were operational, the alliance secured external funding to enhance operational capabilities and expand the project to include University C and six school districts.

The telemedicine alliance with University A is being sustained, but is not growing. The alliance with University B continues to grow and thrive. The alliance with University C was never implemented.

The Five FSP Step Process used to identify and develop these three alliances is described in the case presentation and factors that contributed to the outcomes stated above are discussed. Implications for future practice and research are explored in the discussion.

Methods

A case study format is applied to describe the FSP used to identify and develop strategic telemedicine alliances. The FSP was built on a premise proposed by Luke, Begun and Porter[14] that *loosely coupled* inter-organizational arrangements created to achieve short-term objectives tend to dissolve.[14] In contrast, *loosely coupled* inter-organizational relationships developed for long-term strategic purposes are more likely to last because they are seen by the participating organizations as strategically important.

The process described in the case presentation that follows is intended to ferret out strategic inter-organizational relationships and build on those relationships to develop telemedicine alliances. The FSP is based on eight years of experience in developing telemedicine alliances coupled with on-the-job training and self-study in leadership, change management and community development. Many of the techniques in the FSP use concepts in social exchange theory.[2–10] Following the example of Gagnon and Lamothe *et al.*[18] concepts, theoretical frameworks and practices have been adapted to the specific nature of telemedicine, the healthcare industry and the socio-political environment in which the work described took place.

Participants of the process conducted this study ex post facto. The authors recognize the potential for bias and misinterpretation inherent in self-studies and ex post facto analyses. However, human factor influences on telemedicine utilization and sustainability are largely unexamined. Self-study and ex post facto analysis have been shown to be useful in understanding complex, inter-active or systemic social phenomena, especially relatively innovative and unstudied topics.[19] Case studies are used to identify variables for future study and explore the nature, strength and direction of relationships among variables.[19–21]

Data used in the case study include internal documents – such as grant applications, reports, meeting minutes, internal memorandums and emails – as well as informal interviews and discussions among participants. A review of the literature places the process under study within a theoretical framework and provides a context for discussing the implications of this study for future practice and research.[19]

Case presentation

An FSP used to identify and develop strategic alliances for telemedicine between an academic health science center and health professions programs at three universities is described below. Rationales for undertaking steps and techniques used to accomplish each are explained. The case is then presented and factors that contributed to the case outcomes are proposed.

This process is presented to assist program managers in identifying the key players, designing projects, securing resources, and operating and sustaining telemedicine services. The steps are as follows:

1 build on existing relationships
2 develop co-champions
3 engage the team
4 secure executive commitment
5 gain community support.

Step 1. Build on existing relationships

This step in the process is based on the assumption that the strongest and most lasting telemedicine alliances are often built on existing relationships, the rationale being that there is already a basis for the relationship to exist. Likely, there is a set of shared understandings and a level of trust already established. The relationship may be personal, professional, organizational or community-oriented.

Scan the organization to get a sense of the outreach or community-based activities in which the organization is already involved. These activities may be clinical, educational, research or community service-oriented. Students may be placed in a community practice, clinic or hospital to gain community-based training experience. A good source is an Area Health Education Center (AHEC) or similar community-based organization working to support healthcare professions education. Faculty members may be collaborating on research projects with faculty at another institution. Nursing or allied health programs may be offering distance education degrees at a local college or university. A provider or administrator within the organization may sit on the board of a local company or vice versa.

Questions to be asked are:

- Can the existing relationship be enhanced or expanded with the addition of telemedicine?
- Can that person or organization facilitate introductions to other institutional or community members who may be interested in telemedicine?

Case study scenario 1. Build on existing relationships

University A – prior relationship with HSC well established; attempt to form telemedicine alliance proceeds

In 1994, HSC and the nursing program University A began discussing the feasibility of forming a telemedicine alliance. Eighteen months passed between initial discussions and opening of the clinic in the fall of 1996.[17]

The timing and relationship seemed to be ripe for forming a telemedicine alliance for several reasons. *First*, HSC and University A had been working together successfully for four years to offer the joint nursing degree program (*see* Table 11.2). *Second*, HSC had established a community-based education outreach program – an Area Health Education Center (AHEC) – that opened a regional center in 1991 serving an area encompassing the HSC and University A. Nursing representatives from University A were on the regional center's advisory board and the organizations had collaborated on various education initiatives to the region – including the joint nursing degree program. *Third*, University A had conducted a video-conferencing demonstration in 1993 in cooperation with a public school system. *Fourth*, the nursing program at University A had conducted a needs assessment of public schools in its service area that had revealed the increasing challenge nurses and teachers were facing in coping with the healthcare demands of rising numbers of children with special needs being mainstreamed into the classroom. *Fifth*, the region surrounding University A was a primary source of referrals for the HSC, and specifically, for the pediatric subspecialty interested in providing telemedicine services. *Sixth*, equipment prices had dropped significantly and the state had passed a telecommunications act mandating reduced telecommunication rates for educational institutions and non-profit healthcare.

University B – prior relationship with HSC is guarded; attempt to form telemedicine alliance proceeds after intervention of trusted colleague at University A

HSC and University B initiated a joint nursing degree via video-conferencing immediately following the demonstrations in 1993 (*see* Table 11.2). From the time equipment was installed in January 1994 through the fall 1997, the video-conference system at University B was used solely for the joint nursing degree program. Utilization averaged 25 hours per month or five hours per week for nine months out of the year.

The video-conference system at University B was purchased and managed by the HSC technical group. The dedicated telecommunications line was also paid for by HSC. University B offered to share the cost of the equipment and connectivity, but the HSC declined the offer. The HSC operated and controlled access to the equipment. University B's technical group was refused unsupervised access, prior approval was required before University B could use the system and a fee was invoked if University B wanted to use the system for anything other than the joint nursing degree program. These rules were also applied to the regional AHEC office that operated under a subcontract from HSC to University B. University B housed the equipment and provided classroom space without cost to HSC.

Despite successes with the video-conference demonstration, the joint nursing degree and development of a local AHEC program, policies related to ownership, management, and use of the video-conferencing system inhibited development of additional programs for two and a half years. The rift with the head of nursing at University B was mitigated when the head of nursing at University A shared their success in establishing a telemedicine alliance with the HSC (*see* discussion above). Building on the relationship between the nursing leadership, a telemedicine clinic opened in partnership nursing program at University B in the fall of 1997.

University C – prior relationship with HSC new; attempt to a form telemedicine alliance suspended
HSC and University C initiated a physician assistant[PA] degree program offered via video-conferencing in 1996. The PA program director at University C was approached about forming a telemedicine alliance in 1997. Although one patient was seen through telemedicine, the alliance was never formalized.

The nursing degree and the PA degree were both conferred by the HSC, but the inter-organizational relationships were structured differently. The relationship between the HSC and University C differed from the relationships with the other two universities in *four* ways. *First*, the joint degree program was an undergraduate allied health degree rather than a graduate nursing degree. *Second*, the program director at University C was an employee of the HSC, not University C. In contrast, coordinators for the nursing program at University A and University B were employees of their respective universities *and* students in the joint degree program. *Third*, the PA program was seen as a peripheral program at University C, i.e. members of the health science department did not consider it a part of the university. The nursing degree program was viewed as part of the local nursing units. *Fourth*, University C offered a joint graduate nursing degree with another health science center. University C's nursing program expressed disappointment on learning of HSC efforts to form a telemedicine alliance through the PA program rather than the nursing program – as had been done at the other two universities.

Step 2. Develop co-champions

Identify a power broker and operations leader

Identify two champions in each organization in the proposed alliance. Within the initiating organization, the co-champions should have between them administrative/business expertise, clinical expertise and relationship management skills. In a health provider organization, the champion with clinical expertise is often a physician. This may not be true in non-health organizations such as public schools. The operations leader may come from any part of the organization, but often has community outreach or community development responsibilities.

If the co-champions come from different parts of the organization, they should be able to access the power structure within their respective domains of influence. That is, they should be able to engage the appropriate people from the executive levels of the organization. Also one or both champions should understand or have access to persons with a basic understanding of accepted business practices, clinical operations and technical requirements/capabilities.

Within the target organization, two champions should be identified to assist in alliance development. One champion – referred to as the power broker – should have access to the power structure within the organization and community, again someone who can get the executive level to the table. The other champion should be more oriented towards frontline operations with strong skills and interest in working with patients, students and colleagues – referred to here as operations leader. The two champions must communicate and work well together.

Uncover the value

Numerous meetings, phone calls and/or emails with the power broker may be required to discover the power broker's personal/professional interests in tele-medicine, their organization's interests and the interests of the larger community. They must also understand the potential challenges and opportunities at each of these levels (*see* Figure 11.1).

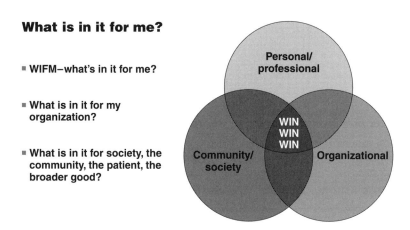

What is in it for me?

- WIFM—what's in it for me?

- What is in it for my organization?

- What is in it for society, the community, the patient, the broader good?

Personal/professional

WIN WIN WIN

Community/society

Organizational

Figure 11.1 Uncover the value.

This is an exploratory process. Often people only have an abstract idea of why they, their organization or community are interested in engaging in telemedicine. Uncovering 'What's in it for me?' (WIFM) at the personal/professional, organizational and community level will help to structure the alliance and design a project that is aligned with the strategic objectives at all levels.

The process of uncovering the value assumes a level of trust, collaborative spirit and creativity among the key players. Each key player should be willing to help others achieve their respective goals. Finding common interests that overlap in personal/professional, organizational and community/societal realms is desirable. The solutions lie where there is a convergence of interests and objectives among the parties and levels.

To uncover the WIFM from others, the co-champions from the initiating organization should reveal theirs first. What attracted them to healthcare, education or public service? How is their role in the organization aligned with their personal values and/or professional aspirations? How might this project support their personal/professional goals while contributing to the organization's mission? Is there an altruistic or public good that will come from the project that is bigger than the individual or organization or community in question? If someone is in academia, are they most interested in teaching, conducting research or providing patient care? How does the organization reward people and for what?

Understand the motivation

The individuals and organizations must be clear about alliance goals (*see* Figure 11.2). Is the alliance being formed to make money? Will the alliance confer prestige or increase individual or organizational power? What is the relative importance of these dimensions of social and economic status to the individual (personally or professionally), to the organization, to the community, region or industry of which the individual and organization is a part?

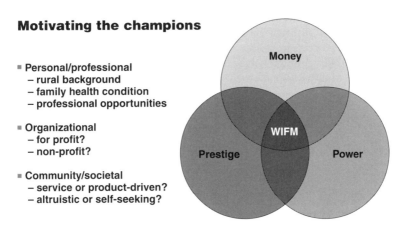

Figure 11.2 Understand the motivation.

As one individual shares their motivation, others will feel comfortable in expressing their own. Everyone has desires and needs. Asking them to explore how this proposed alliance may help them achieve their goals gives legitimacy to their needs while opening the door to engage them in helping find common goals to assure success of the project.

People and organizations are approached differently depending on whether they are interested more by money, power or prestige. Every position, organization and community has varying levels of these dimensions. Each dimension is essential to the success of a project and an alliance.

It is not always necessary to ask what motivates an individual or organization. Sometimes walking into a person's office offers clues as to what they care about. Do they have pictures of powerful people on the wall? Sometimes watching how someone relates in meetings will reveal what they value. Look for cues in conversation. Do they talk a lot about money? About powerful or famous people they know? Again, look for patterns, not isolated instances.

By knowing someone's position title, the relative importance of each of these dimensions can often be inferred. For instance, a chief executive officer (CEO) or chief financial officer (CFO) is probably most concerned about the financial and business impacts of telemedicine, i.e. money or market influence. From the CFO's perspective, prestige and power are likely to be considered only within the context of how these dimensions contribute to the financial picture. A CFO may see telemedicine as simultaneously exposing the organization to the threat of increased competition or expanding market opportunities.

A CEO may be interested in how telemedicine increases the likelihood of recruiting and retaining qualified healthcare professionals. So providing opportunities for collegial exchange, professional consultation, professional education and direct referral access may be important.

Physicians have high prestige, make good money and wield life-determining power. Yet physicians in academia may be more likely to value prestige or power than money. Physicians in private practice may be more motivated by money or power than prestige. Getting to know physicians helps in understanding what they value most.

Do not overlook the technicians, nurses, allied health and administrative staff when exploring motivations. Technicians, for instance, are frequently concerned with control. They are responsible for controlling access to confidential information and guaranteeing reliable service. If they perceive developing a new alliance will create vulnerabilities in their network, they will resist. Many difficulties can be avoided by understanding the interest underlying their resistance.

These dimensions motivate organizations, communities, regions, states and countries as well. It is important to understand how these dimensions drive action in for-profits versus non-profits, economically depressed versus economically prosperous communities, rural versus urban, inner city versus suburbs, academic health centers versus community health centers, young organizations versus established organizations, etc.

Seek to understand, not judge

None of the socioeconomic dimensions (power, money or prestige) are good or bad, or better or worse than each other. The project needs to be visible, well-positioned and solvent. Understanding the relative importance of each dimension for each of the actors – whether the actor is an individual, organization or community – allows for the development of a more strategic alliance, an alliance aligned with the values and objectives of various actors. This will ensure that individuals and organizations are invested in the success of the alliance because the success of the alliance is linked to their success.

Knowing what drives people and organizations also makes it easier to match them to the appropriate role and responsibility within the alliance. Engage those who value prestige in marketing efforts such as newspaper or television coverage.

Engage power brokers in getting upper management support for resources. Engage CFOs in finding the return on investment. Once the 'what's in it for me' (WIFM) in each of these realms (personal/professional, organizational, community/societal) is understood, the champions from initiating and target organizations work together to develop plans formalizing the alliance and implementing the project to meet these interests.

Case study scenario 2. Develop co-champions

Health Science Center co-champions – clinical leader and relationship manager team up to form community alliances

At the HSC, a pediatrician who envisioned using telemedicine to take care of special needs children became the power broker. The operations leader functioned as relationship manager and business leader. The operations leader worked for an HSC outreach organization, Area Health Education Center (AHEC), and had coordinated the three-month demonstration project. The pediatrician participated in the demonstration and concluded that the technology could be used to better serve patients and their families. By the end of the demonstration period, the operations leader had concluded that the technology would be a key strategy for achieving the AHEC mission, which complemented both the educational and clinical goals of the AHEC.

The video-conferencing system purchased by the HSC to support the nursing joint degree program was centrally located on campus and could be used for the pediatric telemedicine clinic. Five hours of clinic per month would be required to meet the need, given the size of the patient population to be served. However, five hours of utilization was too little to justify the investment in equipment and connectivity in the community. Even if the technology investment could be justified, there were no facilities or staff to operate the clinic on the patient end.

Compounding the challenge, the patient population was geographically distributed and was cared for by a variety of independent community providers. A neutral community site was needed to assure that patients of all community providers had equal access.

The relationship operations leader proposed the establishment of the telemedicine clinic in conjunction with the joint nursing degree program. Equipment and a technological link were in place. And the nursing program would not be seen as a competitor to local providers. However, due to the breach between University B and HSC, approaching University B to provide space and staff to operate the clinic was not realistic.

The relationship with University A was good, but they did not have the necessary technology. However, University A was interested in transitioning the ongoing joint degree program from faculty commuting to video-conferencing.

University A co-champions – power broker and operations manager identified; alliance formation proceeds

At University A, the head of nursing served as the power broker. A nursing faculty member who was also a student in the joint degree program was the operations leader.

The head of nursing had been instrumental in bringing the joint degree program to the university and had a vision for enhancing that program by incorporating video-conferencing. The power broker also wanted to start a faculty clinical practice to enhance faculty prestige, maintain faculty practice proficiencies, provide clinical experience for students, and generate revenue and visibility for the institution. The power broker was enthusiastic about providing telemedicine services after recognizing that the telemedicine clinic would provide opportunities for faculty practice and student learning while providing a valuable community service, demonstrating the university's progressiveness and strengthening a valued organizational alliance.

The faculty member who served as the operations leader was enrolled in the joint graduate nursing degree program offered by HSC at University A. With video-conferencing, the learning experience through the distance education program would be enhanced. By running the telemedicine clinic, the operations leader would gain clinical experience and be able to expose nursing students to leading-edge health service delivery technologies. In addition, the faculty member would be an innovative leader among academic peers and within the larger healthcare community.

University B co-champions – power broker and operations manager identified; alliance formation proceeds

At University B, the head of nursing also served as the power broker. As with University A, a faculty member enrolled in the HSC joint degree program at University B served as the operations leader.

Due to the influence of the head of nursing at University A, University B was now interested in initiating a telemedicine clinic. As mentioned earlier, the power broker at University A had brokered initial telemedicine-related discussions between the power broker at University B and the operations leader at HSC. *Second*, the regional office of the AHEC had been working with the head of nursing on health professions education issues. *Third*, the region surrounding University B was a secondary referral area for the HSC, and specifically for the pediatric subspecialty interested in providing telemedicine services. *Fourth*, enough time had passed for the technical group at the HSC to recognize that they needed to remove barriers to access and encourage utilization if they expected the institution and by that time, the AHEC, to continue funding the costs of the connectivity.

The rationale for initiating the telemedicine clinic at University B would differ from University A. The head of nursing at University B saw the telemedicine clinic as an opportunity to strengthen the student service-learning program within the nursing division and to involve all of the health-related programs in the telemedicine alliance.

University C co-champions – operations manager identified, but no power broker; attempts to form alliance discontinued

At University C, the program director for the joint PA degree program was unable to secure a meeting with upper-level administration. As discussions progressed, it became clear that the PA program was peripheral to the health science department, and by association, so was the program director. The peripheral nature of the PA program appeared to be due, in part, to how the PA program was structured within University C. The HSC took total responsibility for the success of the program, including employing separate program staff.

In addition, the nursing program expressed resentment in not being chosen over the PA as the point of contact for forming the alliance and operating the clinic. The long-standing competition between nurse practitioner and PA programs may have accounted for some of the difficulties.

The program director could have functioned effectively as the operations expert. But without a power broker to engage and solidify institutional support, cope with departmental politics between the nurse practitioner and PA programs, and represent community interests and concerns, efforts to develop the alliance were discontinued.

Once the co-champions from each organization are identified, the goals and objectives are clear, and rough estimates of costs are determined, the power brokers from each organization should informally vet the project with each organization's leadership. At this stage the alliance is moving from concept to design. It is important to inform key leadership about the project prior to reaching throughout the organization to pull a project team together. If the leadership has a concern, it should be addressed up front. Also, as a courtesy, the leadership should never be the 'last to know'.

Step 3. Engage the team

Both strategic and business planning was undertaken to provide a long-range, comprehensive approach and optimize all investments in infrastructure, human resources, hardware, software and skills, and to minimize redundancy and waste.[17] Through strategic planning, a common vision, goals and priorities were developed and then communicated among all levels of the telemedicine team, throughout the universities, within the community. Business planning efforts included a thorough needs assessment, early and ongoing user input, and a clear understanding of the existing healthcare delivery system serving the targeted population. In planning for installation and purchase of the technology components, factors considered included: the rapidly changing nature of the technology, the architecture and design of clinic facilities and training for staff utilizing the technology.

The next step involves assembling and engaging the project team. The project team works together to flesh out the implementation plan, clearly articulating what is to be accomplished, how, where, when, by whom and how to sell the project within and outside each of the alliance organizations. Anyone within the alliance member organizations whose role or responsibility will be impacted by the development of the alliance and/or provision of the telemedicine service should be considered a part of the project team. The co-champions at each organization are responsible for identifying the appropriate people and discussing the project with them. If needed, the co-champions will set up a meeting with the other alliance organizations to discuss the project, its impact on their area of concern and the role they will assume or the action needed. People who may need to be involved include technical support as well as anyone concerned with medical records, security and privacy, risk management, contract management, space allocation, etc. However, given the central importance of technical experts to the success of the project, the rest of this section will focus on engaging them. The same principles can be applied to other people who will play a key role in the project.

Each pair of champions should introduce the project to the technical leaders within their respective organizations and ask them to attend a technical planning meeting. The purpose of the technical meeting is threefold. *First*, the co-champions and the technical people at each organization should understand the existing technical capabilities at the other alliance organizations.

Second, the technical people should understand what the co-champions want to accomplish and with whom, so that they can understand the value and the importance of their role. The technical people will be responsible for selecting the technology appropriate to the need, providing cost estimates, purchasing, installing and maintaining the technology once the telemedicine service is implemented. It is not uncommon for the champions of a telemedicine project to bypass the internal technical team. Vendors will cooperate because their interest is in selling their equipment or service. The technical people are then called after the equipment or service is purchased – or worse still – they find out during or after installation when the vendor has gone away and users are experiencing difficulty.

Third, rapport needs to be built between the technical people from each organization in order to become a functional team. Often the difficulties encountered during or after installation are impossible to diagnose in isolation. If the technical teams from the alliance organizations do not have a good working relationship, the project suffers eventually affecting patient care.

Again, the technicians from the telemedicine provider organization should work with technicians at the target organization to increase the knowledge level and expertise at the local level. This enhances the level of technical support available and increases the status of the local technical support within their respective organizations. This person will be invaluable as the project progresses and valuable to the alliance organization and community where there is likely to be a shortage of skilled technicians.

Case study scenario 3. Engage project team

Health Science Center project team

Before arriving at the decision to establish a telemedicine alliance, executive levels at each university and representatives from each of the functional areas of the proposed telemedicine team – from administrators to practitioners to technicians – were engaged in planning efforts. The Area Health Education Center (AHEC) led planning efforts. Once the decision was made to move forward, the project was vetted within the institution. The power broker/clinical champion briefed the clinical department, operations/business leader touched base with the AHEC leadership, and the technical leader contacted the business and finance area. Once the project goals had been well defined and the project had been vetted with key leadership, the technical teams from participating organizations were brought together to put together a more detailed technical plan.

At the HSC, a nurse practitioner and member of the pediatric healthcare team familiar with the healthcare team and the operation of the standard clinic, became key to the success of ongoing clinical operations. Once the clinic was implemented, the nurse practitioner spearheaded day-to-day operations of the clinic. The operations leader continued to focus on managing the interorganizational relationships and developing new applications to increase utilization and strengthen the alliance.

The HSC technical team had gained considerable experience in the year and a half since the video-conference demonstration project. The technical leadership now recognized the need to welcome technicians from away sites onto the team rather than establishing boundaries. The technical team at the HSC provided overall technical design and support, but worked with the technical experts at the universities to integrate the new technology into their environment and realm of responsibility.

University A project team

At University A, the nursing department had a nursing informatics expert interested in the technology. Perhaps more importantly, the informatics expert was interested in how to use the technology most effectively within the clinical and educational setting. Consequently, University A's technical expert became intimately involved in setting up and supporting the clinic and distance education classroom. Once the clinic was operational, the expert continued to be involved in operating the video-conference equipment and managing the cameras until standardized practices were established.

To foster the relationship between the technical groups at the HSC and University A, one of the co-champions at the HSC arranged for University A's technical staff to spend two weeks with HSC technical staff to learn more about the technology and how to provide technical support for telemedicine and distance education activities.

University B project team

At University B, the nursing division did not have dedicated technical assistance. Due to the early breach between the HSC and University B technical groups, the nursing division at University B was never able to engage the technical group at University B in supporting the project. The 'hands-off' policy regarding HSC equipment had become entrenched. Consequently, the HSC continued to provide technical support for the equipment at University A. Given the HSC technical support was limited to making sure the equipment was operational, the nurse operating the clinic was left without a technician to operate the camera. This increased the nurse's stress and resulted in a less efficient clinic.

University C project team

At University C, the technical group was ready and willing. Video-conferencing equipment was already in place for the joint PA degree program. However, because a power broker was never identified, the project never received the necessary blessing from University A's leadership or the broader community. The business champion at the initiating organization felt the power broker was essential to overcoming the barriers within the institution that we discussed earlier and the challenge in the broader healthcare community that will be discussed later.

Once the plan is in place, the target organization's champions convene the remaining meetings. The initiating organization offers support and helps develop strategy, but the local champions spearhead the initiative within their realm of influence. The co-champions from the initiating organization are guests and helpers in the process.

This point is critical and may be difficult to achieve given the relative importance of power, money and prestige to each of the players from the initiating organization. It is difficult to take the second chair when the initiating organization champions believe they know more about telemedicine or have a greater stake in the care to be provided. However, the target organization knows more about the community's healthcare system and local politics. Furthermore, when the initiating organization's champions go back home, someone in the community will need to continue advocating the alliance and its initiatives and troubleshooting when issues arise.

Therefore, the local champions must become the knowledgeable promoters for the alliance within their organization and community. It is the initiating organization's responsibility to position the local champions for this purpose. The local champions must understand enough to approach leadership within their organization and community and be seen as knowledgeable, trustworthy and reliable.

Step 4. Secure executive commitment

Once the champions at both organizations are comfortable with the implementation plan, they arrange for an executive briefing with the leadership inside their organizations. The purpose of the executive briefing is to:

- educate the leadership so they are able to talk knowledgeably about the project with community members
- answer any lingering questions
- introduce leadership to key players and leadership from other alliance organizations
- to get their blessing to move forward.

During this meeting the leadership from the alliance organizations formally and publicly agree to participate. Hopefully, by this meeting, all questions will have been answered so that there will be no surprises. This meeting boosts morale and lifts team spirit as support for the project is demonstrated from the top of the organization down through the operational level. The commitment that is being solidified with this executive briefing could be an agreement to seek funding, deploy infrastructure, expand existing services, etc.

Case study scenario 4. Secure executive commitment

Health Science Center executive commitment

At HSC, the telemedicine initiative grew as a collaborative effort of the clinical department and the Area Health Education Center (AHEC). The clinical department provided the clinical service. The AHEC provided the business acumen and community ties. The technical team was key to project success because they provided the communication vehicle through which services were delivered and the alliance was strengthened. Therefore, commitment was required from all three functional areas. Within the clinical department, the department chair and vice president for clinical affairs approved the project. Within the AHEC, the director of the program and the dean/vice president for academic affairs signed off. For the technical group, the vice president for business affairs agreed to the project. Finally, the president/CEO and/or his representative were included in any key meeting, correspondence or decision. This was done through individual meetings and communications through each key player's chain of command. The pediatrician/power broker and business leader worked together to keep the president's office informed.

University A executive commitment

At University A, representatives from the HSC met with University A's leadership to outline the proposed project, discuss commitments, opportunities and challenges, and gain executive sign off for moving forward. Attendees from the HSC included the pediatrician/power broker, operations leader, technical leader and a spokesperson from the office of the chief executive. Attendees from University A included the dean of nursing/power broker, operations, leader, informatics expert, chief executive leadership from University A's other health-related departments and technical support department, and key leaders up the dean of nursing chain of command, including the chief executive.

University B executive commitment
At University B, the executive briefing was similar to the briefing at University A with a few exceptions. *First*, the power broker and operations leader at University A joined the executive briefing at University B for about 20 minutes via video-conferencing. They spoke to University B's leadership from a common perspective and were able to vouch for HSC intent and integrity. *Second*, given pre-existing equipment and the lack of involvement of the University B's technical group in project planning, only the executive over the technical area was involved in the executive briefing. The technical area executive gave his blessing, but provided no active support.

University C executive commitment

At University C, the project never made it to this stage because a power broker who could get key people to the table was never identified.

Step 5. Gain community support

The last step in alliance formation is gaining the support of stakeholders in the community. The purpose of the community briefing is to gain the support, or understand the opposition, of community members capable of influencing the success or failure of the project. Champions identify relevant community members based on their participation in, or knowledge of, the healthcare community and local politics. The community members are briefed about the project, attempts are made to address any concerns before the project begins and support for the project is sought. Again, the meeting is convened by the local champions with the participation and support of members of the initiating organization if appropriate.

Case study scenario 5. Gain community support

Health Science Center community support

At HSC, the community being targeted was the broader HSC community. An open house was held to celebrate the kick-off of the telemedicine alliance with University A. Representatives from the highest level of the institution were involved, including representatives from the school of nursing, the department of pediatrics and the Area Health Education Center (AHEC). Representatives from University A participated in the open house via video-conferencing. The alliance with University B was announced less formally (emails, phone calls, hallway discussions). The broader HSC community was already familiar with the idea of establishing a telemedicine alliance in conjunction with a distance education program. The technology had been in place and was being used by the nursing school for some years now. Anyone affected by the expansion had been involved in discussions prior to the start of the clinic.

University A community support

At University A, an evening dinner briefing was held where the dean of nursing/power broker invited primary care practitioners in the community – some of whom cared for children being seen by the pediatric subspecialist. Key leadership from University A was present to hear community providers' reactions and communicate support for the project.

The community briefing was held after the equipment had been installed. Consequently, the pediatrician was able to attend by video-conference, which saved the physician travel and served to demonstrate the technology to community practitioners. The nurse practitioner who served as the telemedicine clinic manager at the HSC traveled to University A for the briefing.

University B community support

At University B, the director of nursing/power broker chose to have the operations leader/telemedicine clinic manager and the director from the local AHEC's office visit individually with key practitioners in the community. As with the community briefing at University A, the project was described, questions were answered and any concerns were relayed back to the director of nursing. All physicians visited were supportive and no further action was needed.

University C community support

At University C, this step was never taken. However, regional health system politics played a major role in this project not getting off of the ground. Recall that University C is located in community of 30 000, but a metropolitan area of over 500 000. There are four primary populations centers in the region. Healthcare competition among these four neighboring communities is intense. Because the region is fairly heavily populated but medically underserved, there was a movement in the region to establish a regional academic health center. All four communities were vying for it to be located in their locale. Compounding the politics, three health science centers in the state were vying for the contract to establish the regional academic health center. The HSC attempting to initiate the telemedicine alliance was one of them. While the telemedicine alliance was being undertaken independently of the regional academic health center initiative, University C and community leaders were suspicious. Attempts to further develop the alliance were postponed indefinitely.

Within a year of implementing the second telemedicine clinic, the HSC and the two universities partnered to expand services to two public schools in each of their service regions (*see* Table 11.2). The next year, the HSC and University B partnered again to add mental health, maternal child health and asthma to their activities.

With each expansion, the champion power broker from each of the universities took the lead in developing additional alliances in their regions. As in the initial phase of alliance development, the local champions repeated the FSP. They:

- built on existing relationships in the schools
- identified and developed co-champions within the alliance member organization
- engaged a project team – which at a minimum included a technical member along with the schools' co-champions
- worked with the co-champions to secure executive commitment
- gained community support.

In the project with the schools, community support included parents as well as the healthcare community.

Results

The FSP described in this case study was used to identify and develop strategic alliances for telemedicine among an academic health science center and health professions programs at three universities. Telemedicine services were successfully implemented with two out of the three attempted alliances. The third alliance was never implemented due to the absence of structural mechanisms to support sustainability and lack of strategic alignment between the organizations.

The academic health science center and both alliance members that successfully implemented telemedicine later expanded to include two school systems in each of their regions. The first telemedicine alliance is being sustained, but has not grown since expansion with the schools. The second alliance continues to grow adding mental health, maternal and child health, and asthma programs to their activities in 2000 (*see* Table 11.2).

All five steps in the process were carried out with the two alliances that implemented telemedicine. Development of the third alliance were discontinued in Step 2 (develop co-champions) of the process after it became evident that completing Step 4 (secure executive commitment) and Step 5 (gain community support) was not feasible. The FSP was used again in expanding the alliance to include the local school systems within each of the alliance member's service regions. Each time the process was used, the length of time taken to complete the process was reduced.

Discussion

The FSP is intended to assist program managers in identifying the key players, designing projects, securing resources, and operating and sustaining telemedicine services. Specifically, the process is designed to accomplish two objectives:

identify organizations appropriate for exploring a telemedicine alliance; and guide the development of alliances that assure ongoing telemedicine utilization and assure long-term sustainability.

The process was used to build strategic alliances between an academic health science center and health professions programs at three universities. The first telemedicine alliance is being sustained, but is not growing. The second alliance continues to grow and thrive. Attempts to develop a third alliance were suspended during the second step of the process when it became evident that organizational support could not be engendered for the project.

The process was developed between 1992 through 2000 based on the combined experiences of the authors. Participants of the process conducted this study ex post facto. The authors recognize the potential for bias and misinterpretation inherent in self-studies and ex post facto analyses. However, human factor influences on telemedicine utilization and sustainability are largely unexamined. Self-study and ex post facto analysis have been shown to be useful in understanding complex, interactive, or systemic social phenomena, especially relatively innovative and unstudied topics.[19] It is hoped that this case study will be useful in identifying variables for future study and provide some indication of the nature, strength and direction of relationships among variables.[19–21]

In addition, the organizations studied here are an academic health science center and three health professions education programs in university settings. The authors recognize the establishment of telemedicine clinics in the general academic setting rather than more traditional clinical or hospital settings is novel. The study focused on organizations in the southwestern United States in rural and smaller metropolitan medical markets. The generalizability of this process to more traditional organizational settings, geographic areas and medical markets is an open question.

Nevertheless, the literature review below will reveal that many of the principles behind the FSP have been recognized as important to the development of strategic interorganizational relationships.

Theoretical framework

An amalgamation of concepts from organization,[14,22–24] diffusion,[25–27,29–31] social exchange[2–9] and social stratification theory[2,6,28] form the underpinnings of the FSP. The concepts of inter-organizational relationships, social exchange, intellectual capital, product champions and socioeconomic status are discussed below.

Interorganizational relationships

Luker et al.[14] suggest that loosely coupled inter-organizational relationships developed for long-term strategic purposes are more likely to be sustained than those created to achieve short-term objectives. They refer to this organizational type as a quasi firm.

Quasi firms, they argue, pursue common strategic objectives with the hope of gaining operational efficiencies, capturing advantages of scale, increasing market share, or to segment the market. Cordero-Guzman[23] suggests inter-organizational relationships may be formed to foster organizational learning, acquire status or legitimacy, provide economic benefits, facilitate the management of resource dependencies and provide autonomy for employees.[24]

Referring to Mintzberg,[37] Luker *et al.*[14] point out that if quasi firms are to function effectively, 'they must acquire a capacity for making strategic decisions or, in other terms, they must form a functional strategic apex'. Within the framework of the FSP, the operations leader who primarily focused on relationship management among the organizations formed the strategic apex for the telemedicine alliances formed. Luker *et al.* rightly state that quasi firms require the investment of considerable resources and effort to achieve inter-organizational coordination in the pursuit of strategic objectives.

One of the questions this raises is whether the telemedicine coordinating office should serve as the strategic apex for telemedicine alliances. That is, if the telemedicine coordinating office serves as the structural mechanism supporting strategic decision making, strategy implementation and boundary maintenance, will the continued functioning of the strategic alliances be insured?

Social exchange

Hu *et al.*[7] argue that the motivation for forming intra- and inter-organizational structures in telemedicine can be found in exchange theory. Social exchange theory holds that reciprocity is required to maintain social relationships.[2,6,23] If resources are not mutually and equitably invested, the relationship is likely to end. Extrinsic (money, goods, services) and intrinsic (reputation, love, honor, duty, beauty) assets are recognized as having value in an exchange.[6]

Social exchange theorists recognize that actors – individuals, organizations, societies – are willing to incur costs and imbalances in their exchange relations when those relations are thought to be long-lasting.[3,9] However, mutual trust, understanding and respect are essential to forming long-lasting relationships.[23,24]

Sheppard[32] and Bandura[33] claim that social actors are motivated to commit to a relationship when they perceive that their contributions are identified as being important to the broader community and personally relevant, and that there is a clear relationship between contribution and outcome.[8] Cordero-Guzman[23] refer to Keyes *et al.*[34] in arguing that inter-organizational relationships are more likely to be sustained when there is a long-term relationship of trust and reciprocity, a shared vision among the organizations, mutual interest in the relationship and a financial nexus that ties the groups together. Cordero-Guzman[23] found six reasons inter-organizational relationships were formed in his study of community-based organizations:

- customer demand for increased services
- exchange of expertise
- to provide additional resources
- to reduce and/or share costs
- increased access to opportunities
- to enhance visibility and reputation.

Jackson and Clark[21] examined situational and structural characteristics associated with perceived effectiveness. Situational characteristics used included coalition size, coalition type, resource dependence, awareness, consensus and domain. Structural characteristics included resource flows, formalization, communication frequency and communication quality. They found the best predictors of perceived effectiveness of collaborations were consensus, formalization of agreements and resource dependence.

Cordero-Guzman[23] suggests the following 13 factors are associated with successful inter-organizational relationships:

- selection criteria for participation
- mutual respect, understanding and trust
- inclusive planning process
- members with a stake in the process and outcome
- concrete activities requiring joint effort
- community involvement
- effective consensus-building and conflict resolution strategies
- clear roles and policies
- open and frequent communication that is both formal and informal
- clearly define the service area and population to be served
- visible, early successes
- concrete, long-term goals and objectives
- exit strategy for handling organizational members that leave.

Intellectual capital

Coleman[4] introduced the concept of social capital in exchange theory in 1990.[4,35] According to Coleman, 'Social capital . . . is created when the relations among actors [sic] change in ways that facilitate action'. Social capital is often 'a by-product of activities engaged in for other purposes'. Public goods, which would not be in an actor's self-interest to create, are often created as a by-product of relationships entered into because they have direct rewards for the actor.

Taug[10] incorporated social capital into the concept of intellectual capital. He argues that intellectual capital includes human capital, relational capital – sometimes referred to as *social capital* – and structural capital. Human capital consists of the 'combined skills, experiences, insights and education of organization members'. Structural capital is the 'procedures, norms, routines and rules that make up the organizational system'. Relational capital – or social capital – is the 'web of relations between people and groups of people associated with the organization'. According to Taug,[10] a synergy among two or more intellectual capital resources results in value creation that is greater than the sum of the resources acting alone.

Product champions

The importance of product champions in overcoming barriers and resistance when introducing new products or services into the market has been extensively touted and less often researched.[29–31] The role of clinical champions in the adoption and diffusion of telemedicine has been generally accepted.[20,25] Tanriverdi and Iacono[25] argue that the success of telemedicine programs depends on a champion's ability to lower technical, economic, organizational and behavioral barriers.

In a review of literature on champions, Markham and Aiman-Smith[30] found that the majority of projects have champions and a large percentage have multiple champions. They found product champions are associated with about 80–90% of new product projects. There is a strong positive relationship between project survival and presence of champions. However, product champions do not guarantee market success. Champions support projects when there is a potential benefit to their own department. They may come from any level or functional area of the organization. They materially affect the strategic direction of research and development. They are visionary, calculated, risk takers who are politically astute and attentive to organizational direction and strategy. They gain organizational support for the project along with commitments of resources, space and time. They often provoke antagonists that, if embraced, often force the champion to think though the project, making it stronger. They are sensitive to organizational politics and are likely to become involved in projects that are innovative. The authors put forth some recommendations for managing champions:

- work with champions to assure strategic alignment with subunits of the organization as well as the overall institutional mission
- encourage champions to become involved in relevant professional communities
- seek out an antagonist to balance the champion
- provide champions with training and development in managing interpersonal relationships.

Roure[29] studied the influence of product champions' position and seniority in the highly hierarchical organizations of France versus the flat decentralized organizations of Germany. He found that product champions must have considerable power and prestige in highly hierarchical organizations, but these qualities are less important in flat, decentralized organizations where employees feel close to their superiors.

Reilly et al.[31] suggest the following are desirable personality traits for champions:

- openness (unconventional/curios)
- emotional stability (cohesive; predictable)
- agreeableness (social interaction; cooperation)
- conscientiousness (project management; dependable)
- extraversion (relationship management).

Socioeconomic dimensions

Max Weber introduced the three socioeconomic dimensions of money, power, and prestige in his theory of social stratification.[2] He argued that these dimensions shape a person's choice of, and approach to, work. Phelan and Link[28] found that financial resources, knowledge, power, prestige and social connections are among the mix of social factors that shape a person's health.

These dimensions were incorporated into the framework of social exchange theory and used to understand the motivations of various actors (individuals, organizations, communities, society) in developing strategic alliances. Borrowing from Taug,[10] the FSP creates a knowledge exchange thereby generating shared intellectual capital.

Adoption and diffusion

Helitzer et al.[26] rely on Rogers'[27] theory of diffusion to outline the necessary convergence of decisions from societal, organizational and individual. Gagnon et al.[18] recognize the need to explore individual, professional, organizational and contextual dimensions that have influenced the adoption of telehealth in Quebec. Drake[13] reports that the Institute of Medicine report[36] recognizes the need to consider multiple perspectives in assessing the value of telemedicine. These perspectives include clinical, institutional and system or societal. Tanriverdi and Iacono[25] recognize the economic (societal), organizational and behavioral (individual) barriers that inhibit the adoption and diffusion of telemedicine.

Future research and practice

It is hoped that the FSP, if carried out fully, will lead to the development of strategic telemedicine alliances that result in ongoing utilization and sustainability of telemedicine services. In such alliances, risks will be distributed, resources are shared, and the technology will be used for multiple purposes (administrative, educational, clinical) and across various applications (pediatrics, mental health, asthma). Alliance leadership will understand the risks and opportunities involved, and the people implementing telemedicine will have the resources and commitment to succeed. Whether an individual, organization or community, each actor will understand how telemedicine aligns with respective missions and strategic directions of all of the actors.

Furthermore, this process is not undertaken in isolation of the other *layers of human factor influences* discussed in the editorial commentary of this book.[1] Rather, the process is guided by and draws from the various layers of influence. Therefore, it is necessary to explore how the other layers of human factors influence strategic alliance development.

For alliances to be strategic, the *cultural, institutional and professional contexts* of participating organizations must be considered.[29] *Technological innovations* may not be appropriate for needs, and when they are, organizational resources must be dedicated and new skills developed.[25] *Change management* issues arise with the introduction of technologies and new methods of healthcare delivery, which have consequences for existing policies, procedures, and work practices throughout participating organizations.[25] The *mental model and clinical perspective* of healthcare professionals affect their interest and willingness to participate in telemedicine.[25] They are influenced by organizational incentives or disincentives for participation. Finally, *organizational learning and success* is key to sustaining an initiative as staff turnover and new opportunities arise.[25]

Acknowledgements

The authors thank Paula Simpson for editing a prior version of this manuscript and Jothi Sudhagar Ravindran for assisting with the literature search. Both are with the School of Nursing at Texas Tech Health Science Center. The authors also recognize Michael Chalambaga, Lamar University, for his assistance in developing the project.

References

1 Bangert DC and Doktor R (eds) (2005) *Human and Organizational Dynamics in e-Health.* Radcliffe Publishing, Oxford and Seattle.

2   Coser L (1977) *Masters of Sociological Thought: ideas in historical and social context* (2e). Merton RK (ed.). Harcourt Brace Jovanovich, New York.

3   Homans G (1961) *Social Behavior: its elementary forms*. Harcourt Brace Jovanovich, New York.

4   Blau P (1964) *Exchange and Power in Social Life*. Wiley, New York.

5   Coleman J (1990) *Foundation of Social Theory*. Belknap, Cambridge.

6   Poloma MM (1979) *Contemporary Sociological Theory*. Macmillan Publishing Co., New York.

7   Hu P, Liu S and Wei C (1996) A framework for investigating impacts of telemedicine. *Proceedings of the Americas Conference on Information Systems*, August, Phoenix, Arizona. Available at hsb.Baylor.edu/ramsower/ais.ac.96/papers/hu.htm; accessed 11 March 2004.

8   Tiwana A and Bush A (2000) Peer-to-peer valuation as a mechanism for reinforcing active learning in virtual communities: actualizing social exchange theory. *Proceedings of the 33rd Hawaii International Conference on System Sciences*, 4–7 January, Maui, Hawaii.

9   Scott J (2000) Rational choice theory. In: Browning G, Halcli A, Hewlett N *et al.* (eds) *Understanding Contemporary Society: theories of the present*. Sage Publications, London.

10 Taug J (2003) Reflections on organizational theory, knowledge and relations. Fielding Institute, Santa Barbara, California, Available at www.taug.no/article/articleprint/89/-1/12/; accessed 11 March 2004.

11 Seale D (1995) Golden Crescent Interactive Network: building a rural information super highway. *Texas Journal of Rural Health.* **June**: 78–88.

12 Grigsby J, Rigby M, Hiemstra A *et al.* (2002) The diffusion of telemedicine. *Telemedicine Journal and e-health.* **8**(1): 79–94.

13 Drake DE (2003) Evaluating telemedicine: a literature review. *eHealth International.* Available at ehealthinternational.net/pdf/evaluating_telemed.pdf; accessed 12 March 2004.

14 Luke R, Begun J and Pointer D (1989) Quasi firms: strategic interorganizational forms in the health care industry. *Academy of Management Review.* **14**(1): 9–19.

15 Seale D, Shelton S and Scott D (1993) *UTMB Televideo Demonstration*. University of Texas Medical Branch, Galveston, TX.

16 Robinson S and Seale D (1998) Pediatric telemedicine. In: Viegas S and Dunn K (eds) *Telemedicine: practicing in the information age*. Lippincott-Raven Publishers, Philadelphia, PA.

17 Green A, Esperat C, Seale D *et al.* (2000) The evolution of a distance education initiative into a major telehealth project. *Nursing and Health Care Perspectives.* **March/April**: 66–70.

18 Gagnon M, Lamothe L, Fortin J *et al.* (2004) The Impact of Organizational Characteristics on Telehealth Adoption by Hospitals. *Proceedings of the 37th Hawaii International Conference on System Sciences*, 5–8 January. IEEE Computer Society Press, Big Island, Hawaii.

19 Babbie E (1979) *The Practice of Social Research*. Wadsworth Publishing Company, Belmont, CA.

20 Al-Qirim N (2003) Teledermatology: the case of adoption and diffusion of tele-medicine Health Waikato in New Zealand. *Telemedicine Journal and e-health.* **9**(2): 167–77.

21 Jackson D and Clark R (1996) Predictors of effectiveness of collaborative relationships of the USDA youth at risk coalitions. *Journal of Extension.* **34**(6): 30–7.

22 Weick K (1976) Educational organizations as loosely coupled systems. *Administrative Science Quarterly.* **21**: 1–19.

23 Cordero-Guzman H (2001) *Interorganizational Networks Among Community-Based Organizations*. Community Development Research Center. Robert J Milano Graduate School of Management and Urban Policy, New School University New York, NY.

24   Podolny JM and Page KL (1998) Network forms of organization. *Annual Review of Sociology.* **24**: 57–76.

25   Tanriverdi H and Iacono C (1999) Diffusion of telemedicine: a knowledge barrier perspective. *Telemedicine Journal.* **5**(3): 223–44.

26   Helitzer D, Heath D, Maltrud K *et al.* (2003) Assessing or predicting adoption of telehealth using the diffusion of innovations theory: a practical example from a rural program in New Mexico. *Telemedicine Journal and e-health.* **9**(2): 179–87.

27   Rogers EM (1995) *Diffusion of Innovations.* The Free Press, New York.

28   Phelan J and Link B (2003) When income affects outcome: socioeconomic status and health. *Research Profiles.* **6**. A National Program of The Robert Wood Johnson Foundation. Rutgers, The State University of New Jersey and Institute for Health, Health Care Policy and Aging Research, New Brunswick, NJ.

29   Roure L (1999) Cultural differences in product champions' characteristics: a comparison of France and Germany. *Centre de Recherche DMSP.* Dauphine Marketing Strategie Prospective, pp. 1–24.

30   Markham S and Aiman-Smith L (2001) Product champions: truths, myths and management. *Research-Technology Management.* **May–June**: 44–50.

31   Reilly R, Lynn G and Aronson Z (2002) The role of personality in new product development team performance. *Journal of Engineering and Technology Management.* **19**: 39–58.

32   Shepperd J (1993) Productivity loss in performance groups: a motivation analysis. *Psychological Bulletin.* **113**: 67–81.

33   Bandura A (1995) *Self-Efficacy in Changing Societies.* Cambridge University Press, Cambridge.

34   Keyes L, Schwartz A, Vidal A *et al.* (1996) Networks and nonprofits: opportunities and challenges in an era of federal devolution. *Housing Policy Debate.* **7**(2): 201–30.

35   Frank A (1995) *Supplementary Course Notes on Exchange Theory and Rational Choice Theory for Sociology 333, Contemporary Sociological Theory.* Department of Sociology, University of Calgary. Available at www.ucalgary.ca/~frank/exchange.html; accessed 10 March 2004.

36   Committee on Evaluating Clinical Applications of Telemedicine, Division of Health Care Services, Institute of Medicine (1996) *Telemedicine: A guide to assessing telecommunications in healthcare.* Field MJ (ed.). National Academy Press, Washington, DC, p. 147.

37   Mintzberg H (1979) *The Structuring of Organizations.* Prentice-Hall, Englewood Cliffs, NJ.

Section 6

Mental models and the clinical
perspective in e-health

Chapter 12

Telemedicine in emergencies

Colin F Mackenzie, Yan Xiao, David Lam, Peter Hu and Claudia Oglivie

Introduction

This article reviews the human factors associated with real-time, distributed medical decision making, the telecommunication mode that is likely to occur in wartime or other emergency states. We address two questions, one general to distributed decision making, the other specific to medical application of real-time decision making using telecommunication technology in emergencies. The objectives of describing real-time distributed medical decision making are to:

- characterize the relative importance and priority of certain medical information for remote decision making
- to assess the impact of domain expertise (surgeons, anesthesiologists, nurses) on information gathering and data interpretation
- to determine how medical performance could be evaluated or mentored remotely and identify uncertainties among remote decision makers viewing events through multimedia telecommunication links
- to make recommendations that have implications for the design of medical telecommunications in support of real-time distributed decision making.

Moray has suggested that causes and effects of errors in a system should start with steps that reduce and control the local issue of the workspace layout and ergonomics before tackling more complex and difficult-to-correct issues such as individual and team behaviors. Similarly with telemedicine, the correct images from the observation points must be used with optimal recording of verbalizations before being able to assess individual and team performance. Organizational, legal, societal and cultural pressures are the outer layer of Moray's onion model.[1] This book is designed to present each layer of this onion and to examine its interrelationship with all the other layers.

Review of distributed decision making

Telemedicine provides or supports clinical care at a distance from the provider who is co-located with the patient, by use of electronic communication and information. The provision and support of clinical care is achieved through audio, data and imagery transfer between the co-located provider and the remotely situated provider or supporter of clinical decision making. How distance impacts the abilities of the remotely situated clinical decision maker to perceive the same cues and understand the dynamics and coordination of the co-located providers is unclear. The effects of distance on performance of widely distributed decision making is of importance for situations, such as wartime, disasters, chemical or biologic weapons attack, when dynamic, real-time decision making about medical triage, resource management and coordination of rescue efforts (for example, military, fire, emergency medical services [EMS]) will be needed.

This review of the background of distributed decision making considers the situation when telecommunications will be used dynamically, for remote emergency medical decision making. We believe that in the future, real-time telemedicine communication links will be used for monitoring medical performance, just-in-time training, task-specific telementoring as well as coordination of medical responses (in the broadest sense, for example, triage, resource management, etc.) in wartime, disasters, chemical and biologic attack and other emergencies.

Such distributed decision making is a research paradigm for understanding organizational and group decision making when members are distributed in several senses including: physical location, access to information, authority, expertise and access to resources. Field military medicine missions in wartime, in disasters or secondary to terrorist activity are prime examples of distributed decision making, as collaborating members are distributed in all of these five senses. Telecommunication advances in recent decades have overcome many of the technical barriers to communication over distance and time. Increasingly, telecommunication systems have become an integral part of many professions, enabling remotely located individuals to collaborate on problem solving with expertise unavailable locally. Yet our understanding of how people work together when using communication technologies has been lacking.[2-4] Interesting and challenging research issues arise and surprising uses of telecommunication systems for medical decision making and problem solving occur. For example, the agent used in the Sarin attack in the Tokyo subway was diagnosed by a Japanese physician with knowledge of previous organophosphorous poisonings, seeing the poisoned victims' responses on television news coverage. Telecommunication advances enable remotely situated individuals to collaborate on problem solving with expertise that is not available locally.

Communication and shared mental models

Lack of a shared situational awareness is one of the difficulties in using telemedicine communications to facilitate provision of, or support for, clinical care from a distance. Medical providers co-located with the patient share information through many verbal and non-verbal means. These medical providers have often worked together previously and they know the domain and the context of the current situation, whereas remotely situated decision makers are very unlikely to have trained with the co-located providers or know them, because they may be making the telemedicine communications to this location for the first time. How such remotely situated experts can rapidly get up to the same, or an acceptable level, of understanding to communicate and coordinate activities with the co-located care providers remains uncertain. In order to understand how this can best be achieved from a distance, we first need to understand how such communication and coordination occurs among co-located medical care providers.

The shared mental model[5,6] is an emerging concept to capture how co-located members of a team could function together, often with little overt communication. The underlying assumptions are that team members, through training, experience and communication, achieve congruent mental models of the current situation, choices available, relevant goals and future steps. Xiao *et al.* described several ways in which co-located medical team members were able to coordinate without explicit communication.[7,8] Serfaty *et al.* described the effect of workload on communication processes.[9] Under high workload, team members adopt strategies that reduce the need for explicit communications.

These studies all demonstrate that in highly trained teams with experienced members, communication patterns varied and there are ways for leaders to exert influence without explicit communication. In contrast to many previous studies on leadership, verbal activities are usually the only ways in which leaders function. Such difference would have direct bearing on the potential impact of new communication technologies on leadership.

Verbal communications have often been studied as the major form of coordination process.[10] The concept of 'implicit coordination' was introduced when teams were found to be able to coordinate with reduced communications,[9] especially under high workload situations. To investigate factors promoting implicit coordination, it has been hypothesized that 'shared mental models', or *shared* understanding of goals and tasks, is a key, since division of labor in most work settings may have prevented team members from understanding other people's tasks. Volpe *et al.* tested this hypothesis,[11] and found that cross training, in which team members were trained in other people's tasks, improved team performance by prompting implicit coordination. The concepts of shared mental models and implicit coordination and related empirical data highlight the issue of communication cost. When workload and time pressure are high, reducing the cost or workload related to communication has obvious advantages.[12] If it is important for team members to share an understanding of each other's tasks and goals, which are relatively stable, it is equally important for team members to be aware of task situations and each other's activities, plans and work focus, all of which are changing in dynamic work settings.

Real-time telemedicine distributed decision making in wartime or other emergency states

In the current military, the remote teleconsultant does not give medical direction – the 'guy-on-the-ground' is in charge. However, future military doctrine may change to enable telemedicine communications to be used for real-time telementoring and just-in-time training and decision aiding for emergency responses to disasters, chemical or biological weapon deployment, other terrorist attacks and war.

To assess the needs of telemedicine in such situations, we explored the cognitive demands and information use of decision makers in emergency, real-time medical diagnosis and treatment. Existing videotapes of real trauma patient resuscitation and management at the Shock Trauma Center were used as the stimulus material to recreate dynamic decision making situations where the impact of the telecommunication media on situational awareness and remote decision making could be determined.

There are clearly differences between the military medicine mission environment and a trauma center, but there are similarities in that emergency life-saving medical interventions occur that could potentially be telementored by remotely situated experts.[13] There can be physical deterioration of the field military team members due to fatigue or injury. In the field, unlike the trauma center, there are finite supplies and limited and fixed resources. As a result, there are limited options available to deal with unanticipated events. However, using audio/video records of human processes in real-life trauma patient resuscitation as surrogate material, allows testing the understanding of decision making by remote experts, and examining how these experts view the multidisciplinary teams' function in dynamic and stressful situations. In addition, we used such an approach to identify the information that remote decision makers can extract from audio/video records.

For acute events, human factor resemblances between team members in a military medicine mission and a multidisciplinary trauma resuscitation team are quite strong.[14] The military medicine team has to deal with both the enemy and with many complex and interacting systems within their team. They are required to understand system data in stressful conditions when their capabilities for comprehension can be overloaded with a multitude of signals whose priorities for attention may be ambiguous. During prolonged medical missions, the changing emotions of military team members and anxieties associated with specific tasks or being under enemy attack may result in impairment of decision making and problem solving. Interactions with an expert, but remotely distributed colleague may be able to modulate such stressors and anxieties by providing psychological support and allowing maintenance of cognitive performance.

There is relevance of trauma patient resuscitation to military medical missions for acute events because of performance-shaping factor resemblances between military medicine and a multidisciplinary trauma resuscitation team. The domain of trauma patient resuscitation is high risk; tasks may need to be carried out under severe time pressure with many additional stressors, including noise and uncertainty. The trauma patient resuscitation area (13 feet × 12 feet) is space-limited like military wartime resuscitation areas, so allowing activity monitoring of other care providers and a shared-event space. The trauma team, like the military team, has specific domain expertise. In both trauma resuscitation and military missions, there is a need for a widely shared mental model that allows for diverse, often non-routine decisions to be made with imperfect information. Both the trauma team and military team members have to maintain cognitive performance despite physiological stressors (such as sleep deprivation) and emotional disturbances. For the trauma team, this includes dealing with combative and abusive patients and those with severe injuries.

Like military missions in wartime there are many uncertainties confronting the trauma team decision makers. There are unknowns about the emergency patient (site and extent of intracerebral, thoracic and abdominal injury, past medical history in unconscious patients), and because emergencies are unpredictable, the incoming patient workload is unpredictable. In an analysis of the impact of uncertainty on trauma team performance,[15] in 40 patient resuscitations, we found patient-related and team/organization-related uncertainties. In acute events, similar uncertainties will probably exist for the on-site field military medicine team.

Generalizability of findings to military medicine missions

The domain of trauma resuscitation was used as a 'laboratory' to develop and test general characteristics of how remotely situated decision makers understand events in dynamic domains such as are present during wartime, in disasters, and in chemical or biological attack with weapons of mass destruction. Although the domain of trauma resuscitation is a highly specialized medical domain, it shares many similarities with military medicine missions as described above. In order to understand how real teams function in real stressful situations, the 'laboratory' we studied can be a valuable surrogate to provide insight into the medical environment that might occur in war and other emergencies. We paid special attention to the underlying theoretical concepts, such as task urgency and uncertainty so that our results can be generalizable.

These data yield insights into the cognitive processes involved in skilled performance and decision making during distributed decision making in trauma resuscitation. They have interest to the military and the medical community because urgent diagnosis and treatment of medical problems and coordination of medical resources by telecommunication links will need to occur in wartime, disasters and as a result of chemical or biological attack with weapons of mass destruction.

Our previous findings[14] suggest the possibility that the involvement of a remote expert, depending on the information available to them, may assist the on-site team in avoiding certain pitfalls. For example, some errors in this task environment have been attributed to the team fixating inappropriately on suspected instrumentation problems, at the expense of continued observation and physical examination of the patient.[8] A remotely located expert might be less prone to being caught up in such inappropriate allocations of collective attention. Trauma teams functioning in high-stress emergency cases have been shown to take procedural short cuts, which can be counterproductive, e.g. failing to make use of available instrumentation. Remote experts, to the extent that they retain a 'big picture' perspective of the case, might more readily detect procedural oversights or other errors that are due to the stress of the moment rather than to lack of knowledge. Likewise, it may be easier for the more detached, remotely located expert to focus on trends in patient vital signs, and to formulate diagnostic conclusions there while the on-site decision maker may be burdened with concurrent tasks to the extent that they only have the working memory capacity to monitor moment to moment.

Research effort questions for distributed decision making

This effort addresses two research questions, one general to distributed decision making and the other specific to medical applications of dynamic distributed decision making, such as would occur during wartime or other emergencies, e.g. disasters, chemical or biological attack with weapons of mass destruction.

As a first general question, the effort was directed at answering the question 'What information is used by a remote decision maker?' For a decision maker to participate in a decision making process effectively, a prerequisite is to be able to assess the situation and problems at hand. In a distributed decision-making context, this requirement means that the decision maker has to rely on telecommunication links (e.g. computer, telephone and video networks) to achieve situation assessment and to understand problems to be tackled. This requirement may be fulfilled relatively easily when events evolve slowly, but it can be difficult to satisfy when situations change rapidly.[16] Little empirical data have been reported on how people can assess dynamically changing situations and problems through telecommunication links. Therefore, there is little empirical basis existing to guide the design of telecommunication systems in support of distributed decision making.

A second question, specific to medical applications of distributed decision making, is also addressed: 'How should we make use of remote expertise?' This question is related to a broadly defined field of telemedicine. With the development of technologies, many of the long-time desires of medical practice seem to come true: the physicians can see and talk to the patient over long distances, physicians themselves can use video teleconferences to save travel costs. Much of the efforts on telemedicine have been driven by technology and have been based on untested assumptions about the impact of technology. As evidenced in the research on the impact of technology and on the use of video teleconferencing systems in organizations,[17] each use of technology is an experimentation with unexpected outcomes and it creates a new work environment with new tasks and requirements. New modes of errors and new patterns of workload will result when technology is deployed, sometimes seemingly innocently replacing or automating a component in the work environment.

It is unclear what information a remote medical decision maker requires to manage medical emergencies and how effective remote management is at producing appropriate and timely diagnosis and management of humans with medical problems. It is also not known how different types of medical subject matter experts (surgeons, anesthesiologists, nurses) function as independent remote decision makers and, third, how the response of the on-site trauma patient managers affects the remote decision maker is also uncertain.

As a preliminary step to address these research questions, our project examined the ability of trauma experts to remotely manage trauma patients through telecommunication links and identify how telecommunication systems should be designed to facilitate such tasks. Important features of the domain of trauma patient resuscitation are that the patient's condition changes rapidly and is often uncertain, and that the resuscitation effort is carried out by a multidisciplinary team. Apart from being used as a research 'laboratory', trauma patient resuscitation could benefit from telecommunication because in many situations injured patients are spatially remote from expert care providers.

Specific aims

We used our existing videotapes and database (*see* below, under 'Video library'), including transcriptions of reviews of the management by participant and non-participant subject matter experts (SMEs), summaries of diagnostic and surgical findings, and laboratory and radiological data.[18] From these data, we examined the following specific aims.

- **Specific aim 1:** characterize the importance of various information-providing factors in remote decision making for the emergency management of the trauma patient. These results would address questions about the relative importance of patient vital signs (heart rate, blood pressure, oxygen saturation, etc.), and physical examination in determining appropriate emergency medical management of the trauma patient.
- **Specific aim 2:** assess the effects of different types of subject matter experts (surgeons, anesthesiologist, trauma nurse) functioning independently as the remote decision makers. This specific aim would examine how strategies of information-gathering data interpretation and integration differ among medical subject matter experts working independently.
- **Specific aim 3:** determine how team coordination and breakdowns in coordination might impact on the decision making of a remote expert and identify what remote experts were uncertain about when viewing events through multimedia telecommunication links.

The studies were carried out by the National Study Center for Trauma and EMS investigators working at the R Adams Cowley Shock Trauma Center of the University of Maryland. This facility is a Level One trauma center that is regarded as one of the pre-eminent facilities of its kind in the world and is the Primary Adult Resource Center for the State of Maryland trauma system. As such, it serves as a training ground for trauma anesthesiology and surgery residents and faculty from all over the world.

Video library

Audio/videotapes in the library were earlier developed in this real shock trauma environment under a grant funded by the Office of Naval Research (ONR#N00014-91-J-1540) and supplemented by video clips as a result of other funding sources (NASA grant #NCC2-921, ARI Grant #DASW01-99-K003 and AHRQ grant #U18HS-11279-01).

A unique feature of the video recordings was that the video images contained overlaid patient vital signs (Figure 12.1). The images in the video-acquisition systems network (VASNET) are overlaid with patient vital signs obtained from a serial interface on the patient's monitors.[19] These vital signs are essential to understanding of the decision making process of the resuscitation team. They include heart rate, oxygen levels in the patient's blood (SpO_2), measures of ventilation (end-tidal CO_2) and blood pressure, temperature and filling pressures of the heart. Such a recording method makes video analysis efficient as trauma resuscitation activities are initially guided by the goals of diagnosis of the causes of abnormality in the vital signs and normalization of vital signs.

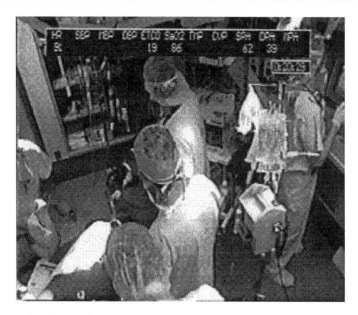

Figure 12.1 Video image of trauma patient resuscitation. This patient had a flail chest and major intra-abdominal bleeding. Vital signs show: heart rate (HR) 91/min on extreme left; end-tidal $CO_2 = 19$ mmHg, O_2 saturation $= 86\%$, and non-invasive BP $= 62/39$ shown on the right side of overlay. Time code is shown beneath BP.

The audio/video acquisition system has been in operational use for more than 11 years and it is reliable and easy to use. Our research team established rapport among the care providers in the Trauma Center for audiovideo taping. The system is turnkey operated and we believe this does not interfere with patient care, nor does the videotaping from cameras affixed to the ceiling appear to influence the behavioral aspects of the trauma team. The trauma team members expressed their lack of remembrance that they were being videotaped on review of the events. Rather, they were concentrating on the tasks at hand. One of the useful parts of videotape review was that the participants noted events that during resuscitation they had not recognized because of their selective attention to other aspects of care.

Using the VASNET system, we have established a video library of team performance during trauma patient resuscitation. The video library contains over 200 cases of real trauma patient resuscitation. These existing videotapes and other materials were used as stimulus material in this study of distributed decision making. Aside from video and audio recordings, medical records (e.g. patient admission records, anesthetic and surgical records, discharge summary, vital signs and blood chemistry) were also collected. After patient identifiers were removed, these were copied and became part of the database. A majority of these cases were reviewed by SMEs, both neutral (i.e. not in the recorded cases) and participant (i.e. in the recorded cases). It was this database that was used to examine the three specific aims.

Experiments on real-time distributed decision making in emergencies general methodology

The general methodology adopted in the experimentation was to present the subjects with video segments of reallife trauma patient resuscitation from our video library. The subject's ability to assess the status of the patient and the progress of the resuscitation effort was then measured. Experiment subjects were all SMEs. The video presentation was to *simulate* remote diagnosis through telecommunication in which experts would be provided with live video images. Patient history on admission to the Shock Trauma Center was given to the SMEs at the start of each experiment. During the course of the presentation of the stimulus materials, stop points were inserted, at which the subjects filled in questionnaires specially designed to capture their understanding of patient status and resuscitation activities contained in the stimulus materials. The questionnaire contained open questions and was generic (i.e. the same across all stop points and not case-specific).[20]

Stop points were chosen in each case segment based on the stages in the resuscitation effort. For each stop point, one to three items of description were generated, based on the analysis results, to represent the ideal understanding of the status of the patient and of the resuscitation activities, and these items were used to score the questionnaires filled by the subjects (Table 12.1). Thus even though questionnaires were generic, the scoring items were dependent on the specific stop point (*see* Figure 12.2).

Four case segments (5–8 minutes each) were used in the experiment; with three to four stop points in each case segment. These case segments were selected to represent a wide range of trauma patient resuscitation scenarios, and they were relatively complex.

Table 12.1 Questions in the questionnaire used in the experiment to measure the subjects' understanding of remote events and activities

---

1 I would describe the current patient status as (list up to 5 most important descriptors, in order of decreasing importance)
   The following is unclear to me (list up to 3 most important, specific areas, in order of decreasing importance)
2 I would describe the current team activities as (list up to 3 most important descriptors, in order of decreasing importance)
   The following is unclear to me (list up to 3 most important, specific areas, in order of decreasing importance)
3 I would describe the decisions just made by the team as (list up to 3 most important decisions, in order of decreasing importance)
   The following is unclear to me (list up to 3 most important, specific areas, in order of decreasing importance)
4 The team at the moment should consider the following differential diagnoses (list up to 5 most important differential diagnoses, in order of decreasing importance)
   The following is unclear to me (list up to 3 most important, specific areas, in order of decreasing importance)
5 I am anticipating the following immediate patient problems (list up to 3 most important, specific problems, in order of decreasing importance)
6 List, in priority order, 3 most important objectives of the team and the instructions you would give to achieve the objectives
7 List, in priority order, 3 decisions that the team could be making next
8 List, in priority order, 3 most important pieces of information you would like to obtain, and the reasons why you need them
9 Please rate your responses to the following statements on the 5-point scale:
   • I am comfortable with giving instructions to the team
   • Given the opportunity, I would obtain more information
   • I know the tasks being carried out by the team

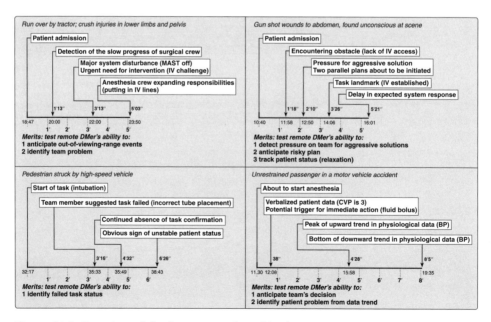

Figure 12.2 Overview of the four cases selected in the experiments (top row: case 1 and case 2); bottom row: case 3 and case 4).

Methods for experiments performed

Experiment 1

Three subjects went through a total of 12 experiment sessions (four case segments each subject). An overview of these cases is shown in Table 12.2. There were four stop points when questionnaires were completed. Two subjects had one year and one ten years of shock trauma experience. This experiment was designed to address what cues were detected and missed by experienced subjects.

Table 12.2 Items used for scoring questionnaires at stop points (SP 1–4) for the four case segments (case 1–4)

Case	Stop points	Time	Scoring items
Case 1	SP 1	1'13"	Detected the acute hemorrhage
			Anticipated 'MAST[a] off' event
			Detected the slow progress of the surgeons
	SP 2	3'13"	Detected 'MAST off' event
			Detected the urgent need for rapid infusion
	SP 3	5'03"	Detected ACPs[b] effort in establishing IV accesses
Case 2	SP 1	1'18"	Detected the pressure on ACP to intubate
			Detected the lack of IV[c] access and obstacles to intubation
	SP 2	2'10"	Detected nasal intubation and IM[d] injection in the tongue
			Anticipated possible patient vomiting
	SP 3	3'26"	Recognized IV established
	SP 4	5'21"	Detected the delay in achieving patient muscle relaxation
			Put forward differential diagnoses for the delay
Case 3	SP 1	3'16"	Identified cues for missed intubation
			Identified cues for confirming correct ETT[e] position
	SP 2	4'32"	Detected the lack of positive ETT position confirmation
			Put forward differential diagnoses for the lack of positive ETT position confirmation
	SP 3	6'26"	Detected the need to remove ETT
Case 4	SP 1	0'38"	Detected the need for IV bolus
	SP 2	4'28"	Detected the increasing, very high BP[f]
			Detected the need for intervention
	SP 3	8'05"	Detected the decreasing, very low BP
			Detected the need for intervention

[a] MAST = military anti-shock trousers; [b] ACP = anesthesia care providers; [c] IV = intravenous; [d] IM = intramuscular; [e] ETT = endotracheal tube; [f] BP = blood pressure.

Experiment 2

Four trauma nurses, four trauma anesthesiologists and four trauma surgeons participated in this experiment to assess the effect of experience background on remote diagnosis. This experiment followed up a hypothesis that was generated from Experiment 1 as the reason why cues were missed.

The stop point questionnaire asked SMEs to describe current patient status, current team activities, anticipated patient status and anticipated team objectives. Written or audio-recorded responses were used and answers divided into:

- airway
- breathing
- circulation
- patient status and injuries
- team activities
- other.

Experiment 3

Twelve subjects, four attending trauma anesthesiologists, three attending trauma surgeons, three experienced trauma nurses and two medically naive graduate students (control) participated in this experiment. An eye tracker was worn by the subjects to evaluate video as a medium to convey information, to assess domain expert visual scanning patterns during remote diagnosis and to compare information gathering from the same scenarios viewed by anesthesiologists, surgeons and nurses. Two measures of visual scanning patterns were analyzed: fixation and dwell. A fixation was described as a cessation of eye movement; a dwell as a consecutive sequence of fixations within a given area of interest. The dwell time (start of first fixation to end of last) was taken as an indication of how focused the subjects were on a particular area of interest of the videotaped scenarios.

Experiment 4

In this experiment, we assessed team coordination and breakdowns to examine how a remote decision maker could collaborate as an important member of the distributed trauma resuscitation team. The first part of the experiment examined how the trauma team coordinated and when coordination breakdowns occurred. The second part of the study examined uncertainty in resuscitation and team communication. This experiment was driven by the fundamental question of how it was possible for the trauma team to function so smoothly most of the time with so little apparent effort spent on coordination. Three types of critical incidents were included in the stimulus material. These were decision points, high workload periods and apparent problems in team coordination. The qualitative data were reported in two areas. First, task coordination or the distribution and delegation of tasks and information flow; and second, the passage of information regarding patient status and contingency plans.

Experiment 5

This experiment was conducted to determine the impact of uncertainty on team performance. Using previous reviews of the stimulus material videotapes from those present during the real patient management and commentary provided by SMEs not involved as participants in this experiment, we categorized uncertainties in the case segments as follows:

- mechanism and extent of injury
- patient's prior medical history
- working status of patient monitors
- the effect of treatment
- availability of team members
- task distribution among team members
- intentions of team members
- availability of resources (e.g. operating room, radiology)
- what occurred during transport
- the status of the patient during field management.

Findings of experiments

Experiment 1 investigated what cues were detected and what was missed by remotely situated expert decision makers

The results showed that missed cues occurred for several reasons, including:

- degradation of verbalizations and verbal communications because of background noise interference[21]
- viewing range for the remotely situated subject was restricted with a fixed camera location
- visual access from this fixed location was not secure because care providers moved in and out of the camera line of sight and sometimes obstructed the view at critical moments when the cue was presented
- typical video imagery used showed the activities of three to five crew members of the trauma team working on patient resuscitation and such multiple actions appeared to overwhelm the remotely situated expert decision makers causing visual information overload.

Some clues were not picked up by all remote decision makers. Difficulties in recognizing these cues included:

- lack of an adequate dynamic mental model of patient status because they had not participated in patient care and were therefore cognitively 'out of the loop' in regard to their information seeking[22]
- there was lack of context information in comparison to the on-site providers – it was not as obvious to the remotely situated person what other team members were doing or how to extrapolate their intentions
- because not all concurrent activities could be simultaneously followed.

Experiment 2 addressed the question: what is the effect of the remote decision makers experience background on the capability to extract information from these audio/video sources?

Nurses', surgeons' and anesthesiologists' understanding of the identical audio/video material was compared by responses to questions about the current patient status, team activities, future patient status and team objectives. The analysis of nurses', surgeons' and anesthesiologists' responses compared performance of correct answers against an ideal understanding of the cases and content of the answers categorized into airway, breathing, circulation, patient status and injuries, team activities and other.

The performance analysis showed that anesthesiologists performed better than the other two groups. Performance-scoring items that presented difficulties included detection of conflicting plans and anticipation of nursing plans. Surgeons and nurses did poorly in determining task status of placement of a breathing tube, traditionally the responsibility of the anesthesiologists.

Content analysis showed that the distribution of answers across the six categories (above) among all three groups of subjects was similar. The surgeons provided more general comments; the anesthesiologist subjects used a higher proportion of phrases describing airway-related issues, whereas the nurses were consistently more focused on teamwork.

All subjects experienced, at one time or another, similar difficulties to those in Experiment 1. An explanation for why anesthesiology subjects outperformed the nurses and surgeons is that the videotapes selected for this experiment all contained the activities of airway management, a role performed by anesthesiologists on the trauma team. The traditional divisions of labor within the trauma team may have constrained the nurses and surgeons and prevented them from detecting critical cues. The nurses performed better than surgeons; this may have been motivational. The surgeons may have used different types of descriptions than nurses, but in general, surgeons provided fewer written and verbal responses than nurses or anesthesiologists.

These results suggest that experts with different experience backgrounds may appreciate different aspects of events and activities presented in audio/video sources.

Experiment 3 used an eye-tracking device to determine visual scanning patterns of domain expert observers

Information extracted from video was identified by use of the eye tracker. Nurses, surgeons, anesthesiologists and medically naive undergraduates (control group) participated. They provided verbal comments and answered questions about the current patient status and team activities and future patient status and team objectives, as in Experiment 2, while wearing the eye-tracking device.

All subjects spent the majority of the time looking at the head and faces of the care providers on the video. The eye movements of the control group were rapid over large areas of the video in comparison to the expert subjects. Subjects with different experience backgrounds among nurses, surgeons and anesthesiologists had different visual scanning patterns. The distribution of total time spent on the area surrounding the patient's head was just over 40%, and on the care providers under 40% of the total viewing time. The nurse subjects scanned more around the patient and the anesthesiologists looked most at the airway manager. Viewing of the vital signs data occupied about 10% of the total viewing time.

The eye-tracking data corroborated the hypothesis of the effect of experience background on information extraction during remote diagnosis.

Experiment 4 was conducted to understand team coordination

As a result of understanding team coordination, a remote decision maker might be able to identify decision points, high workload periods and problems in team coordination.[23]

Videotapes were reviewed and several non-communication task coordination activities were noted including:

- following the protocols
- following the leader
- anticipation of future events
- activity monitoring the task status of team members.

Explicit verbal communications regarding situational assessment and future plans were relatively rare in comparison to non-verbal communication. When team members voluntarily provided their views, it occurred when the team was clearly at a decision point. There was considerable variation among team leaders in plan verbalization, with some leaders providing clear intentions, while others appeared to let the events drive the team actions and the goals were inferred by these actions.

Coordination breakdowns occurred in a number of crisis situations including when:

- extreme difficulties or unexpected patient responses were encountered, which prevented the implementation of routine procedures
- the team was under pressure to seek alternative solutions
- there were unexpected attempts to adopt novel solutions to acute emergency situations.

These breakdown situations compromised the abilities of the supporting team members to provide assistance because of their lack of anticipation of the need. Coordination breakdown occurred when the patient was so unstable that the treatment plan had to be abandoned; such changes in plan occurred during crisis and under great time pressure, and required the team to change their process from diagnostic activities (hypothesis seeking) to action activities (hypothesis testing) rapidly.

Verbal communication was viewed as only one of many ways teams use to coordinate their activities. Other communication media include:

- activities
- workspace
- events
- focus of attention of team members.

In most circumstances, team coordination was achieved with a minimum of explicit verbal communication.

Experiment 5 – analysis of uncertainty in resuscitation events and team communications

Forty videotaped cases were reviewed from our video library that identified a wide range of sources of uncertainty. A total of 76 uncertain items were identified by examining verbal communications and SME reviews. These uncertainties were categorized as patient-related uncertainty (26%), including reports provided by distributed pre-hospital team members, effect of treatment interventions and mechanism of patient injury; and team/organization-related uncertainty (41%), including task distribution among team members, interaction of other team members, status of team members' task accomplishment, and resource availability and schedules. Many of these factors would also probably be causes of uncertainty for the military medicine team. It seemed that lack of communication among team members and among personnel work in nursing, surgery and anesthesiology contributes to many of the uncertainties identified. In addition, technological issues such as signal interference of patient vital sign monitors cause uncertainty in many crisis situations because patient factors (low blood pressure, combativeness, etc.) cause signal detection failures.[18] Last, because of overlap in task distribution among team members, uncertainties occur about who should do what and when.

Conclusions and recommendations on real-time distributed decision making in emergencies

The cases on which this chapter is based were selected to allow testing of the participating subjects as remote decision makers. This meant that out-of-viewing range events were included to determine if these could be anticipated. Non-optimal case management situations were used as stimulus material to determine whether coordination failures could be identified. Risky interventions were included to see if the remote decision maker could anticipate the hazards of such plans when not co-located. Patient status after an intervention is part of what a care provider does to follow-up the outcomes. The ability of the remote decision maker to seek follow up without direct participation in the intervention was sought in another of the cases, to determine whether they could track patient status dynamically over a period of time (about three minutes). Whether or not remote decision makers can detect some of the subtleties of local and peer pressures within a team was also assessed with cases where there was pressure to aggressively intervene, and situations where a team mate failed to identify the task status or the co-located team recognized positive or negative cues for task status. Whether a remote decision maker can prospectively anticipate the same decisions that the team ultimately made, or whether they could identify patient problems from trends (patterns) of patient vital signs, was also tested with the cases used in this chapter.

Understanding both verbal and non-verbal communications is an important part of real-time distributed decision making. Capture of optimal verbal signs can be achieved both by tools such as standardized communication or call-back protocols, as well as technological solutions including individual microphones, directional microphones, and noise cancellation technology. Non-verbal communications cues can be captured by using multiple cameras to record the same event, including both close up and general environmental views. Multiple cameras also minimize restrictions in viewing range and access to non-verbal communications. The fixed camera provides a general overview of the entire area of activity and allows both identification of who is coming and going, and also some context for the team events. The shared-event space, shown on such overview images, is an important media for non-verbal communication. The workplace designs should avoid interference with the function of the space.

In dynamic events with a multidisciplinary team, where simultaneous actions are part of the coordinated effort, it is easy to miss important interventions. Cues to prompt a remote observer may be useful to focus their attention on specific events or performance of particular parts of task performance when multi-tasking is occurring. A framework of prototypical sequences of tasks (e.g. ATLS protocols for resuscitation of trauma patients) can provide useful reference points to allow a remote decision maker to understand what is occurring even though they may not have the same familiarity as the co-located team with their surroundings. Training of remote decision makers in observation of events outside their usual domain of expertise can be helpful in ensuring maximal information input into their decision. Multiple domain expertise among multiple remote observers may be the only available means of ensuring real-time expertise for dynamic tasks. Training or cueing remote teleconsultants to systematically scan video sources may overcome the difficulties associated with rapidly evolving events.

The most straightforward, but most difficult to implement, strategy for keeping a remote decision maker informed and avoiding uncertainty is explicit verbalization of plans prospectively. Increased communication among the team, even defined communication protocols for certain tasks with call-back by other team members confirming their understanding can be very useful. Improved reliability and artefact reduction among signals from monitoring technology would increase their decision-support usefulness, e.g. patient vital signs monitoring technology. Check lists of tasks to be completed in a sequence can help avoid omission and commission errors. They may be restrictive in dynamic and complex domains, as one of the characteristics of expert teams is that they can adapt their behavior to changing circumstances and so often do not follow predictable or prescribed pathways.

Implications

This paper has addressed the core of the onion by examination of issues directly related to optimal observational analysis of remote events through video, audio and data links using multiple sources of information from a single remote location. The paper examines team performance and does not propose any outcomes such as learning or success. Rather, it recommends a way that quantitative and qualitative data can be collected that might be used to confirm such outcomes.

Acknowledgement

Work performed under MRMC Contract DAMD 17-01-1-0758 of the Army Medical Research and Material Command, Fort Detrick, Maryland. The opinions expressed in this chapter are those of the authors and do not represent the opinion of the Department of Defense.

References

1 Moray N (1994) Error reduction as a systems problem. In: Bogner MS (ed.) *Human Error in Medicine*. Lawrence Erlbaum, Hillsdale, NJ.

2 National Research Council (1990) *Distributed Decision-Making*. National Academy Press, Washington, DC.

3 Rasmussen J (ed.) (1991) *Distributed Decision Making: cognitive models for cooperative work*. Wiley, Chichester.

4 US Congress, Office of Technology Assessment (1995) *Bringing Health Care Online: the role of information technologies (OTAITC624)*. US Government Printing Office, Washington, DC.

5 Orasanu J (1990) *Shared mental models and crew decision-making*. Technical Report 46. Cognitive Science Laboratory, Princeton University, Princeton, NJ.

6 Orasanu J and Salas E (1993) Team decision making in complex environments. In: Klein GA (ed.) *Decision-Making in Action: models and methods*. Ablex, Norwood, NJ.

7 Xiao Y, Mackenzie CF, Orasanu J et al. (1998) Visual scanning patterns during remote diagnosis. *Proceedings of Human Factors and Ergonomics 42nd Annual Meeting*, pp. 272–6.

8 Xiao Y, Mackenzie CF, Patey R et al. (1998) Team coordination and breakdowns in a real-life stressful environment. *Proceedings of Human Factors and Ergonomics 42nd Annual Meeting*, pp. 186–90.

9 Serfaty D, Entin EE and Volpe C (1993) Adaptation to stress in team decision-making and coordination. *Proceedings of Human Factors and Ergonomics Society 37th Annual Meeting*, pp. 1228–32.

10 Kanki BG, Folk VG and Irwin CM (1991) Communication variations and aircrew performance international. *J Aviation Psychology*. 1: 149–62.

11 Volpe CE, Cannon-Bowers JA, Salas E et al. (1996) The impact of cross training on team functioning: an empirical investigation. *Human Factors*. 38: 87–100.

12 Segal LD (1994) Actions speak louder than words: how pilots use nonverbal information for crew communications. *Proceedings of the Human Factors and Ergonomics Society 38th Annual Meeting*, pp. 21–5.

13 Teich JM, Wagner MM, Mackenzie CF et al. (2002) The informatics response in disaster, terrorism, and war. *J Am Med Informatics Assoc*. 9: 97–1104.

14 Mackenzie CF, Jaberi M, Dutton R et al. (2000) Overview of simulation in comparison with telementoring for decision-making. *Am J Anes*. 27: 186–94.

15 Xiao Y and Mackenzie CF (1997) Uncertainty in trauma patient resuscitation. *Proceedings of the Human Factors and Ergonomics Society 41st Annual Meeting*, pp. 168–71.

16 Allely EB (1995) Synchronous and asynchronous telemedicine. *J Med Systems*. 19: 207–12.

17 Finn KE (ed.) (1997) *Video-Mediated Communication*. Lawrence Erlbaum Associates, Mahwah, NJ.

18 Mackenzie CF, Jefferies MJ, Hunter WA et al. (1996) Comparing of self-reporting of deficiencies in airway management with video analysis of actual performance. *Human Factors* 38: 623–35.

19 Mackenzie CF, Hu PF-M, Xiao Y et al. (2003) Video acquisition and audio system network (VAASNNET®) for analysis of workplace safety performance. *Biomed Instr. Tech*. 37: 285–91.

20 Xiao Y, Mackenzie CF, Orasanu J et al. (1999) Information acquisition from audio-video data sources: An experimental study on remote diagnoses. *Telemedicine J*. 5: 139–55.

21 Donchin Y, Gopher D, Olin M *et al.* (1995) A look into the nature and causes of human errors in the intensive care unit. *Crit Care Med.* **23**: 294–300.
22 Endsley MR and Kins EO (1995) The out-of-the-loop performance problem and level of control. *Human Factors.* **37**: 381–94.
23 Xiao Y, Hunter A, Mackenzie CF *et al.* (1996) Task complexity in emergency medical care and its implications on team coordination. *Human Factors.* **38**: 636–45.

Chapter 13

Telehealth advances for diabetes

Nancy Johnson, Rita Webb, Steve Moser, Rosanne Harrigan and Jean A Pezzoli

Introduction

Implementing a diabetes monitoring and management delivery system that reaches a large rural population and results in behavioral change is a significant challenge. Telehealth strategies including e-health (i.e. via the Internet) may enhance access to the individual patient. Telehealth strategies may also assist the patient's family and support system in their home environment.

Specific aims

This qualitative and quantitative clinical study sought to explore the relationship between e-health interventions and the progression of renal disease in diabetics with native Hawaiian ancestry.

Research question

Are e-health interventions significantly associated with the progression of renal disease in diabetics with native Hawaiian ancestry compared to control patients who received regular physician care without e-health augmentation?

Background and significance

Rapid increases in the aging population – 34 million today in the USA and 70 million projected by the year 2030[1] – signify a substantial increase in the demand for services from those with chronic illness. The proportion over age 65 is expected to increase from 12.4% in 2000 to 20% by 2030. In addition, minority populations will increase from 16.4% to 25.4%, with the largest increase (285%) occurring in Asians and Pacific Islanders.[1]

e-Health

Telehealth tools such as videophone, video teleconferencing and Internet need to be explored to manage disease, promote health and reduce healthcare costs for elderly persons with chronic disease. Studies document that elders with adequate support have an increased potential to remain in their homes.

One form of telehealth is using the Internet (e-health) for the delivery of healthcare.[2] Although there is extensive literature on telehealth and its applications, there is limited research documenting clinical outcomes associated with e-health intervention.[3] The data-based research related to telehome care, the most commonly used term for delivery of care in the home using telehealth technology, is summarized below in relationship to the major themes addressed: cost, satisfaction, access and outcomes.

Cost

The literature indicates cost savings associated with the implementation of telehome care in both maternal-child and elder populations.[4] Cost comparisons of traditional care with telehome care provision for mothers with preterm labor documented significant cost savings ($14 459) per pregnancy.[4] In another study, cost comparisons for outpatient services for patients with chronic disease did not vary significantly. However, the investigation took place over 1.5 years; if equipment costs were amortized over a longer period of time, a greater cost saving for the telehome group would result. Hospital costs for the telehome group were less ($1087 compared to $1940).[5]

Satisfaction

Patient satisfaction and nurse satisfaction with telehome care were consistently high.[6–9] Although one investigation documented initial provider resistance, the intensity of the resistance improved over the duration of the investigation.[5]

Access

Access to medical care can be defined as the ability of an individual to obtain healthcare services. In the early stages of telemedicine, consultations by a specialty physician were provided to rural communities, overcoming the barriers of distance, travel time and costs.[10] The same advantages can be realized with e-health when patients have access to providers via the Internet without leaving their home.

From those initial telemedicine projects to the current use of e-health in the home setting, patient access is enhanced when the healthcare provider has improved access to the data needed to evaluate patient progress and responds more quickly with treatment. Efficacy of telehealth to expand access to care has been demonstrated in a variety of patient populations: maternal-child,[4] chronic disease[5] and the elderly.[7] Enhanced access to diabetic disease management via telehealth with the goal of altering progress of renal disease has not been studied.

Outcomes

Many investigations did not specifically report outcome data. However, Morrison's study regarding management of preterm labor using telehome methodology clearly documented reduced numbers of infants admitted to the neonatal intensive care unit. It should be noted that significant differences were found between study groups in this trial for marital status and race. It is possible that these differences rather than methodology could have explained the differences in outcome. The analysis did not reveal any negative clinical outcomes.

Clearly a need exists to further evaluate the efficacy of e-health interventions to reduce health disparities related to diabetes, especially in populations with health disparities such as native Hawaiians, Asians, Filipinos and other Pacific Island people. Sample sizes for the few investigations that exist are relatively small. Many investigations are retrospective in design and measurements of clinical outcomes are inconsistent. At the time of this study there is no clear evidence base for e-health practice related to care of any clinical population, including diabetes. However, the findings suggest that this methodology could improve health outcomes especially for those with chronic disease.

Diabetes

Comprehensive data are sparse on type 2 diabetes mellitus for Pacific Islanders. Yet, the incidence of diabetes is considerably higher for those with Filipino and Pacific Islander ancestry.[11] The prevalence rate for pure Hawaiians is nearly 50 per thousand, which is twice the rate of Caucasian residents of Hawaii.[12,13] Further data show that native Hawaiians die of diabetes at a rate of 117 per 100 000 – more than double compared to the average rate of 53 per 100 000 for other ethnic groups.[14]

The cardiovascular and renal complications of diabetes significantly increase the incidence of chronic disease in Hawaii.[11] The Behavioral Risk Factor Surveillance System reports a rate of 52 per thousand of all adults in Hawaii ever having been told they have diabetes, a number twice as high as the Healthy People 2000 goal.[15]

Regarding type 1 diabetes in children, where the overall rate is 1.16 per 1000,[16] higher rates are displayed in some ethnic groups in Hawaii than in others. The rate for type 1 diabetes in part-Hawaiian children is 2.5 times as high as Caucasian children and ten-times higher than the rate for Japanese children in the same environment.[17]

Despite these alarming discrepancies, emphasis on type 1 diabetes is overshadowed by the rapidly increasing rates of type 2 diabetes in Pacific Islander populations in Hawaii. Indeed, the age-adjusted prevalence rates for type 2 diabetes in Hawaiian Polynesians are among the highest reported for any Polynesian or part-Polynesian population in the world.[16] Furthermore, mixed Hawaiian ancestry has not diminished the risk of type 2 diabetes, unlike in other native American populations. This discrepancy may be due to inaccurate ethnic self-reporting or because the mixed ancestry includes other ethnic groups with known high rates of type 2 diabetes.[16]

An increasingly Westernized and sedentary lifestyle is correlated with the increasing prevalence of diabetes in other populations and may be a factor in the high diabetes rates in native Hawaiian populations. A study comparing Japanese-American men who maintained either traditional Japanese or a modern American lifestyle demonstrated the influence of a Western lifestyle on diabetes risk. The more traditional Japanese-American men had lower rates of diabetes than did the Japanese-American men who were more acculturated to a Western lifestyle.[17] Other literature suggests that traditional cultural beliefs about the caretaking of ill family members and the concept of the spiritual unity of a person with the environment may prevent individuals from taking preventive measures and/or from seeking conventional medical care.[18]

The Hawaii Department of Health indicates that 50% of the people with kidney failure in Hawaii have diabetes, and the rate of newly diagnosed end-stage renal disease (ESRD) in 1994 was more than three times higher in Hawaii than the national average.[19] According to the Center for Disease Control, the direct (medical care) and indirect (lost productivity) costs of diabetes in Hawaii was $613 million in 1993.[20,21]

Individuals with diabetes mellitus are at high risk for many complications that are gradual, insidious and may be irreversible. An example is diabetic ESRD. Once symptoms of ESRD present, the individual has kidney failure. It is only a matter of time until hemodialysis is required to sustain life. The need for dialysis has a profound impact on the cost of healthcare and the individual's quality of life.

Diabetic patients and their families must understand that diabetes is a chronic illness and there is no cure: only adherence to diet, exercise and medication can modulate the impact of diabetes. Through stringent self-monitoring blood glucose (SMBG), blood pressure (BP) and adherence to diet, exercise and medications, diabetic ESRD and other complications can be minimized.[22] A ten-year study conducted by the American Diabetes Association on type 1 diabetics entitled Diabetes Comprehensive Control Trial (DCCT) found that diabetes mellitus complications could be stabilized or reversed with tight daily glycemic control within normal range.[23] These recommendations were incorporated into the Hawaii State Practice Recommendations for Diabetes Mellitus. The Advanced Practice Nursing protocols developed for this investigation are based on these recommendations.

Locus of control

Health behavior is thought to be a function of belief about the degree of control individuals believe they have over life events. Wallston *et al.* suggest that health locus of control is useful for predicting some health behaviors but not others.[24] Pima Indians with internal locus of control were more physically active than those with an external locus of control.[25,26] The Wallston locus of control scale proposed three components of control: internal, powerful others and chance. Given the potential for understanding an individual's decision about disease management, these three measures of locus of control were included in the data collected.

Research design and methodology

This qualitative and quantitative clinical trial monitored the progression of renal disease in two groups of diabetics with native Hawaiian ancestry. The experimental group received e-health teleconferencing visits two times per week, in addition to usual care by their physician. The control group received usual care by their private physician. No attempt was made to control 'usual care'. 'Usual care' included routine screening and diabetic education by physicians. Differences in frequency of patient follow-up with physicians were not evaluated.

Sample

Study participants were of native Hawaiian ethnicity, 18 years of age or older, with a medical diagnosis of diabetes mellitus.

Letters were sent to private physicians and community groups inviting referrals into the project. These physicians and groups were provided screening questionnaires and consent forms. Potential participants were identified. At the time of initial consent, participants were told they would be assigned to either the experimental or control group. Patients were assigned to groups by pulling numbers out of a hat.

Participants were contacted via phone or mail with additional program information, entry questionnaires and an invitation to the orientation class. During the orientation class, participants provided informed consent and received instruction on use of the computers, software and peripheral devices (glucometers and blood pressure cuffs). Appointments were made for installation of the computers in participant homes. Study computers were password-protected and all patient data were maintained by a numerical coding system.

Procedures

Written evidenced-based advanced practice nursing protocols were developed including monitoring, education, counseling, support and referral components. The focus of the interventions was on lifestyle modification resulting in healthy adaptation reflected by decreased progression of diabetic disease.

Three advanced practice registered nurses (APRNs) participated in development of the protocols based on published evidence to assure face validity. Reliability was assured because only these three APRNs provided care using e-health methods. Validity was affirmed by having the protocols reviewed by a nephrologist. The protocols are available from the principal investigator. The clinical trial procedures and consent forms were evaluated and approved by the University of Hawaii Office of Research Services, Committee on Human Subjects.

The experimental group received e-health teleconference visits once or twice per week by the APRN, in addition to usual care by their physician. The e-health visits included a diabetic education protocol that focused on patient and family education, support, medication management and monitoring of health measures.

An Internet website was created for the project. The site included pictures of project staff, diabetes information, instructions on use of the glucometer, icons for obtaining diabetic information on the Internet and use of email.

Equipment and technical support

The e-health visits were conducted using home computer technology (NEC 466 Cache Pentium PC computers with 64 MB memory purchased at a local retail store) and modem connection to the Internet. Inexpensive Intel Cameras and free NET Meeting software allowed video-conferencing. The technology support team consisted of community college students enrolled in the computer technology program. The students provided technical support to both practitioners and patients, and made telephone, video-conferencing and home visits.

Monitoring

Blood pressure, weight and blood sugar were reported by the patient and evaluated by the nurse at each e-health visit. Downloadable Lifescan glucometers were used to measure blood glucose. Weight and blood pressure were self-reported following the orientation program and demonstration of reliability.

Instrumentation

Physiologic, experiential and behavioral variables were measured pre and post treatment to assess the dependent variable of progression of renal disease. Urine microalbumin (reported as ratio of microalbinuria/urine creatinine-specific) evaluated the progression of renal disease. Standard laboratory analyses were used to measure urine microalbumin. Microalbumin is a valid objective measure of progression of renal disease and indicates the degree of blood sugar control for the diabetic patient over a period of time.

Experiential data included qualitative assessment (questionnaire) of computer competence, satisfaction, ability to use diabetic Internet resources and locus of control measured using a 15-item health locus of control scale.[27] Demographic data, lifestyle information (questionnaire) and beliefs towards healthcare (questionnaire) were collected at the onset and at the conclusion of the study.

The locus of control questionnaire was administered to patients in the experimental group at the onset of treatment (pre) and re-administrated at its conclusion (post). Pre and post scores were tallied for the 16 resulting patients on each of the three locus of control beliefs:

- internal – the extent to which one believes that internal factors are responsible for health or illness
- chance – the belief that health or illness is a matter of fate, luck, or chance
- power – the belief that one's health is determined by powerful others such as a health professional.

Each measure was based on a five-point scale, where '5' indicated the highest level of that factor.

A four-item satisfaction questionnaire was administered to experimental patients at the conclusion of treatment to assess participant affect on the e-health approach.

Results

Demographic

The initial control group included 34 individuals with roughly equal males to females (53% male). At the conclusion of the study, researchers were able to locate and obtain data for 11 of the control subjects, for a retention rate of 32%.

The experimental group included 30 individuals with comparable gender distribution (50% male). Twenty-one of the experimental patients participated in the project for the entire year, for a 70% retention rate. Sixteen[16] completed the locus of control post test. Seventy-five percent of the experimental subjects did not have a computer or Internet access prior to the study.

Microalbinuria/creatinine ratio

Pre and post scores for microalbumin (mg/l), creatinine (mg/dl), microalbumin/ creatinine ratio (mg/alb) and percentage change in ratio were evaluated for the experimental and control groups. A negative value in the percentage change indicated the customary progression of renal disease, whereas little change reflects stabilization of the disease and a positive value signified reversal of the disease and improved health.

Progression of renal disease as measured by an increase in the microalbumin/ creatinine ratio was observed in a greater proportion of the control patients ($n = 7$, 63.6%) compared to the experimental group ($n=11$, 52.4%). Additionally, the average increase in ratio was considerably higher in the control group (1,315%) compared to that of the experimental group (90%).

Some patients in both groups demonstrated improvement, but the experimental group had a greater proportion showing improvement ($n=\tilde{N}0$, 47.6%) compared to the control ($n=7$, 36.4%). The average decrease in microalbumin/ creatinine ratio was 54.2% in the experimental group and 53.2% in the control group. However, the experimental effect is spuriously dampened by the post urine microalbumin scores of four experimental patients which were so low (< 3 mg/l) that the ratio could not be calculated. Such decrease in microalbumin may signify a lack of progression of renal disease. This is a goal of tight control of blood sugar in the diabetic patient.

To test the significance of the difference between experimental and control group means, a chi-square analysis was performed on the average onset and post ratios. As seen from Figure 13.1, the average onset ratios for the experimental and control groups were 71.2 and 171.6 respectively. (A t-test showed these pre-test means did not differ significantly, $p \leq 0.34$). At the conclusion of the treatment period, the average post ratios were higher for both groups, at 94.7 and 365.6 respectively. However, the control group average was 247.3 points higher, compared to only +23.5 points for the experimental group.

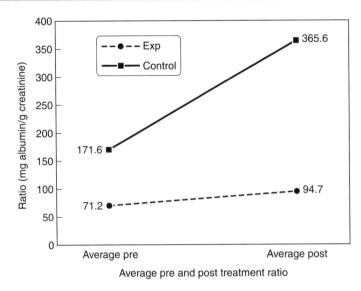

Figure 13.1 Pre and post ratios for e-health (experimental) and traditional (control) treatments.

The chi-square test for independence supports rejection of the null hypothesis that the average ratio is independent of treatment ($\chi^2 = 2.7$, df $= 1$, 2-tail test, $p \leq 0.01$). The post ratio score appears to depend on the treatment. The rapid ascent of the post mean found under the control group suggests that the standard treatment will result in progression of renal disease, which may be significantly slowed by intervention of e-health visits.

Locus of control

The most consistent change in locus of control was seen on the internal scale, where post scores decreased for 11 of the 16 patients (68.8%) who completed both pre and post surveys. As seen from Figure 13.2, the average pre score at 3.9 was on the high end of the five-point scale, and the average post score was lower at 3.6 points. A *t*-test conducted to determine the significance of the difference between the two means approached the acceptable level of ≤ 0.05, but reached only $p \leq 0.08$ on a 2-tailed test.

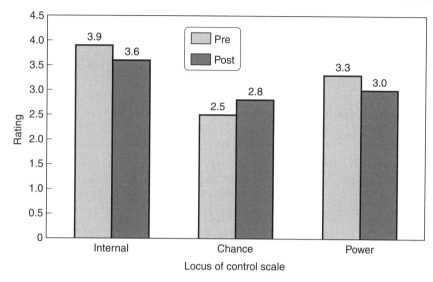

Figure 13.2 Locus of control pre and post comparisons.

On the chance scale, the mean pre score (2.5) was at the midpoint of the scale. The post mean of 2.8 was higher. The t-test, however, did not find this difference to be significant ($p \leq 0.22$). Individual variance was rather high on this measure, with post scores going up or down about equally among the 16 patients (down $= 7$, 43.8%; same $= 1$, 6.3%; up $= 8$, 50.0%.)

Little change was also found on the power scale. Here the mean score went down from 3.3 to 3.0. An equal number of patient post scores went down as up. The t-test did not find a significant difference between the means ($p \leq 0.20$).

Satisfaction

Satisfaction with the e-health protocol was assessed from responses of 15 patients to a four-item questionnaire that evaluated access, technical support, comfort with e-health, and overall satisfaction.

Table 13.3 shows patients were quite favorable towards the e-health treatment. Practically all responses were high ranks of 4 or 5 on all four dimensions of satisfaction.

Table 13.3 Satisfaction questionnaire responses

Item		*Disagree*			*Agree*	
	1	*2*	*3*	*4*	*5*	
I was able to contact my nurse when I needed to				30%	70%	
I was able to obtain technical support when I needed it			7%	7%	86%	
I felt comfortable visiting by televideo				15%	85%	
Overall, how satisfied were you with your e-health visits?		6%	6%	13%	73%	

Further analysis was conducted using the overall satisfaction item to ascertain whether a relationship exists with a patient's locus of control. If it were determined that a questionnaire could adequately predict which patients would be least satisfied with telehealth treatment, then a survey could be used before treatment to select patients who would have the greatest likelihood of benefiting. On the overall satisfaction item, the mean rating was 4.5 from the 15 patients who responded. High ranks of 5 or 4 were awarded by practically all (87%) participants (11 = 5-rank; 2 = 4-rank). Only the two remaining participants assigned a rank of 3 and 2, respectively. This lack of variability in ratings precluded administration of a test of significance on the correlation between measures of satisfaction and locus of control. As an aside, however, it is interesting to note that both participants who expressed the lower levels of satisfaction had relatively high scores (4.6 and 4.2) on the internal scale.

Access

The e-health intervention provided access to health information and guidance for subjects, their families and their friends. A positive outcome of the study was the participation in e-health visits by members of the subject's 'ohana' (family group). This access provided the practitioner with important instructional opportunities with the ohana.

All experimental patients reported that the nurse involved them in their plan of care, and 93% shared information gained during the project with family and friends. When asked, 'Did you feel that this care delivery system invaded your privacy?' all experimental patients answered with no. A large percentage (93%) indicated they would recommend this program to other diabetics, and two-thirds (66%) indicated they wanted to continue in the program in the future.

Technical support

Technical support was important to the success of the program. Most patients utilized technical support for questions and assistance. Most (86%) indicated they were able to obtain the technical support they needed and 93% indicated their questions were answered adequately. Most subjects indicated they utilized technical support six or more times over the one-year period. The majority of the technical support requests were during the first three months of the study.

It is important to note that even though technical support was essential, the services were provided utilizing cost-effective college students and sometimes, in the home, the children or grandchildren of the patients.

Conclusions

This study demonstrates a successful utilization of e-health to impact healthcare outcomes. The use and acceptance of the e-health visits by both nurse practitioners and patients with little computer experience illustrates the potential for peeling the layers of the onion to dramatically change healthcare delivery. Early in the study, alliances developed between the project technician and the most computer-savvy individual in each home. The impact of these alliances on stability of the e-health intervention is demonstrated by the 70% retention rate for patients in the experimental group.

Effectiveness

Diabetic subjects of native Hawaiian ancestry who received usual physician care experienced significantly greater progression of renal disease (measured by ratio of microalbinuria/creatinine) indicating poorer control of blood sugar over the study period, compared to experimental subjects who received regular care augmented e-health educational protocols.

Locus of control

The locus of control analysis found the relatively high Internal scores at the onset dropping after treatment. This drop approached significance ($p \leq 0.08$) with the sample size of just 16 subjects. Further research conducted on a larger sample might find support for a hypothesis that e-health monitoring attenuates high levels of Internal control. Would it be plausible that attenuated Internal control indicates patients became more accepting of the challenges of their diabetes and the importance of disease management?

Satisfaction

Telehealth in the form of e-health video-conferencing visits was well accepted by patients, who had little prior computer experience.

Increased access and decreased costs

Among the more interesting findings of this study was confirmation that patients could receive effective medical/health interventions without leaving their home. The e-health methodology proposes a number of features that promulgate a conclusion that the future of medicine will incorporate telehealth practices as a way of improving patient access.

- Cost of equipment is not a barrier. The e-health methodology used a standard computer with Internet access found in many homes today. The software is downloadable free from the Internet with new features to manage privacy issues.
- Less mobile elders and those with conditions making it difficult to get around can switch on a computer to access medical monitoring, in lieu of physically getting to a provider's office.
- Rural patients need not travel long distances, and instead gain access to medical monitoring on the computer just an arm's reach away.
- Seniors and others who no longer drive can circumvent problems of securing rides to the doctor's office.

- Inclement weather, blocked traffic and treacherous roads are not barriers to receiving medical attention.
- Travel time and mileage expense are eliminated for both patients and providers, who no longer need to travel to reach each other's office or home.

Future research

While the results did affirm the association of nursing telehealth intervention with improved patient outcomes, the sample size was small and the comparability of groups was not assured. The effectiveness of nursing telehealth strategies in supporting patient management of chronic diseases must be further validated using randomized controlled clinical trials with larger further samples. The aging population and the inadequate supply of healthcare providers demands the use of cost-effective strategies to manage diabetes and other chronic diseases. Telehealth strategies devised by advanced practice nurses may address this need.

References

1   Administration on Aging, Future Growth. Retrieved from: www.aoa.dhhs.gov
2   Bangert DC and Doktor R (eds) (2005) *Human and Organizational Dynamics in e-Health.* Radcliffe Publishing, Oxford and Seattle.
3   The eHealth Landscape – A Terrain Map of Emerging Information and Communication Technologies in Health and Health Care. Retrieved at: http://www.rwjf.org/publications/pubDetail.jsp?pubCode=146
4   Morrison J *et al.* (2001) Telemedicine: cost-effective management of high-risk pregnancy. *Managed Care.* **10**(11): 42–6, 48.
5   Johnston B (2000) Outcomes of Kaiser Permanente tele-home research project. *Archives of Family Medicine.* **9**(1): 40–5.
6   Allen A (1996) Home health visits using a cable TV network: user satisfaction. *Journal of Telemedicine & Telecare.* **2**(Suppl. 1): S1: 92–4.
7   Shaul M (2000) What you should know before embarking on telehome health lessons learned from a pilot study. *Home Healthcare Nursing.* **18**(7): 470–5.
8   Rooney E (1997) A model for nurse case-managed home care using televideo. *Journal American Geriatric Society.* **45**(12): 1532–3.
9   Naylor M, Brooten D, Campbell R *et al.* (1999) Comprehensive discharge planning and home follow-up of hospitalized elders. *JAMA.* **281**(7): 613–20.
10 Baldwin LP and Clarke M (2005) Using ICT to better support the fragmentary nature of healthcare. In: Bangert DC and Doktor R (eds) *Human and Organizational Dynamics in e-Health.* Radcliffe Publishing, Oxford and Seattle.
11 Hawaii Department of Health Diabetes Facts. Retrieved from: www.hawaii.gov/health/resource/diabetes/hp-dcbur.html
12 Grandinetti A, Chang H, Mau M *et al.* (1998) Prevalence of glucose intolerance among native Hawaiians in two rural communities. *Diabetes Care.* **21**(4): 549–54.
13 Anon (1996) Hawaiians. *Public Health Rep.* **111**(2): 53–5.
14 Maskarinec G (1997) Diabetes in Hawaii: estimating prevalence from insurance claims data. *Am Public Health.* **87**(10): 1717–20.
15 Hawaii Department of Health (2000) *Adult Diabetes in Hawaii: a surveillance report, Hawaii State Diabetes Control Program.* Honolulu, Hawaii.
16 Department of Business, Economic Development and Tourism (1996) *Hawaii Data Book, 1996.* Honolulu, Hawaii.

17   Patrick S, Kadohiro J, Waxman S *et al.* (1997) IDDM incidence in a multiracial population: the Hawaii IDDM registry. *Diabetes Care.* **20**(6): 983–7.

18   Huang B, Rodriguez B, Burchfiel C, Chyou P, Curb J and Yano K (1996) Acculturation and prevalence of diabetes among Japanese American men in Hawaii. *Am J Epidemiol.* **144**(7): 674–81.

19   Hawaii Diabetes Data Network: Final Report, Pacific Health Research Institute. January 1998. Honolulu, Hawaii. Transpacific Renal Network, Annual Report, 1994. ESRD Network #17.

20   National Diabetes Fact Sheet. Retrieved from:
www.cdc.gov/diabetes/pubs/estimates.htm

21   American Diabetes Association (1998) Economic consequences of diabetes mellitus in the US in 1997. *Diabetes Care.* **21**(2): 296–306.

22   Wang C, Abbott L, Goodbody A, Hui W and Rausch C (1999) Development of a community-based diabetes management program for Pacific Islanders. *The Diabetes Educator.* **25**(5): 738–46.

23   The Diabetes Control and Complications Trial Research Group (1993) The effect of intensive treatment of diabetes on the development and progression of long-term complications in insulin-dependent diabetes mellitus. *N Engl J Med.* **329**(14): 977–86.

24   Wallston BS *et al.* (1976) The development and validation of the health related locus of control (HLC) scale. *Journal of Consulting and Clinical Psychology.* **44**: 580–5.

25   Wallston KA and Wallston BS (1982) Who is responsible for your health? The construct of health locus of control. In: Sanders GS and Suls J (eds) *Social Psychology of Health and Illness.* Lawrence Erlbaum Associates, Hillsdale, NJ.

26   Gregg E *et al.* (1996) Relationship of locus of control to physical activity among people with and without diabetes. *Diabetes Care.* **19**(10): 1118–21.

27   Wallston B (1981) What are the questions in psychology of women? A feminist approach to research. *Psychology of Women Quarterly.* **5**(4): 597–617.

Chapter 14

Evaluating the human dimension of primary care telemedicine encounters

Robert J Bulik, Sherry Wulff, Kathleen K Bultman and Thomas J Pfeil

The initial debate about telemedicine was primarily centered on connectivity issues – for the most part, technology is no longer the major concern. When other questions such as cost-effectiveness of telemedicine have entered the discussion, the reviews seem to be mixed. In a systematic review of studies on cost-effectiveness, few have conclusively demonstrated any cost benefit data.[1] Yet, when human factors are considered, such as lost productivity resulting from employees who miss work to obtain outpatient medical care or to return for a routine follow-up visit with their primary care provider, telemedicine at a large worksite has been shown to provide significant cost savings and increased productivity.[2] Another branch of research has centered on the critical factor of physician acceptance of telemedicine. Using the Technology Acceptance Model (TAM) developed by Davis[3] to assess *intention to use*, Hu *et al.* found that a positive perception of the technology's usefulness for physicians was crucial, while *ease of use* was reported to be not as important.[4]

There is no doubt that discussions on connectivity and cost issues will continue. However, we believe the paramount focus in telemedicine is shifting to a consideration of the patient–provider relationship, and becoming centered on communication issues. In looking at primary care telemedicine, we believe that issues of communication are one example of themes that cross the dimensional characteristics (individual, technology and organizational context) of the TAM model. Because traditional healthcare is most often a face-to-face interactive process between provider and patient in a closed-door examination room, a major issue centers on how distance and technology affect the patient–provider relationship during a telemedicine visit.

While our research does not attempt to investigate the full TAM application, we do seek to understand patient and healthcare provider perceptions of telemedicine, as well as to determine potential techniques and strategies for enhancing communication in primary care telemedicine encounters. Consequently, we believe that primary care telemedicine provides us with an authentic setting for considering the various aspects of communication that make up the patient–provider transaction in an electronically mediated clinical encounter.

In this chapter, we discuss an inclusive and positive approach for investigating patient–provider relations and perceptions of communication quality – the *human dimension* in primary care telemedicine by:

- targeting central communication issues
- developing a working description of *transactional presence* as an approach for supporting effective patient–provider relationships
- describing a telemedicine communication matrix which visually represents components associated with technologically mediated communication events
- reporting on five research projects that we conducted on aspects of the human dimension of primary care telemedicine.

The primary care setting

Primary care is considered to consist of three generalist medical disciplines: family medicine, general internal medicine and general pediatrics. The American Association of Family Medicine provides the following definition of 'primary care' on its website:

> *Primary care is that care provided by physicians specifically trained for and skilled in comprehensive first contact and continuing care for persons with any undiagnosed sign, symptom, or health concern (the 'undifferentiated' patient) not limited by problem origin (biological, behavioral, or social), organ system, or diagnosis.*[5]

In a face-to-face encounter between a healthcare provider and patient in a generalist physician's office, the opportunity for promoting effective communication and for developing a healthcare partnership usually begins with the 'visit', which typically includes a complete health history (or *focused* health history on returning patients) and physical exam. Taking a patient's health history contributes to a process of developing interpersonal *social presence*, i.e. interpersonal awareness, interaction and relational appreciation. At the same time, taking a patient's health history is often viewed as a form of transactional communication, i.e. an interaction or conversation with a purpose – to gather information from the patient, to establish a trusting and supportive relationship, as well as to offer health information and counseling to the patient.

Not only is good communication essential in a face-to-face encounter between patient and provider, but effective communication is integral to optimal healthcare. For example, poor communication can impact the ability of physicians and patients to form true decision-making partnerships through:

- patients' inability to elucidate their health history and physicians' inability to solicit accurate information
- physicians' inability to adequately explain a diagnosis, prognosis, and quality of life choices
- patients' lack of recognition of the need and value of healthcare choices and understanding of test results.

Yet the patient–provider relationship is considered central in patient care,[6] and US biomedical ethics are based on a model that emphasizes patient autonomy and self-determination emphasizing informed consent.[7]

Interestingly, a 2003 advertising campaign for a midwestern healthcare clinic captured current social concerns related to the fundamental role of communication in the patient–physician relationship. The advertisement begins as follows: 'I want doctors who listen. Doctors who discuss. Doctors who care'.[8] The text succinctly captures several important communication concerns and needs of patients seeking high-quality interactions with healthcare providers.

While the face-to-face encounter between a healthcare provider and patient may be considered the ideal for promoting effective communication, it does not necessarily guarantee successful communication or the feeling of social and psychological *presence*. Moreover in a telemedicine encounter, psychological and technical 'filters' impose upon and challenge the development of perceived *presence*. We believe that two-way communication between a patient and their healthcare provider in which both feel *present* with each other during a face-to-face (or telemedicine) clinical encounter are more likely to develop into a successful primary care partnership.

Communication issues in primary care telemedicine

Technologies, such as telemedicine systems, have the mediating capacity to bring people together in real time, even though they are physically separated by distance. Yet, because communication and the presence–distance dichotomy is mediated by technology, there are additional factors and filters that can impact a healthcare provider's ability to attend actively and dialogue with the patient, to empathize, to diagnose accurately, and to establish and sustain a primary care partnership. For example, if video images and sound quality are poor, then providers may not be able to detect and diagnose health problems associated with physical appearance, such as abnormal skin coloration, or they may not be able to pick up on patients' health concerns conveyed through vocal expression. Concurrently, these same factors and filters can affect patients' perception of connection, satisfaction, confidence and efficacy, as well as influence their ability to interact effectively and build a successful primary care partnership with their primary care physician.

In developing our research into *transactional presence*, we considered the communication theory of Jurgen Habermas.[9,10] One of the basic distinctions in his work is between: (a) strategic forms of communication where the purpose is using language in order to have certain effects; and (b) communication oriented towards understanding. What the communication processes in both of these basic distinctions have in common is that they can be considered to be directional – both aspects of the dichotomy have the intent of moving the listener in a particular direction.

Habermas's framework for communication, when applied to a primary care telemedicine encounter, provides us with some potential insights into understanding the dynamics of the patient–provider dialogue in terms of developing *transactional presence*. Here we consider the patient–provider relationship in terms of a bond or trust that needs to be established within a communicative relationship. While the Habermasian view centers on an open-ended communicative process to achieve understanding and an equality of respect, 'participants' also have a responsibility to similarly give and receive (qualitatively) within the context of the telemedicine encounter. Patients have the responsibility to 'move' the dialogue along toward an answer to their medical questions so that they develop an understanding of the issues; physicians have the responsibility to 'move' the discourse toward a resolution of the presenting problem.

Research issues

The issues of technologically mediated communication and the communication presence–distance dichotomy, raise a set of research questions for investigating patient and provider perceptions of primary care telemedicine encounters. These include, but are not limited to the following:

- How might a consideration of human, technological and environmental dimensions inform an understanding of communication presence and lead to a working definition of *transactional presence*?
- What are the central human, environmental and technological communication factors and filters associated with patient and provider perceptions of presence and/or distance in primary care telemedicine?
- How might the perceptions of patients and providers about communication *transactional presence* influence their evaluation of primary care telemedicine?
- How might the cultivation of *transactional presence* and the monitoring of *transactional distance* increase patient and provider perceptions of satisfaction, efficacy, and partnership in primary care telemedicine?

Transactional distance

Within the context of distant education, Moore centered on developing a concept of *transactional distance* – the perceived distance in student-teacher learning relationships, as well as the influence of communication mediated by technology.[11–13] Moore's concept holds possibilities for application to studies connected to perceptions of physical and psychological distance in telemedicine encounters, and extends to a consideration of how these perceptions might influence communication in patient–provider relationships. More importantly, *transactional distance* implies a reciprocal, and perhaps more positive concept for considering communication and perceived relationships in telemedicine visits, i.e. *transactional presence*.

Based on the work of Moore, Bischoff *et al.* (1996, p. 5) constructed an operational definition of *transactional distance* as ' . . . the perceived interpersonal closeness between the teacher and student, among students, and between students and the teacher, as perceived by the student respondents'.[14] Two elements associated with transactional distance, *dialogue* and *structure*, have been important discussion points concerning student–teacher transactions in traditional classrooms.[15] These concepts have been associated with inquiries into connecting teacher–student transactions to learning outcomes,[16] and have developed into significant themes in distance education since the early 1970s.

For example, when faculty deliver content through a one-way lecture format, interpersonal distance between teacher and student is generally increased by linear structure, limited dialogue and spatial distance. In contrast, small group discussions and problem-based learning (PBL) environments typically represent close or small transactional distance by decreasing the linear structure of the student–teacher interaction, increasing human dialogue and decreasing perceived interpersonal spatial distance.

From classroom to clinic

Translating the concept of *transactional distance* from the discussion of the classroom to a telemedicine encounter allows for some parallel observations. First, the smallest transactional distance possible is desirable; and second, the structure of the telemedicine encounter is critical. Additionally, transferring the points made concerning transactional distance to primary care telemedicine raises potential implications for developing and sustaining good patient–provider relationships.

Despite technological advances, history taking and the physical examination remain a major component of a clinician's diagnostic ability. Previous studies estimated that 50–70% of diagnoses were dependent on the quality of data collection and integration,[17] and that faulty data collection or integration accounted for many diagnostic errors.[18,19] It may be the solid presence of the patient and provider dialogue that will be the lynchpin for determining effective telemedicine. If there is a breakdown in patient–provider communication, if technology 'filters' the provider's questions or the patient's responses, or if patients only pretend to understand the primary diagnosis and plan of care, errors will occur and optimal healthcare will not be provided, resulting in poorer clinical outcomes and avoidable problems.[20]

For optimal healthcare to occur, technical, environmental and human factors that serve as positive communication channels, conduits or supports for good dialogic interaction need to be identified, developed and sustained. In a similar manner, technical, environmental and human factors that serve as communication constraints or filters with negative impact need to be eliminated or at least reduced. For example, a video-conference system that consistently channels 'true' (as close to physical reality as possible) visual images and sound contributes to a physical impression of presence necessary for interpersonal interaction. Depending on non-verbal cultural codes, human factors such as frequent patient and provider eye contact may add to personal interpretations of physical and psychological presence.

In other words, facilitating close, mediated feelings and perceptions of inter-personal presence in a primary care telemedicine encounter means that we must account for and yet move beyond the physical dimensions represented by distance and technology. Supporting effective primary care telemedicine interactions rely on, we believe, creating guidelines for developing a personal *presence* in a telecommunicated event.

From *transactional distance* to *transactional presence*

Moving the initial debate about telemedicine from connectivity issues to human factors focusing on communication is a commonsense evolution. We have

developed rather objective assessment measures, which can be used by technicians for a wide variety of variables from sound to picture quality. We have asked
patients and providers about the quality of the picture transmission and audio
levels, and looked to professional TV newscasters for tips on dressing for 'prime
time'. However, it is the interpersonal relationship developed between a provider
and their patient, traditionally in a face-to-face, closed-door encounter, that is the
evolving focus in primary care telemedicine.

Garrison and others began to expand on the utility of constructs other than
connectivity issues in electronically mediated spaces when they characterized
four phases of cognitive presence: evocative, inquisitive, tentative and committed.[21] Their model focused on higher-order thinking skills, and depicted
interaction in an online learning environment as coordinated and synergistic,
not undirected, unreflective or as random exchanges of opinions. The primary
care telemedicine encounter exhibits a variation of the four cognitive phases of
presence as well as patient and provider interactions that appear at times
synergistic. Likewise, Social Dynamic Theory informs us that social spaces are
those places in which individuals interact-transact, influencing one another to
take certain actions.[22] Originally conceptualized as interactions occurring within a
defined physical space, the theory has expanded to include the mediated space
provided by video-conferencing. While not physical in the purest sense of the
term, video-conference space offers a different meeting place for patient and
provider to interact and transact. This 'different' space-place suggests a growing
concern for immediacy – 'the degree of perceived physical or psychological
closeness between people'.[23] In our discussion, we continue this dialogue to
explore a potential 'umbrella' for discussions of human factors – the construct of
transactional presence.

Presence (being engaged with another) may simply be described as 'being
with'. How do patients and healthcare providers achieve 'being with' one
another in a traditional clinic encounter? Being physically, emotionally and
cognitively 'present' and engaged in a face-to-face clinical encounter is a goal
of primary healthcare providers – achieving that same level of interactivity in
a primary care telemedicine encounter requires an even higher level of
engagement, or attention to those mediating factors and filters imposed by
technology.

Lombard and Ditton[24] synthesized the literature on non-mediated presence
from such fields as communication and psychology to inform their understanding
and representation of technology mediated presence. They found six conceptua-
lizations linked to presence; five of the six are especially pertinent for considering
the development of presence in primary care telemedicine:

1 social richness – the feeling of authentic togetherness, which supports patient–
   provider relationship construction
2 realism – the perception of physical accuracy, which not only assists diagnosis,
   but human bonding
3 transportation – the feeling of being there, here or together, contributing to
   patient–provider perceptions of immediacy and the quality of their social
   interaction
4 immersion – the feeling of full involvement, which leads to successful
   healthcare transactions

5 medium as social actor – the perception of and response to cues given by the medium, such as healthcare providers use of a close-up image (of themselves) to prompt in the patient a response feeling of provider concern.

Social presence has been defined as the degree of awareness of another person in an interaction and the consequent appreciation of an interpersonal relationship, and includes factors such as facial expression, direction of gaze, posture, dress, non-verbal cues and vocal cues.[25] Social presence in an online learning environment was defined as a measure of the feeling of community (being a part of, being together) that a learner experiences and is represented by three dimensions:

- social context – task orientation, privacy, topics, recipients/social relationships and social process
- online communication – attributes, application, and perception of the language used
- interactivity – those cooperative activities and communication styles used by online learners.[26]

When social presence, through diverse forms of dialogic interaction, is encouraged and supported, then a close social transactional distance can be imbedded and developed in 'distance' learning relationships.[27]

In a similar manner, social presence in a telemedicine primary healthcare encounter can be described as a measure of patients' and providers' feelings of being together in a social-professional context that is defined by or constructed through mediated interactivity.

An important dimension of that interactivity is the seamless integration of a provider's interpersonal communication and interviewing skills. Brammer and MacDonald constructed a set of seven skill clusters to guide and develop effective communication in professional 'helping relationships' such as primary care events. The skill clusters are:

1 listening
2 leading
3 reflecting
4 challenging
5 interpreting
6 informing
7 summarizing.[28]

These present an important framework for providers to consider as they cultivate presence within the communication domain of primary healthcare, whether that care is given in a traditional face-to-face or in a telemedicine encounter.

Even with this discussion as background, the telemedicine primary healthcare encounter requires a deeper probing into the concept of *presence* – the idea of 'being with' is mediated by technology and suggests a social identity. The script and subsequent narrative of the patient–provider interaction is not only influenced by human factors, but conversely it is also mediated by technological and environmental factors such as equipment functionality and the physical attributes of at least two healthcare sites (the site where the patient is located and the provider's site). Described succinctly, *transactional presence* in a telemedicine primary healthcare encounter is *purposeful human action-interaction within mutual (patient–provider) perceptions of being fully involved and engaged with one another and the technological factors affecting the telemedicine encounter itself.*

In primary care telemedicine encounters, the construct of *transactional presence* helps to prioritize the idea of a purposeful 'being with' in which patients and providers are brought together by/through the video-conference medium for the purpose of effective healthcare. It also incorporates the concepts of social presence and richness, immediacy, realism, transportation, immersion and medium as influencing factors – the focal point of this discussion.

Telemedicine Communication Matrix

The Telemedicine Communication Matrix (TCM) represents the complexity of a technologically mediated primary care telemedicine encounter, and provides a way of visualizing the components of *transactional presence* (Appendix A). At the same time, the matrix suggests a paradoxical simplicity. The matrix is arranged into three 'umbrella' dimensions, followed by categories and finally factors. Moreover, each section (from dimensions to factors) increases in complexity. It would be difficult indeed for any one person to monitor all aspects of the elements represented in the matrix. Yet if we are mindful of the dimensions, categories and factors, we believe that the likelihood for communication effectiveness (and improved healthcare outcomes) will increase. The matrix offers a set of *dimensions*, *categories* and *factors*, to support considerations of how best to construct and/or analyze and evaluate a mediated communication event.

Research methods

Our research design and survey questions are based on prioritizing the human dimension of medicine; specifically, by focusing on categories and factors that influence the perception of patients and providers of *transactional presence* in a primary care telemedicine encounter.

We began the chapter by disclosing our belief that connectivity was no longer the major issue in telemedicine. We strive to achieve the best connections possible with the highest quality sound and visual displays – the reality is that telemedicine may take place in subideal conditions. For example, for some indigent patients, telemedicine may be the only clinical care available through a county clinic. That county indigent clinic may have a converted exam room serving as the telemedicine 'space' – the exam room may be very adequate for face-to-face primary care encounters but lacking in terms of lighting or acoustics for telemedicine. However, the county budget is no doubt insufficient to 'fix' the space used for telemedicine. Thus, providers need to develop personal skills to overcome sub-ideal conditions in order to provide care to populations that: (a) do not have a county healthcare provider available; and (b) can't afford transportation to a state hospital or clinic. Consequently, while it might be desirable to paint the room or upgrade otherwise adequate lighting, primary care telemedicine will often be conducted in subideal, but functional, technical environments. Therefore, we focus our research on the *human dimensions* of the TCM in order to consider how providers can overcome the 'filtered' visual and verbal elements.

For our research, we videotaped four telemedicine clinical encounters between the University of Texas Medical Branch (UTMB) in Galveston, TX, and several distant clinics that have existing contracts for telemedicine services. Three different healthcare providers and four different patients formed the subject matter for this study of *transactional presence* and patient–provider communication.

1 *Telemedicine encounter 1*: provider on-site at UTMB and white female at a distant clinic for follow-up on allergy medication. Overall encounter time: 7 minutes.
2 *Telemedicine encounter 2*: provider on-site at UTMB and white female at a distant clinic with gastro-intestinal pain as her presenting problem. Overall encounter time: 28 minutes.
3 *Telemedicine encounter 3*: provider on-site at UTMB and black male (with wife and child in attendance) at a distant clinic for follow-up/adjustment of seizure medication. Overall encounter time: 17 minutes.
4 *Telemedicine encounter 4*: provider on-site at UTMB and white female at a distant clinic with skin irritation as her presenting problem. Overall encounter time: 20 minutes.

The videotapes were digitized and transcripts were made of the verbal interaction that took place during the encounters. In addition, two groups of patients – those who had previously experienced at least one primary care telemedicine encounter and those who only viewed the digitized telemedicine encounters described above, were included in these studies. Patient and provider permissions were obtained in accordance with the IRB protocols established for this project (International Review Board (IRB) #01-223 and #03-364).

This research study occurred at two separate locations (University of Texas Medical Branch, Galveston, TX, and Alverno College, Milwaukee, WI) and used different evaluation approaches as described below; however, the findings of our research are combined and reported by the themes that emerged.

Study group 1: telemedicine patients (UTMB, Galveston, TX)

Patients who had experienced at least one telemedicine primary care encounter were asked to respond to a set of questions designed to assess the effect of telemedicine on the patient–provider relationship ($n = 20$). While telemedicine patients routinely complete a satisfaction survey at the conclusion of their visit, this survey was the first attempt to evaluate the impact of telemedicine on patient–provider relationships. This group completed a survey and responded to interview questions at their remote site immediately following their telemedicine visit. Participants answered numerous questions relating to concerns about trying telemedicine, the relationship they have with the doctor and their overall satisfaction.

Study group 2: primary care patients (UTMB, Galveston, TX)

A focus group made up of patients who had no experience with a telemedicine encounter, were asked to view the digitized tapes and then to respond to a set of structured questions specifically looking for elements of providers' verbal and non-verbal behaviors that encouraged (not inhibited) the development of patient–provider relationships ($n = 7$). Prior to viewing the tapes, this group was first challenged to recall their last clinic visit with their primary care provider and to describe what physician behaviors encouraged the development of a close patient–provider relationship. Viewing of the digitized tapes followed this discussion. During the focus group, one of the tapes was replayed a second time with the sound turned off in order to assess the non-verbal interaction between patient and provider.

Study group 3: primary care (telemedicine) providers (UTMB, Galveston, TX)

A focus group of primary care providers who are regularly scheduled to conduct telemedicine 'visits' to remote clinics were asked about their perceptions of communication factors and preferences association with quality patient–provider interactions ($n = 5$). Providers were initially asked to reflect on what occurred during their face-to-face clinic visits with patients, and then to compare the differences and similarities to telemedicine visits. The healthcare providers (physicians, physician assistants and registered nurses) were asked questions regarding their decision-making abilities, the relationships with patients and their comfort level with telemedicine.

Study group 4: undergraduate and graduate students (Alverno College, Milwaukee, WI)

Two groups of students were asked to complete the *Transactional Presence Research Project* (TPRP): a qualitative research approach that focused on gathering and investigating students' perceptions of *transactional presence* between provider and patient based on the textual transcript of one taped telemedicine encounter. Specifically, the textual (transcript) analysis focused on the *human dimension, verbal category* and *language factor*, i.e. the actual 'transcripted' dialogue between patient and provider during the telemedicine encounter. The broad intent centered on identifying patterns and considering implications for developing and/or increasing *transactional presence* in primary care telemedicine encounters. The visual response shifted to the *technological dimension* of the TCM, the *communication tool category* and *medium factor*, i.e. video image display conveyed through camera field of view (extreme long shot: ELS – the 'full' person(s) and a lot of the room can be seen; long shot: LS – the 'full' person(s) and some of the room can be seen; medium shot: MS – person can be seen from waist or chest up; close up: CU – the person can be seen from neck up or a specific part of the person can be seen; and, extreme close up: ECU – part of the person's face or a specific part of the person can be seen).

Undergraduate professional communication students were asked to complete the TPRP ($n = 10$). They completed a textual analysis of the transcript, identifying within the patient–provider dialogue moments of *transactional presence*, if any. In pairs, students discussed and came to agreement on key moments of perceived *transactional presence*. Then each pair of students prepared a storyboard with field-of-view camera shots, depicting the patient and provider during the key moments of *transactional presence*. After all storyboards were completed, students viewed a digitized version of the telemedicine event, compared the actual field-of-view camera shots with their storyboard representations, noted any differences in their perceptions of presence, and ranked (high, medium, or low) the perceived quantity and quality of *transactional presence* in the telemedicine encounter. In a debriefing session, students discussed their analyses and perceptions, and offered suggestions for increasing *transactional presence* in similar telemedicine encounters.

Graduate instructional design students were also asked to complete the same *Transactional Presence Research Project* ($n = 12$). Additionally, the graduate students were asked to make written recommendations for developing and/or increasing *transactional presence* in primary healthcare telemedicine encounters.

The textual-transcript analyses, storyboards, recorded discussions and written recommendations from both groups were examined and compared for interpretation and response patterns linked to quality factors associated with *transactional presence*.

Study group 5: undergraduate nursing students and registered nurse monitors (Alverno College, Milwaukee, WI)

Undergraduate nursing students and registered nurse monitors were asked to complete a textual (transcript) analysis designed to gather perceptions about language content (verbal/non-verbal) from the respective perspective of novice and experienced healthcare providers ($n = 7$).

The design for the transcript analysis drew on communication skill set clusters from Brammer and MacDonald[28] to identify perceptions of presence between patient and provider in a primary care telemedicine encounter. Specifically, they were asked to code the following skill set clusters: listening, reflecting, confronting and interpreting, along with an 'other' category. The coding was analyzed to determine participates' perceptions of patient–provider *presence*. The transcript survey for nursing education participants also focused on the TCM *human* dimension. Based on a close reading of the transcript, participants considered the factors of (verbal) language, (relational) roles and types of actions/transaction that occurred.

The overall intent of this part of the project was twofold – to identify communication patterns that were effective when using a teleconferencing medium; and to identify specific skill clusters that were perceived as valuable in a primary care telemedicine encounter.

Findings and discussion

The TCM provided the organizing structure for our studies, and we will point to outcomes within the *Dimensions*, *Categories* and *Factors* wherever relevant. Our research design utilized quantitative and qualitative methods. Follow-up interviews, written surveys and focus groups provided some significant insights into the primary care telemedicine encounter. We grouped the overall findings from these five discrete studies by themes. Analysis of the perceived impact of telemedicine on patient–provider communication, and development of relationships during primary care clinical encounters, were the focus of study groups 1, 2 and 3. Study groups 4 and 5 used the verbal transcripts to discover moments of *transactional presence*, and confirmed their findings with the digitized videotape.

Written response surveys – a starting point

In the written survey, patients rated their overall *comfort* level with telemedicine as 95.25%, while providers ranked this item as 92.5%. When both groups were asked to then compare their telemedicine experience to a traditional face-to-face visit, patients reported a *satisfaction* level on that question of 61.25%, while providers reported 71.07%. On a global question of satisfaction, all participants rated their satisfaction level at 90% or above. Patients in this survey all felt that telemedicine did not affect the interpersonal relationship with their healthcare provider. Healthcare providers judged that telemedicine did not impact the relationship with patients; and all reported spending about the same amount of time with patients using telemedicine as with patients in the clinic.

Focus groups – in-depth follow-up

We then took these survey results to a focus group in order to help us understand the difference between the high global satisfaction with telemedicine and the discrepancy that appeared when the question was phrased: 'compared to a regular visit . . .'. It was during these conversations with patients and healthcare providers in study groups 2 and 3 that we discovered the impact that specific behaviors – the human element – had on primary care telemedicine encounters. In addition to the survey results, we utilized the videotaped telemedicine encounters to set the context and further stimulate discussion.

Focus group participants first commented on the impact of everyday non-verbal behaviors that usually go unnoticed, but became amplified through the telemedicine encounter. Participants pointed out how patients in the videotapes seemed more animated, and distractions appeared 'on tape' where they wouldn't be noticed in day-to-day meetings; for example, a healthcare provider 'played' with her hair during conversations with the patient and 'busy-ness' of hands and shifting posture of the patient became annoying. They further observed that eye contact appeared to be very low in comparison to a face-to-face encounter. While providers often refer to the patient's chart during a face-to-face clinic visit, that behavior became extremely distracting 'on tape'. The focus group discussion continued concerning the amount of reduced visual information that a provider receives on a patient through the camera, and therefore relies more heavily on the patient's medical record. Conversely, a patient 'sees' less and has fewer visual cues to assess what is actually taking place. These discussion tracks lead to an expression of underlying feeling of potential abandonment by patients. Although no specific examples could be cited, patients felt that they could possibly be cut off at any time by the provider, and/or the technology.

Perhaps most insightful were comments on the patient–provider interaction itself. Focus group participants again commented on the reduced 'information' available from visual sources during a telemedicine encounter (compared to a face-to-face visit). Consequently, they felt that first impressions were often reserved until after the verbal interactions began – the sound of the provider's voice, and the manner and kinds of questions were most important to patients when considering *transactional presence*. Yet patients also observed less 'small talk' and reduced socialization processes during telemedicine visits – providers appeared to 'get down to work' almost immediately. Additionally, the focus group participants were split on the perceived need for a 'physical' connection with the provider. For example, a patient/provider handshake at the beginning of a clinic visit, or a patient being handed a prescription (the physical giving and receiving of a slip of paper) at the conclusion of the visit.

Focus group participants who were healthcare providers (study group 3) commented that they behaved more conservatively when utilizing telemedicine – they felt less in control of both their time and the direction of their history taking; they felt they talked 'differently' (and less) to telemedicine patients; they explored fewer collateral issues apart from the presenting problem; and, they felt they couldn't afford to 'open a can of worms' because they only had 'verbal control' (versus verbal and non-verbal control) over the direction of the visit. Additionally, providers acknowledged that they ordered more tests and provided more referrals when seeing patients through telemedicine encounters than in face-to-face visits. The final comment by one of the physicians summed up the observations of this group: 'I think it is a matter of knowing which patients and conditions are appropriate for this type of service.'

Transactional presence – *assessing interactions*

Despite the personal concerns expressed by both patients and providers during this critical analysis, we found objective evidence of *transactional presence* in each of the videotaped primary care telemedicine encounters.

In critical readings of the telemedicine transcripts, both the undergraduate and graduate students (study group 4) identified four to six moments of 'agreed upon' perceived *transactional presence* within the patient–provider dialogue. Overall, compiled team ratings for the perceived quantity and quality of *transactional presence* in the telemedicine encounter averaged a medium rating (neither high nor low). Sketches of the camera's field of view indicated that key affective moments of transactional presence, i.e. moments of emphasis, were optimal when the camera allowed for 'bonding' through a CU display image – the person can be seen from the neck up – and when eye contact was sustained – the provider looking at the camera and not the monitor. Other key moments of *transactional presence* that were more casual, i.e. with less emotional under/ overtones or less emphatic, were typically sketched with a MS display image – the person can be seen from waist or chest up.

Similarly, study group 5 coded the transcript of the third telemedicine encounter, in an effort to identify communication behaviors used by the healthcare provider to establish and sustain a working relationship with the patient (and in this scenario, his wife). There was a sure sense of engagement evident in the communication behaviors that were used throughout the patient appointment.

Listening skills: the healthcare provider used active listening phrases in response to the patient's description of his medical problem, and questions were asked in a reflecting mode in order to gather information that was more descriptive and to check the accuracy of perceptions of the meaning of the information. For example, early in the interaction the healthcare provider questioned whether the patient might have forgotten to take his medication. He responded that he had taken it as ordered. His wife added information that he had also taken a second prescription medication and she wondered if that was a correct thing to do.

Reflecting skills: the healthcare provider heard the response, presented her interpretation of the behaviors and then allowed for perception-validation when she stated '. . . and I think taking (the drug) before you go to bed, if that's helping . . . that's good . . .'. Later in the interaction, the patient asked about an intervention he saw on television. The healthcare provider listened to the idea and then used reflection and interpreting behaviors to respond.

Confronting skills: the healthcare provider suggested some reasons why the TV therapy would not be feasible in this instance and returned to the patient's use of the previously discussed medication and interpreted how it worked in managing the patient's symptoms.

Interpreting skills: there was some discussion of the need to increase the medication and that brief exchange appeared to be used by the patient's wife as an invitation to ask about a concern she had in taking care of her husband. The healthcare provider asked a question or two (suggesting listening) and then stated, 'Well I'm thinking though . . .', as she went on to interpret the information in relation to the client's medical condition and presenting needs. It is at this point in the telemedicine encounter, a little more than mid-way through the appointment, that the interaction suggested a real sense of *transactional presence*. The healthcare provider, patient and his wife exchanged ideas, reinforced each other's suggestions and responses, and developed a workable plan that was agreeable to all. A tangible sense of partnership was reflected in the dialogue of the interaction at this point and was sustained to the end of the appointment.

Summary

Once optimal technical connectivity is accomplished between patient and provider sites, and the most favorable clinic environment is established to conduct primary care telemedicine, there remains the human dimension of the transaction to consider. 'Simply' replicating what transpires in a face-to-face primary care office visit, during a telemedicine encounter, will most often lead to a lowered satisfaction level for both patients and providers. Consequently, in addition to technical connectivity, we feel that consideration needs to be given to the visual, auditory and social filters associated with the technology that affect the patient–provider relationship. In addition, we believe that the dialogue between patient and provider is the lynchpin to the effective delivery of primary care telemedicine. As we stated earlier, we find this concept is embodied in the framework developed by Habermas[9,10] in which communication is considered directional – patients have the responsibility to 'move' the dialogue along toward an answer to their medical questions so that they develop an understanding of the issues; physicians have the responsibility to 'move' the discourse toward a resolution of the presenting problem.

The Study of Human Factors model (Doktor and Bangert – *see* Introduction, p. 7) provides a framework to address the complexity of providing telemedicine in diverse environments. The model proposes layers of considerations influencing human dynamics in an e-health context. In each of the layers of the 'onion' are imbedded mental models, supposition and expectations – exposing, exploring and examining each in turn, along with the *dimensions, categories* and *factors* that cross the boundaries of those layers, will bring about thoughtful consideration of the significance of telemedicine. Striving for a close transactional presence between patient and provider in a primary care telemedicine encounter emphasizes the importance of the human dimension of telemedicine.

From our exploration of *transactional presence* and consideration of the overall patient–provider relationship, we make the following prescriptive observations that could improve communication, develop true patient–provider relationship, and overcome technological and environmental 'filters' in a primary care telemedicine encounter.

- *Verbal categories*: social 'small talk' at the beginning of the telemedicine encounter provides an opportunity to develop a conversation between patient and provider, and to overcome the sense of potential abandonment identified by telemedicine patients. Specific attention to verbal interaction: tone of voice, style of questions asked and 'wait time' – a meaningful pause to allow a patient to respond – are approaches to enhancing patient–provider relations.
- *Non-verbal categories*: ensure camera placement allows for patient eye contact even as the provider looks at the monitor to 'see' the patient rather than looking into the camera. Utilize close-up shots of the patient as well as of the provider to support diagnosis and a sense of 'bonding'. Additionally, being *present* was interpreted as a forward-leaning posture; being *distant* was interpreted as sitting back, unengaged and giving the impression of 'let's finish this'.
- *Relational categories*: providers should acknowledge to patients that 'I'm looking at . . .' when consulting an off-camera electronic medical record or other patient chart. Similarly, since *all* behaviors are amplified during a telemedicine encounter, a provider should acknowledge to a patient that 'I'm thinking about . . .', instead of reflecting in silence. This directionality in communication includes the patient in the process, thereby improving *transactional presence*.
- *Actions/transactions categories*: conscious attention to the basic characteristics associated with active listening provide a sense of purposeful 'being with', essential behaviors for the development of *transactional presence* and the patient–provider relationship.

The human dimension of telemedicine is, we believe, the most important of the various elements in the TCM – it is the component of the transaction over which healthcare providers have some measure of control. We associate our TCM dimensions primarily with the 'Actors, network and alliance layer; of the Study of Human Factors model. The concepts of 'Actor' and 'Alliance', when aligned with the human dimension of the TCM, suggest that healthcare providers may find it beneficial to 'view' themselves in the lead role of the healthcare narrative. By doing so, providers can begin a reflective and pragmatic consideration of how their character and performance influence patient perceptions of 'being with' during primary care telemedicine encounters. They may also begin to recognize and to encourage a reciprocal response from their telemedicine patients. The TCM offers a framework for designing the telemedicine 'stage', choreographing the human performance and constructing the healthcare narrative. Consequently, we believe ongoing research is needed to further examine the role and to evaluate the influence of the specific factors in the Telemedicine Communication Matrix as one means for determining appropriate mental models, for exploring the full range of telemedicine suppositions, and for improving overall acceptance and utilization rates. The goal is to create guidelines for creating a personal *transactional presence* in a telemedicine encounter.

References

1 Whitten P, Mair F, May C *et al.* (2002) Systematic review of cost-effectiveness studies of telemedicine interventions. *BMJ*. **324**: 1434–7.
2 Raimer B, Bonin S, Hermstein S *et al.* (2002) Telemedicine in the workplace can increase productivity and reduce costs. *Telemedicine J.* **8**(2): 195.
3 Davis F (1986) A technology acceptance model for empirically testing new end-user information systems: theory and results. Dissertation, Sloan School of Management, MA.
4 Hu P, Chau P, Liu heng *et al.* (1999) Examining the technology acceptance model using physician acceptance of telemedicine technology. *J Management Information System.* **16**(2): 91–112.
5 American Association of Family Physicians (2004) definitions. www.aafp.org/x6034.xml; accessed 1/26/04.
6 Blanchard C and Ruckdeschel J (1986) Psychosocial aspects of cancer in adults: implications for teaching medical students. *J Cancer Educ.* **4**: 237–48.
7 Marshall P, Thomasma D and Bergsma J (1994) Intercultural reasoning: the challenge for international bioethics. *Camb Q Health Ethics.* **3**: 321–8.
8 Aurora Health Center (2003) I want doctors who listen [advertisement]. Shorewood Herald, Shorewood, WI.
9 Habermas J (1976) *Communication and the Evolution of Society*. Beacon Press, Boston, MA.
10 Habermas J (1984) *Theory of Communication Action, Vol I: reason and the rationalization of society*. Beacon Press, Boston, MA.
11 Moore M (1972) Learner autonomy: the second dimension of independent learning. *Convergence.* **5**(2): 76–7.
12 Moore M (1990) Recent contributions to the theory of distance education. *Open Learning.* **5**(3): 10–15.
13 Moore M (1993) Theory of transactional distance. In: Keegan D (ed.) *Theoretical Principles of Distance Education*. Routledge, New York.
14 Bischoff W, Bisconer S, Kooker B *et al.* (1996) Transactional distance and interactive television in the distance education of health professionals. *Am J Distance Education.* **10**(3): 4–19.
15 Apps J (1989) Foundations for effective teaching. In: Hayes E (ed.) *Effective Teaching Styles*. Jossey-Bass, San Francisco, CA.
16 Chen Y and Willits F (1998) A path analysis of the concepts in Moore's theory of transactional distance in a video-conferencing learning environment. *J Distance Education/Revue de l'enseignement a distance*. http://cade.athabascau.ca/vol13.2/chen.html accessed 1/26/04.

17   Schmitt B, Kushner M and Wiener S (1986) The diagnostic usefulness of the history of the patient with dyspnea. *J Gen Intern Med.* **6**: 386–96.

18   Gruppen L, Wolf F and Billi J (1991) Information gathering and integration as sources of error in diagnostic decision making. *Med Decis Making.* **11**: 233–9.

19   Bordage G (1999) Why did I miss the diagnosis? Some cognitive explanations and educational implications. *Acad Med.* **74**(10 Suppl): S138–43.

20   Davis T, Michielutte R, Askov E *et al.* (1998) Practical assessment of adult literacy in healthcare. *Health Education & Behavior.* **25**: 613–24.

21   Garrison D, Anderson T and Archer W (2001) Critical thinking, cognitive presence, and computer conferencing in distance education. *Am J of Distance Education.* **15**(1): 7–23.

22   Littlejohn S (2002) *Theories of Human Communication.* Wadsworth, Belmont, CA.

23   Richmond V and McCroskey J (2000) *Nonverbal Behavior in Interpersonal Relations.* Allyn and Bacon, Boston, MA.

24   Lombard M and Ditton T (1997) At the heart of it all: the concept of presence. *J Computer-Mediated Communication.* www.ascusc.org/jcmc/vol3/issue2/lombard.html; accessed 1/26/04.

25   Short J, Williams E and Christie B (1976) *The Social Psychology of Telecommunication.* Wiley & Sons, London.

26   Tu C (2002) The measurement of social presence in an online learning environment. *International J on E-Learning.* **1**(2): 34–45.

27   Wulff S, Hanor J and Bulik R (2000) The role and interrelationships of presence, reflection, and self-directed learning in effective world wide web-based pedagogy. In: Cole R (ed.) *Issues in Web-based Pedagogy.* Greenwood Press, Westport, CT.

28   Brammer L and MacDonald G (2003) *The Helping Relationship: process and skills.* Allyn and Bacon, Boston, MA.

Appendix A   Telemedicine Communication Matrix

Dimensions	Categories	Factor
Human Individual: patient and provider Interpersonal: between patient and provider, which may include advocate and/or mid-level presenter with the patient and a primary care provider	Verbal (spoken and written)	Specific language (conventions, word choice, message structure, etc.)
	Non-verbal	Appearance, movement and expression (touch, gesture, facial, eye, vocalic, etc.)
	Relational	Roles and culture (socially prescribed, individually enacted)
	Actions/transactions	Type and sequence (specific behaviors that create a healthcare narrative, including intuition-based behaviors)
Technological (tools)	Medical artefacts/tools (diagnostic, e.g. stethoscope, records)	Quantity, quality and use (amount, types and functionality)
	Communication artefacts/tools (video-conference, computer, telephone systems)	Quantity, quality, use and medium (amount, types and functionality, image-sound display, qualities and integration, etc.)
Environmental (places integral to the telemedicine event)	Physical place (two or more sites associated with healthcare event)	Pragmatic and affective (use of space, appearance, temperature, comfort, etc.)
	Medicated place (social context)	Immediacy and presence (physical presentation and psychological perception of togetherness)

Developed by Sherry Wulff. Funding was provided, in part, by the SBC Telehealth Center at the University of Texas Medical Branch, Galveston, TX.

Section 7

Organizational learning and success in e-health

ICT-supported cooperative work: healthcare and the concept of learning organizations

IH Monrad Aas

Introduction

Many countries in the world are in a process of great historical change. The changes have been proposed to be larger than those of the industrial revolution. Information and communication technology (ICT) plays a fundamental role in these changes. The changes in society are many, and many sectors are changed by the technology. Some sectors have already seen great organizational changes, e.g. the bank sector. Other sectors are in the early stages of the changes the future may bring. The health sector is one example. An essential trait of the industrial revolution was the mass production of goods. In post-industrial society, the knowledge and information society, this is replaced by production of knowledge, information and services.[1]

With a society changing rapidly, citizens may be a part of lifelong learning processes. Learning will become important in the new society. There is talk about learning organizations[2,3] and even a learning society.[4] The capital of organizations is not only financial, but also the human capital.[5] It is possible to speak about a *learning system* within organizations. The *learning system* may play a role not only for more formal job training and education, but also for distribution of knowledge and skills among employees, re-engineering of production processes and the quality of healthcare.

In healthcare, information has already become easily available to patients with the Internet. Many doctors have experienced patients coming to the visit with information found on the Internet.[6] The situation is more demanding for the doctors' professional competence. Remote education is already an important part of telemedicine in Norway[7–9] and in other countries.[10–14] When modern telecommunications make learning less dependent on place, we may speak about *anywhere learning*.[4] When what needs to be learnt maybe changed, we may also speak about *flexible learning*.

In Norway, the organizations of healthcare are widely dispersed, as is the population. This does not make the dissemination of knowledge either easier or less important. Dissemination of knowledge and experience may be a tool for improved patient care.[15] Dissemination of knowledge does not only occur as a result of programs for education, but communication in the work situation also plays a role. Healthcare employees may be participants in informal networks. In such networks, some doctors may be especially influential and important for learning.[16] Learning may occur on an individual basis, for work groups, organizations and organizations in networks. In the study of IT and human factors, organizational learning has a central role. The onion model used in this book illustrates this, where organizational learning is found at the core of the onion.[17] Working with telemedicine has been proposed to result in learning.[18–21] Such possible connection between communication technology and learning in healthcare is little investigated.[20,22,23] In the present study, four qualitative questions were asked to obtain information about actual learning from tele-medical work, consequences of this learning, what could be done to promote people's learning and how participants had learnt to use the telemedical equipment.

Methods

The work presented in this chapter is a part of a larger study and the methods have been described previously.[22,24–29] Sampling was done by first contacting a local hospital where telemedical work was being undertaken. Those directly involved in the telemedical work gave details of persons and organizations with which they had telemedical cooperation. These people were in turn asked to provide details of others working with telemedicine. All who were identified were contacted and asked to participate in a qualitative interview. The data were collected in the period from September 1998 to April 1999. The interviews were tape-recorded and the larger investigation consisted of 39 hours and 20 minutes of recorded interviews. On the basis of transcripts, all information considered to be of interest was coded and, to ease the review,[30] transferred to a statistical package, i.e. SPSS (SPSS Inc., Chicago, USA). In all, 960 elements of information were recorded; for the present chapter, 67 were examined. These related to four questions within the interview concerning learning.

Results

Two of the 32 contacted persons refused to be interviewed due to lack of time, giving a response rate of 94%. The 30 respondents worked for 13 organizations (seven hospitals, four municipalities, one county-owned health center and one private general practice), all located in the five northernmost of Norway's 19 counties. For each of the 30 respondents, mapping was performed of whom they cooperated with. In total, there were 28 telemedical networks, which were different by at least one respondent, and seven telemedical networks, which were totally separate, with no respondent in common. A summary of the responses to three of the four qualitative questions is given in Table 15.1.

Table 15.1 Summary of answers to three of the qualitative questions

	Yes		No	
	N	%	n	%
Have you learnt anything new by using telemedicine?	25	83	5	17
Have you started to perform tasks yourself which you previously were seeking assistance for?	10	33	20	67
Can anything be done in telemedical work which promotes your own learning?[a]	20	67	9	30

[a] One (3%) did not know.
$n = 30$.

The respondents' distribution on the four types of telemedical work and their experience with telemedicine was as follows.

- Twelve worked in psychiatry – three psychiatrists, one general practitioner (GP), three psychologists, four psychiatric nurses and one assistant nurse with training in psychiatry. They had worked with telemedicine for an average of 3.9 years and had performed an average of 41 such remote consultations.
- Six worked in dermatology – three dermatologists and three GPs. They had worked with telemedicine for an average of 4.2 years and had performed an average of 638 such remote consultations.
- Ten worked in a frozen-section pathology service – four pathologists, three surgeons and three laboratory technicians. They had worked with telemedicine for an average of 4.3 years and had performed an average of 43 such remote consultations.
- Two worked in otolaryngology – one otolaryngologist and one GP. They had worked with telemedicine for an average of 3.5 years and had performed an average of 450 such remote consultations.

The hypothesis of age differences in the answers was analyzed. The median age of the 30 respondents was 45.5 years, Q_1 quartile $= 42$ years (25% of the respondents have a lower age than the Q_1 value) and the Q_3 quartile $= 52$ years (25% have a higher age than the Q_3 value). The sample was split according to age in two ways. The answers of those above and below median age were compared. The answers for those below the Q_1 quartile and above the Q_3 quartile were compared. For both ways of splitting age, differences in the answers to three of the qualitative questions were difficult to identify. For the question 'Have you started to perform tasks yourself which you previously were seeking assistance for?', age difference in the answers was suspected. Further analysis showed those who answered 'yes' to the question to have a mean age of 44.6 years and those who answered 'no' a mean age of 46.9 years, but this is not at statistically significant difference $(p < 0.05)$.

Seventy percent $(n = 21)$ of the respondents were men and 30% $(n = 9)$ women. The material was split according to sex, but there were no obvious sex differences in the answers to the four questions.

The hypothesis of the answers to be dependent on volume of use was analyzed. Median for the number of remote consultations was:

- telepsychiatry $= 22.5$
- teledermatology $= 525$
- telepathology frozen section service $= 22.5$.

Quartiles for the number of remote consultations were:

- telepsychiatry $Q_1 = 4.8$ and $Q_3 = 72.5$
- teledermatology $Q_1 = 169$ and $Q_3 = 1125$
- telepathologic frozen-section service $Q_1 = 20$ and $Q_3 = 65$.

With only two respondents in teleotolaryngology values for median and quartiles are not given. For all four types of use the sample was split in high and low volume of use. For telepsychiatry, teledermatology and telepathology the sample was split in two ways. The answers above and below median number of remote consultations were compared. The answers of those below the Q_1 quartile and above the Q_3 quartile were compared. For the different ways of splitting volume of use, there were no obvious differences in the answers.

The four qualitative questions on learning with answers

'Have you learnt anything new by using telemedicine? If yes, what?'

Of the five respondents working in teledermatology who answered 'yes', all three GPs said they had learnt more dermatology. Two said they had learnt more about technology and one specialist said that: 'use of two different settings makes me reflect over the methods we use'.

All 12 working within telepsychiatry said that they had learnt something new. Seven said that they had learnt more psychiatry. Each of the following was mentioned by one respondent:

- learnt each time (e.g. from the psychiatrist, how to ask and from different angles being represented)
- learnt from the instruction
- learnt that planning is important
- learnt how to behave in front of a camera
- learnt more technology.

Also within psychiatry one said that use of two different settings gives reflection over the methods used. Each of the following factors were mentioned by one respondent:

- learnt about cooperation with the patients, about measures concerning patients' social setting, and strengthening of self care
- learnt from working in a group with other professionals
- learnt from cooperating with the specialist in psychiatry
- learnt from participating in remote education
- learnt from using telepsychiatry.

Within the telepathology frozen section service, seven respondents were of the opinion that they had learnt something new. Three said that they had learnt about the frozen section service. Two said that they had learnt more about making sections for microscopy. Each of the following answers was given by one respondent:

- learnt more pathology
- have got a repetition of pathology
- in the start I learnt from cooperating with other professionals like engineers and sociologists
- gives a basis for reflection on what we stress in diagnostic work with less information in the images
- telepathology is a new way of diagnosing although it is quite similar.

The one in teleotolaryngology who answered the question with 'yes' said that he had learnt more otolaryngology and technology.

'Have you started to perform tasks yourself which you previously were seeking assistance for?'

Within dermatology, the three GPs answered that they now did more themselves within the discipline. One said that he now sent fewer patients to the hospital with a dermatology department.

Of the five respondents within psychiatry who answered the question with 'yes', each of the following factors were mentioned by one respondent:

- I have got more difficult patients
- I am frequently used in other connections too
- only to be in control of the technology
- to a certain degree, but still leaves much to the specialist.

Within the telepathology frozen section service, one surgeon at a local hospital said that they admitted fewer patients to the university hospital.

Within otolaryngology, one respondent said only to a certain degree, but that he still left much to the specialist.

One of those who answered the question with 'no' said: 'No, but maybe I become more confident and dare to diagnose on my own'.

'Could anything be done in telemedical work to promote your own learning?'

Within dermatology, two GPs answered that they could learn more by extending telemedicine to include other areas of medicine. One GP was of the opinion that other GPs who referred patients to him for teledermatology could themselves participate in the studio, and that this would have better learning effects for them. One said that more is learnt about communication by working via a screen.

Within psychiatry, two said that more teaching should occur by telematics, and two were of the opinion that they could learn more if the instruction was done by telematics. Two psychiatrists said that they could have learnt more by telemedicine meetings with specialized expertise. Two were of the opinion that there was a need to summarize and describe the experiences with telemedicine. One GP who worked within telepsychiatry found that he could learn more by extending the use to other medical fields. Each of the following factors was mentioned by one respondent:

- bring along other therapist in the studio as observer
- more frequent use leads to more learning
- greater possibility for bringing in external competence
- more experience with telemedicine.

Within pathology, two pathologists and one laboratory technician mentioned that they could learn more with more experience. One of the laboratory technicians would have liked to visit the department of pathology more for learning. One surgeon said that if the technology had been better they could have had more remote teaching. Another surgeon wanted the pathologist to speak out about what he saw during the telemedical sessions and that (the name of an experienced pathologist) give a course. One of the pathologists would have liked to have telemedical discussion groups for pathologists.

'How did you learn to use the telemedical equipment?'

Nineteen said that when they were new to telemedicine they received instructions on how to use the equipment. Eight said that they received no education or organized education. Eight said they had access to a technician. Three had learnt by trial and error. Only two had attended a course. Each of the following was reported by one respondent:

- had three hours with instruction during a few afternoons
- have participated in the development of the equipment
- responsibility for the telemedicine equipment has been given to the responsible for the studio. Do not feel this to be our responsibility.

Within the telepathologic frozen section service, the three laboratory technicians had been trained at a department of pathology to prepare frozen sections for telepathology, and two had also learnt by visits from the department of pathology.

Discussion

In previous publications the methodology used to obtain the empirical data has been presented and discussed in more detail, with issues like qualitative versus quantitative studies, sampling, bias and the reporting of qualitative data.[29]

In a study of IT it was proposed that older employees might find changes in the work situation more difficult, view implementation of IT as a threat, and have problems with the understanding of functions, manuals and IT terminology.[31] Such findings may be related to a lower educational level of older employees.[31] Many of the present users were of a quite mature age. A previous study showed increasing age to be significantly correlated with decreasing anxiety for using the telemedicine technology.[24] In the present study, age differences in the answers could not be found, but splitting of the sample gives small subgroups. In the present sample, higher age is also associated with higher educational level (14 were specialists in medicine) and with more experience. In a study of IT, it was proposed that women might find it easier than men to learn how to use IT.[31] In the present study, no sex differences in the answers could be identified, but splitting of the material into subgroups based on sex gives small sample sizes.

The average experience with telemedicine should be enough to answer the questions. The variability in telemedicine experience in the material is not necessarily negative. Also in the future users will use the technology to different degrees. If respondents were split into two groups – those with a high number of consultations and those with a low number of consultations – we found no difference in their answers to our questions between the high and low groups. But such splitting of those working within the four disciplines results in very small subgroups. In future, larger use of the system may allow more comprehensive answers to these questions.

From empirical basis to learning organizations

The present organization of the health sector is the result of an historical process, and medical technology is often assumed to have had a basic influence on organization. But it is important to be aware that technology and organization may interact and constitute a complex phenomenon. Organizational consequences of technology do not mean that a simple cause and effect relationship exists. It may be easy to see the organizational potential of the technical infrastructure, but organizations may behave according to their own logic. To obtain information about real organizational consequences, empirical research is necessary. For the present contribution empirical data represent the core.

A previous study showed that joint consultations outside of telemedicine might lead to substantial educational gains for participants.[18] A disadvantage with such joint consultations is the need to travel for the joint consultation.

Lifelong learning is not the product of healthcare education. Renewal and further development of knowledge are necessary. With four of five in the present study saying they had learnt something new, the main impression is that learning does occur in telemedicine.

The limited time used on teleconsultations per week is of clear educational value. Such diffusion of knowledge contributes to learning in the organizations and may improve services offered to the patients. The result may also be fewer return visits to the GP after a joint consultation between GP and specialist.[18]

It is known that employees working with telemedicine may share their experiences with each other.[25] The social capital (knowing one another) of the organizations may improve. The transfer of knowledge from one organization to another may give organizational learning, creating a collective memory across organizational borders.

Learning need not result in the performance of new tasks, but nonetheless a third of the respondents reported such effects. The learning potential of telemedicine had not been fully realized, though: two-thirds of respondents indicated that something more could be done in the telemedical work to promote their own learning.

If similar learning is found for other applications of telemedicine, the term 'learning organizations' will be relevant for future healthcare. When healthcare organizations are connected by systems for ICT-supported cooperative work, they also connect for ICT-supported cooperative learning. The learning effect in itself may constitute an argument for implementing telemedicine, and in future the thinking concerning formation of organizational networks may even take into consideration the question of which network has the best learning effects. In such a situation telemedicine may influence organization, and organizational design considerations will be more focused on organizing around the electronic networks and take other considerations less into account.[32] In telemedicine, health care providers have more opportunities to be exposed to: 1) expertise of colleagues and 2) diversity of patient admits. It is possible that increased contact with specialized care will lead to faster and more widespread adoption of new diagnostic and treatment measures.

In future, work organizations may become important arenas for learning and may have to focus on learning.[33] The many possible applications of telemedicine[34,35] may be implemented in one and the same health service, and distance education may play a greater role. Leaders may have to develop a leadership facilitating organizational learning. Management to promote the intellectual capital of the organization may include a management of relationships between employees to promote knowledge sharing and to develop a learning organization culture and infrastructure.[36,37] In telemedicine, learning may be an unplanned by-product, but in learning organizations the learning becomes a part of an organized effort. It has been proposed that a clearly hierarchic organization may represent a hurdle for the flow of knowledge in organizations, and that this is often the case in healthcare.[2,5,38] The answer may be decentralization of functions, change in organizational structure to a less centralized form, and delegation.[39] Use of multidisciplinary teams may also promote learning.[38,40]

When telemedicine is more a failure than a success, it becomes important to understand why. The explanation may be found in factors such as organizational design, culture and decentralization status.[41] Development of local champions and support from top management may also be important.[42] Organizations with learning cultures may be keener to adopt new things, including new technology.[41] Perhaps re-organization needs to occur prior to, or during, implementation of a new technology, rather than after the implementation.

'Have you learnt anything new by using telemedicine? If yes, what?'

Trial and error is a well-recognized way of learning, but in healthcare such learning may have severe consequences for the patients and result in malpractice.[20,43] With telemedicine, personnel in rural areas may learn from medical specialists directly without running special risks. Thus, 83% of the respondents say they have learnt something new by working with telemedicine. Most frequently the respondents improve their knowledge of the specialties in which they are involved. They may also learn other things, e.g. about technology and cooperation. It has been proposed that remote consultations, with GPs and specialists as participants, may result in considerable learning.[18] Questions to Scandinavian hospital leaders showed 59% to be of the opinion that telemedicine gives better education of GPs.[44] It should be noticed that all GPs in the present study said they had learnt something new. The learning effect for GPs is clearly confirmed. The GPs' professional isolation may be reduced,[45] and a decentralized development of competence promoted. The one-to-one, student (GP) to mentor (specialist) relationship tested by the telemedicine encounter may be an important aspect in enhanced learning.[45] The specialist and GP form a coach and apprentice relationship to take care of the patient. Other categories of personnel also learn, e.g. nurses and psychologists. Even the specialists may learn when they work with telemedicine.

In the present study all GPs in teledermatology said they had learnt more dermatology. Learning by the GPs in teledermatology has also been proposed by others.[19] Also the new work situation may be interesting for the specialists, and one specialist said: 'use of two different settings makes me reflect over the methods we use'. In psychiatry, the technology provides considerable potential for learning. Health services could take advantage of this to a greater degree. All those involved in telepsychiatry said they had learnt something new. Some even said they learnt something new every time they worked with telepsychiatry. Most of the ten respondents working within the telepathology frozen-section service were of the opinion that they had learnt something new, and even the specialists reported learning. Surgeons may be reminded of some aspects of cytopathology, and for the pathologist the new situation gives a basis for reflection on what to stress when there is less information in the images.

This chapter gives information about learning for four types of use of tele-medicine. If similar learning is found for other applications, expansion of telemedicine could result in considerable learning.

'Have you started to perform tasks yourself which you previously were seeking assistance for?'

In future, a situation may be created where work organizations require employ-ees to become more flexible and adaptable in terms of the diversity of tasks they undertake. Informal, flexible work systems have been proposed to become the dominating organizational form of the 21st century.[46] The unit 'one person-one function' (or specific set of functions) may constitute a basic building block for organizations. But such organization limits the flexibility and adaptability to new situations. An extension of employees' roles would make healthcare organ-izations more flexible, e.g. to changes in demand. It is not only changes in technology that may play a role for learning, but also organizational factors. It is a common opinion among Scandinavian hospital leaders that telemedicine means that local doctors can perform more precise diagnosing.[44] Learning in telemedi-cine may give local participants the necessary knowledge to take decisions without consulting specialists. When two of three respondents in the present study did not report having an extended professional role, this suggests limits to learning from telemedical work. For those involved in the telepathology frozen-section service there may be less opportunity for an extension of professional roles. When the telepathology frozen-section service is excluded from the sample, 45% (9/20) reported having an extended role.

In the present study, one of three GPs in teledermatology said he sent fewer patients to the hospital dermatology department, and all GPs answered that they now did more themselves within the discipline. In a study of teledermatology it was proposed that learning benefits for GPs could result in an average reduction of referrals of 20%.[21] Making fewer referrals and solo performance of tasks they previously sought assistance for are examples of consequences of learning. The learning leads to changes, with clear importance for economic analysis of telemedicine. It has been proposed that GPs working with remote consultations become semi-specialists.[47] The specialists function as role models for how work within a specialty should be performed.[47] If a semi-specialist is someone able to take care of 50% of the patients without referral to a specialist, calling GPs semi-specialists may be going too far.

In Norway, supply of psychiatric expertise is limited. Telepsychiatry may improve access to the limited resource. When personnel perform tasks they previously needed assistance for, the total capacity of a mental health service increases. Discharge of patients to their local community may improve quality of life.[48] Follow-up may occur via telepsychiatry, and an extended role for local personnel would reduce the daily dependency on outside psychiatric expertise. Extended roles may also improve job satisfaction.[24]

It has been proposed that teleotolaryngology will lead to a better quality of examination technique on the part of the GP, and that this will decrease demand for expert services.[45] In the present study, the GP performing otolaryngology work mainly continued with remote consultations, rather than taking care of the patients alone.

'Could anything be done in telemedical work to promote your own learning?'

The alternative to delivering the expertise by telemedicine could be to develop competence at local sites. The problem is that such training would cost more, and it takes time to develop competence. Economies-of-scale considerations may make such a way of proceeding questionable. Demand at local sites may be too low to fully exploit the competence. In such situations using telemedicine can solve the problem.

The more informed patients, as a result of the Internet,[6] place greater demands on the healthcare personnel's competence. In the remote consultation, the specialist and GP work at the same time, with the same patient, have the same information about the patient, and there is only one teacher and student. For clinical learning, this may be a good situation. The technology may contribute to more seamless care and the healthcare personnel come into direct contact with the patient for more of the total episode of care.

Two-thirds of respondents answered this question with 'yes'. Telemedicine seems to represent a potential for learning not fully exploited. Learning could be promoted by extending the use of remote consultations to other areas. In addition to the four disciplines studied here, a number of other disciplines have employed telemedicine successfully,[34,35] such as geriatrics, acute medicine, rehabilitation, surgery (e.g. guidance during surgery), gastroenterology (endoscopic examination) and ophthalmology. Extended use of the remote consultation may occur for example between primary care and hospitals, home healthcare and hospitals, nursing homes and hospitals, and local hospitals and university hospitals.

When all respondents within psychiatry say they learn, systematic exploitation of telemedicine should be considered. This can be done by including teleconsultations with a remotely located mentor in the ordinary education of personnel, organizing the availability of specialized expertise from central locations and by arranging telemeetings about treatment of patients. In psychiatry, multidisciplinary teams may have a role to play (e.g. when patients are discharged from mental hospital to local community), but it may be difficult to find time for a common meeting for people from different organizations and locations. The technology makes it easier to arrange meetings for multidisciplinary teams and more such meetings may promote learning.

In general, more distance education is wanted. With the technology, lectures by leading experts, previously attended by few people, can be made available to many. Transfer of knowledge from one organization to another may lead to greater similarities in competence, ease communication between organizations and enhance quality. For quality assurance, more participative, open and enhanced feedback of results may play a positive role, together with greater decentralization giving the professionals power to review and implement changes.[41]

The cooperation between specialists and generalists may develop social ties and encourage them to share some professional and cultural values. This could promote the cooperation and the learning further. Merging organizations, on different sides of the networks, would give a common management possibility to influence the situation by strengthening the ties and similarities even further. When organizations cooperating by telemedicine are separate, management may also want to develop stronger network relationships between those involved on both sides. Relationships can be developed, for example by arranging common meetings of social and professional character. In future more could be required from healthcare organizations when it comes to developing network relationships.

Diffusion of technology is influenced by characteristics of the technology, organizations, communication, economics and regulations (e.g. legislation, financing methods). Some work may be required for both sites to find time for each session of remote consultation. In practice, such extra work may represent a barrier for diffusion of remote consultations and result in patients waiting longer for treatment. The alternative could be that a primary healthcare center and a specialist department decide, for each coming half-year, a day and time for telemedicine sessions. Based on knowledge about consumption this could be, for example, one half-day per week for dermatology patients.

'How did you learn to use the telemedical equipment?'

For Electronic Patient Records adequate skills for system users have been identified as important, and we find ideas about improving computer education for health personnel on a larger scale in the European Computer Driving Licence Health Supplement.[49] In the present study, 90% said that they found the technology easy to use.[24] This in spite of few having learnt to operate the equipment by attending courses. The finding may in part be explained by some health personnel having access to a technician. There does not seem to be a need for more extensive training in how to work with the technology. Initial instruction may be enough. The equipment can be switched on as the light is switched on. Calling a hospital can be done by pressing a button with the name of the hospital on. Still the belief that operation of the equipment is difficult may represent a barrier to its use, and it is possible that more information could overcome this perception and contribute to a more rapid expansion of telemedicine. The further expansion of telemedicine could also be promoted by economic incentives, such as a per consultation method of payment.[50]

Conclusions

Learning by telemedicine more than lives up to expectations. Telemedicine work undoubtedly results in learning. More than four of five of the respondents say that they have learnt something new by working with telemedicine. Most frequently the participants learn about the specialty in which they are involved. When two out of three respondents said that more could be done in telemedical work to promote learning, this demonstrates the potential for learning by telemedicine. The remote consultation can be used in a higher number of disciplines and between several levels of care. When all within psychiatry learn, taking full advantage of this, e.g. by including telepsychiatry in teaching programmes, should be considered. More remote education is wanted and could improve competence and quality. Lectures by leading experts could be made available for many, irrespective of their location.

All GPs learn, and so do nurses, psychologists, other categories of personnel, and even medical specialists. The learning does not necessarily change behavior, as two-thirds of the respondents cannot say that what they learnt made them capable of performing tasks they previously needed assistance for. It may be an exaggeration to claim that GPs become semi-specialists by working with remote consultations – the volume of patients they take care of on their own is hardly that large.

To start working with telemedicine some initial instruction seems to be enough, and more extensive teaching programmes are not necessary.

In future, with more telemedicine, work organizations may become important arenas for learning, and leaders may have to focus on learning. The term 'learning organizations' may become important. Learning organizations may be designed to promote learning in the organizations, to keep pace with the rapid increase in medical knowledge, increased quality requirements, more demanding patients, and make technology implementation more successful. For healthcare organizations essential questions will be: What kind of learning is wanted? Which organizational measures can be taken to influence learning?

References

1   Castells M (2000) *The Rise of the Network Society* (2e). Volume 1. Blackwell Publishers, Oxford.
2   Nikula RE (1999) Organisational learning within healthcare organizations. *Medical Informatics.* **56**: 61–6.
3   Davies HTO and Nutley SM (2000) Developing learning organisations in the new NHS. *British Medical Journal.* **320**: 998–1001.
4   Gates B (1999) *Ledelse med t@nkens hastighet* [Business @ The Speed of Thought]. Egmont Hjemmets Bokforlag, Oslo.
5   Nordhaug O (1993) *Human Capital in Organizations. Competence, Training, and Learning.* Scandinavian University Press, Oslo.
6   Hjortdahl P, Nylenna M and Aasland OG (1999) Internett og lege – pasient – forholdet – fra 'takk' til 'hvorfor?' [Internet and the doctor–patient relationship – from 'thankyou' to 'why?']. *The Norwegian Medical Journal.* **119**: 4339–41.
7   Vaagland O (1999) Nasjonale satsinger innen fjernundervisning [National efforts in remote teaching]. *Proceedings for Norsk Telemed '99,* 13–15 Oktober, Tromsø, p. 62.

8   Bach B (1999) Møteplassen for helseutdanninger [The meeting place for healthcare education]. *Proceedings for Norsk Telemed '99*, 13–15 Oktober, Tromsø, p. 67.

9   Aasebø U, Opdahl R, Strøm HH *et al.* (1998) Decentralisert spesialistutdanning i lungesykdommer [Decentralized education of specialists in pulmonary diseases]. *Nordisk Medicin.* **113**: 237–9.

10 Fulmer J, Hazzard M, Faan SJ *et al.* (1992) Distance learning: an innovative approach to nursing education. *Journal of Professional Nursing.* **8**: 289–94.

11 Orusild E (1999) Undervisning på distans av AT- och ST läkare – ett telemedicinskt pilotprosjekt på Visby lasarett och Huddinge sykehus' [Remote teaching of AT- and ST doctors – a telemedicine pilotproject at Visby and Huddinge hospitals]. *Proceedings for Norsk Telemed '99*, 13–15 Oktober, Tromsø, p. 68.

12 Sherwood GD, Armstrong ML and Bond ML (1994) Distance education programs: defining issues of assessment, accessibility, and accommodation. *The Journal of Continuing Education in Nursing.* **25**: 251–7.

13 Sixsmith A, Beer M and Green S (1999) An occupational therapy Internet school. *Proceedings of Telemed 99*, 28 November–1 December, London, pp. 175–7.

14 D'Souza R (1999) A pilot study of an educational service for rural mental health practitioners in South Australia using telemedicine. *Proceedings of Telemed 99*, 28 November–1 December, London, pp. 187–9.

15 Danielsen HE (1997) Telemedisin – kostnad og nytte [Telemedicine – costs and benefits]. *The Norwegian Medical Journal.* **117**: 1582–3.

16 Anderson JG, Jay SJ, Perry J *et al.* (1994) Modifying physician use of a hospital information system. In: Anderson JG, Aydin CE and Jay JS (eds) *Evaluating Healthcare Information Systems. Methods and applications*, pp. 276–87. Sage Publications, Thousand Oaks, CA.

17 Bangert DC, Doktor R and Valdez M (eds) (2005) *Human and Organizational Dynamics in e-Health*. Radcliffe Publishing, Oxford and Seattle.

18 Harrison R, Clayton W and Wallace P (1996) Can telemedicine be used to improve communication between primary and secondary care? *British Medical Journal.* **313**: 1377–80.

19 Jøsendal O, Fosse G, Andersen KA *et al.* (1991) Fjerndiagnostisering av hudsykdommer [Remote diagnosing of skin diseases]. *The Norwegian Medical Journal.* **111**: 20–2.

20 Robinson DF, Savage GT and Campbell KS (2003) Organizational learning, diffusion of innovation, and international collaboration in telemedicine. *Health Care Management Review.* **28**: 68–78.

21 Wootton R, Bloomer SE, Corbett R *et al.* (2000) Multicentre randomised control trial comparing real time teledermatology with conventional outpatient dermatological care: societal cost-benefit analysis. *British Medical Journal.* **320**: 1252–6.

22 Aas IHM (2002) Learning in organizations working with telemedicine. *Journal of Telemedicine and Telecare.* **8**: 107–11.

23 Bangert D and Doktor R (2000) Implementing store-and-forward telemedicine: organizational issues. *Telemedicine Journal and e-health.* **6**: 355–60.

24 Aas IHM (2000) Working with telemedicine: user characteristics and attitudes. *Journal of Telemedicine and Telecare.* **6**(Suppl. 1): 66–8.

25 Aas IHM (2001) A qualitative study of the organizational consequences of telemedicine. *Journal of Telemedicine and Telecare.* **7**: 18–26.

26 Aas IHM (2001) Telemedical work and co-operation. *Journal of Telemedicine and Telecare.* **7**: 212–18.

27 Aas IHM (2002) Changes in the job situation due to telemedicine. *Journal of Telemedicine and Telecare.* **8**: 41–7.

28 Aas IHM (2002) Telemedicine and changes in the distribution of tasks between levels of care. *Journal of Telemedicine and Telecare.* **8**(Suppl. 2): 1–2.

29   Aas IHM (2003) Organizing for remote consultations in healthcare – the production process. *Behaviour & Information Technology.* **22**: 91–100.
30   Qureshi H (1992) Integrating methods in applied research in social policy: a case study of carers. In: Brannen J (ed.) *Mixing Methods: qualitative and quantitative research,* pp. 101–25. Avebury Ashgate Publishing, Aldershot.
31   Solberg LA, Natvig H, Endestad T *et al.* (1998) IT-endringer i Norske Bedrifter: IT-kvalitet og brukeres mestring av ny teknologi [IT changes in Norwegian firms: IT quality and users' mastering of a new technology]. STF 78 A98405, SINTEF Unimed, Oslo.
32   Aas IHM (1999) *Styring av helsetjenesten. Mangfold og muligheter* [Managing the Health Service. Many alternatives and possibilities]. Kommuneforlaget, Oslo.
33   Harman WW (1979) *An Incomplete Guide to the Future.* WW Norton & Company, New York.
34   Aas IHM and Geitung JT (1998) Telemedisin: Teknologi med mange anvendelsesområder. Del 1: Introduksjon, fysiske nettverk, kliniske anvendelsesområder, medisinske servicefunksjoner [Telemedicine: technology with many applications. Part 1: Introduction, physical networks, clinical applications, medical service functions]. HMT Tidsskrift for Helse Medisin Teknikk, No. 6, pp. 24–8, 30–31.
35   Aas IHM and Geitung JT (1999) Telemedisin: Teknologi med mange anvendelsesområder. Del 2: Extramural anvendelse, kompetanseutvikling, administrasjon og styring, organisatoriske konsekvenser [Telemedicine: technology with many applications. Part 2: Extramural applications, development of competence, administration and management, organizational consequences]. HMT Tidsskrift for Helse Medisin Teknikk, No. 1, pp. 20–3, 26–9.
36   Snow CC, Lipnack J and Samps J (1999) The virtual organization: promises and payoffs, large and small. In: Cooper CL and Rousseau DM (eds) *Trends in Organizational Behaviour. The Virtual Organization,* vol. 6, pp. 15–30. John Wiley & Sons Ltd, Chichester.
37   Senge PM, Kleiner A, Roberts C *et al.* (1994) *The Fifth Discipline Fieldbook. Strategies and Tools for Building a Learning Organization.* Doubleday, New York.
38   Stead WW (1998) The networked health enterprise: A vision for 2008. *Journal of the American Medical Informatics Association* **5**: 412–15.
39   Aas IHM (1997) Organizational change: decentralization in hospitals. *International Journal of Health Planning and Management.* **12**: 103–14.
40   Øvretveit J, Mathias P and Thompson T (1997) *Interprofessional Working for Health and Social Care.* Macmillan Press, London.
41   Bangert DC and Doktor R (2005) Organizational learning and culture in the managerial implementation of clinical e-health systems: an international perspective. In: Bangert DC, Doktor R and Valdez M (eds) *Human and Organizational Dynamics in e-Health.* Radcliffe Publishing, Oxford and Seattle.
42   Seale DE, Robinson SS, Green A *et al.* (2005) Developing strategic alliances for telemedicine. In: Bangert DC, Doktor R and Valdez M (eds) *Human and Organizational Dynamics in e-Health.* Radcliffe Publishing, Oxford and Seattle.
43   Aas IHM (1991) Malpractice. *Quality Assurance in Health Care.* **3**: 21–39.
44   Danneskiold-Samsøe B, Hatling M, Arnlind M *et al.* (1998) Telemedicine in the Nordic countries – attitudes and diffusion. NIS-report 4/98, SINTEF Unimed, Trondheim.
45   Pedersen S, Hartviksen G and Haga D (1994) Teleconsultation of patients with otorhinolaryngologic conditions. A telendoscopic pilot study. *Archives of Otolaryngology: Head & Neck Surgery.* **120**: 133–6.
46   Heydebrand WV (1989) New organizational forms. *Work and Occupations.* **16**: 323–57.
47   Akselsen S and Lillehaug S-I (1993) Teaching and learning aspects of remote medical consultations. *Telektronikk.* **89**(1): 42–7.

48 Dobson R (2000) Psychiatric patients enjoy better life in community. *British Medical Journal.* **320**: 1228.

49 Rigby M (2004) Protecting the patient by promoting end-user competence in health informatics systems – moves towards a generic health computer user 'driving license'. *International Journal of Medical Informatics.* (in press).

50 Aas IHM (1995) Incentives and financing methods. *Health Policy.* **34**: 205–20.

Chapter 16

Organizational learning and culture in the managerial implementation of clinical e-health systems: an international perspective

David C Bangert and Robert Doktor

The problem

Organizational culture is recognized as a key component of knowledge manage-ment and organizational learning.[1] However, organizational culture is signific-antly influenced by national culture.[2] Further, for organizational culture to function effectively as a managerial control mechanism, the organizational culture and the formal organizational structure must be harmoniously inter-related.[3] Thus, the structure and culture of an organization must be aligned with the demands and predispositions of the environment in which the organization operates,[4] noting that a significant aspect of that environment is the national culture in which the organization is embedded.[2]

Modern healthcare organizations are confronted with a steady stream of new clinical e-health technologies, many of which have significantly enhanced the quality of clinical practice. Some of these technologies have also offered the potential of increasing access and/or reducing the overall societal costs of healthcare.[5,6] Yet, early evidence suggests great difficulty in implementing some of these new technological advances in the US.[7]

Telemedicine is a good example of this challenge. Bashshur discusses how the second generation of telemedicine has the requisite technology, but faces such uncertainties as lack of long-term sustainability plans, lack of mature programs that can be the basis of definitive cost-benefit analyses, and limited acceptance of telemedicine by health providers and health administrators.[5] Telemedicine was originally conceived as a two-way video-conference between a primary care provider and patient at one end, and a specialist at the other end. It has evolved into a clinical information technology subsystem inclusive of multimedia email, Web-based applications and real-time consultation transfer of detailed clinical patient information that flows between healthcare providers and often to/from patients. This development holds the potential for enhanced patient access to better healthcare, reduced total healthcare costs and, as a consequence of easy access to the most appropriate specialist expertise, higher overall quality of the healthcare delivered.[8] Despite the great promise of clinical e-health solutions such as telemedicine, successful implementations with high utilization have been rare in the US.[9]

There are many reasons for poor implementation performance:[10,11] often legal barriers prevent telemedicine's use across political boundaries; the issue of reimbursement to healthcare providers (HCP) often presents a barrier to utilization; and sometimes the technology does not perform as promised. While these issues are real and relevant, they do not explain what we believe to be one of the primary causes of the problem: organizational dynamics.[12,13]

Most modern healthcare delivery organizations in the US are conceived, designed and structured to promote effectiveness and efficiency of a bygone era – a time when quality was assured by formal authoritarian control, iron-clad rules and a one-best-way mentality. In some national cultures, such an organizational approach is still appropriate. However, we contend that in many national cultures around the globe, successful adoption of an e-health strategy requires a more organic and less mechanistic organizational culture and structure. For healthcare organizations of such national cultures, a more organic form will better match the cultural and knowledge/learning predispositions of the organization's members. The acceptance of the highly disruptive technology by the members is fundamental to its successful adoption.

When the organizational culture and structure are in harmony with the predispositions and demands of the national culture within the organization's environment, then it is our contention that the organization is primed to be a fast learning organization.

All organizations learn. Some organizations learn more quickly than others. A key determinant in the speed with which an organization analyzes its environment and changes its behavior to be more adaptive to that environment (i.e. *learns*) is its culture. With other things being equal, such learning depends on the underlying harmony between the organization's national culture* on the one hand, and its organizational culture and structure, on the other. The greater this harmony, the speedier is the learning. The speedier the learning, the greater is the effectiveness of implementations of new technologies.

Healthcare systems need to adapt to changing environments, draw lessons from past success and failures, detect and correct errors of the past, anticipate and respond to impending uncertainty, and realize images of a desirable future. There is a virtual consensus among leaders in healthcare as to the 'learning imperative', and in the world of healthcare organizational practice organizational learning has become an idea in good currency.[14]

But not all organizations, in healthcare or in other industries, learn at the same speed or in the same way. Different organizations have different learning styles.[14] Some organizations are best at adaptive learning (sometimes referred to as

---

* Multinational organizations exist in many cultures concomitantly. Some multinationals retain their parent national culture throughout. In these cases, it is the parent national culture which we refer to when speaking of national culture. Other multinationals encourage each subsidiary to embrace the national culture in which that subsidiary is embedded. In these cases, by national culture vis-à-vis organization structure and culture, we mean the national culture in which the subsidiary is embedded.

single-loop learning), i.e. changes made in reaction to changed environmental conditions. Other organizations have a learning style often referred to as proactive learning, i.e. organizational changes made in anticipation of a desired end-state. That is, the organization has a systemic model of its interaction with the environment and a forecasting model of the environment's future behavior. Based on these models, the organization generates actions designed to interact with the environment's future behavior in a manner to produce the organizationally desired end-state. Proactive learning is often referred to as double-loop learning[14] or generative learning.[15]

We contend that for organizations embedded in some national cultures, the most appropriate organizational culture and structure is that which achieves its speediest and most effective learning performance through an adaptive organizational learning style. In other organizations, embedded in different national cultures, the most harmonious organizational culture and structure need to promote proactive learning; and, although more complex than an adaptive organizational learning style, such a proactive organizational learning style is actually speedier and more effective for these organizations.

In what follows, we discuss certain dimensions of national culture which drive the development of organizational culture and structure that are most appropriate for an optimal organizational learning style. We focus on healthcare delivery organizations; we relate their organizational learning effectiveness to their competency in implementing and utilizing new clinical e-health technologies.

We assert that cultural analyses have shown that what works in one culture may not be appropriate in another.[2,7] Specifically, we will discuss how the capacities of a successful healthcare delivery organization depend on the values of the society it serves, and, accordingly, that one solution to the e-health implementation problem does not fit all situations.

Relationship to other chapters in this book

In the literature review that follows, the reader will notice many 'layers of the onion' analyzed as separate literature. As noted in the introduction to this book, the chapter demarcations are artificial categories there only to serve readers' cognitive habits of linear information processing,

Along those lines, this contribution best fits in the last section of the book which is devoted to organizational learning and e-health utilization. Nonetheless, there are strong interrelationships with many of the articles in preceding chapters. The layers of the onion are not independent and instead are integrally connected, each to all others; that connection is manifest in the pages that follow.

In this section of the book, the chapter by Aas discussed the significance of organizational learning to the utilization of telemedicine. He showed how telemedicine utilization interactively effects and enhances organizational learning in his study in Norway.

The literature

Cross-cultural organization literature

We find the work of Geert Hofstede[2,16–18] insightful when considering the organizational designs for successful e-health implementation. Hofstede has argued that organizational systems work best when their design is consistent with the underlying values and culture of the society in which they function.[17] In particular, Hofstede has pointed out that American management practices may not be appropriate or successful when implemented in societies with cultural values that differ from those held in the US. Critics of Hofstede's work believe that he takes too simplistic a view of the multifaceted, complex dimensions which comprise the notion of culture. However, for our purposes, Hofstede's defined basic dimensions are exceedingly useful theoretical constructs.[2] Hofstede's five dimensions of cultural variability are:

1 power distance
2 uncertainty avoidance
3 individualism-collectivism
4 masculinity-femininity
5 Confucian dynamism (long versus short-term orientation).[2]

Each of these dimensions is rather complex; we refer the reader to Hofstede for a complete analysis.[2] However, it is the second basic dimension, uncertainty avoidance, which seems most relevant to our analysis of the relationship of organizational design to organizational learning and, in turn, to successful e-health implementation.

Uncertainty avoidance refers to the extent to which people feel threatened by and avoid uncertain or unknown situations. Cultures with high uncertainty avoidance value predictability and stability. They create formal rules and believe heartily in their relevance. They prefer fixed structures and clear interpretations. They like things black and white, not gray. They dislike experimenting with unknown outcomes.

We maintain that societies high in uncertainty avoidance create environments that strongly favor mechanistic organization. They do so to achieve the organizational learning necessary for such changes as the successful implementation of disruptive technology – and we suggest that the obverse may be true for low uncertainty avoidance cultures.

Hofstede's measurement of national cultures reveals that such countries as Japan, France and South Korea have high uncertainty avoidance.[2] Examples of middle-level uncertainty avoiding national cultures are Italy and Taiwan. National cultures scoring low on uncertainty avoidance include Singapore, US and Great Britain. The complete ranking of countries is in Table 16.1.

Table 16.1 Scores on five cultural, national dimensions for 53 countries or regions

Country	Power distance		Individualism/collectivism		Masculinity/femininity		Uncertainty avoidance		Confucian dynamism	
	Index	Rank	Index	Rank	Index	Rank	Index	Rank	Index	Rank
Argentina	49	18–19	46	31–32	56	33–34	86	39–44	–	–
Australia	36	13	90	52	61	38	51	17	31	9–10
Austria	11	1	55	36	79	52	70	29–30	–	–
Belgium	65	34	75	46	54	32	94	48–49	–	–
Brazil	69	40	38	27–28	49	27	76	32–33	65	18
Canada	39	15	80	49–50	52	30	48	12–13	23	4
Chile	63	29–30	23	16	28	8	86	39–44	–	–
Colombia	67	37	13	5	64	42–43	80	34	–	–
Costa Rica	35	10–12	15	8	21	5–6	86	39–44	–	–
Denmark	18	3	74	45	16	4	23	3	–	–
Ecuador	78	45–46	8	2	63	40–41	67	26	–	–
Finland	33	8	63	37	26	7	59	22–23	–	–
France	68	38–39	71	43–44	43	18–19	86	39–44	–	–
Germany, FR	35	10–12	67	39	66	44–45	65	25	31	9–10
Great Britain	35	10–12	89	51	66	44–45	35	6–7	25	5–6
Greece	60	26–27	35	24	57	35–36	112	53	–	–
Guatemala	95	51–52	6	1	37	11	101	51	–	–
Hong Kong	68	38–39	25	17	57	35–36	29	4–5	96	22
Indonesia	78	45–46	14	6–7	46	23–24	48	12–13	–	–
India	77	43–44	48	33	56	33–34	40	9	61	17
Iran	58	24–25	41	30	43	18–19	59	22–23	–	–
Ireland	28	5	70	42	68	46–47	35	6–7	–	–
Israel	13	2	54	35	47	25	81	35	–	–
Italy	50	20	76	47	70	49–50	75	31	–	–
Jamaica	45	17	39	29	68	46–47	13	2	–	–
Japan	54	21	46	31–32	95	53	92	47	80	20
Korea, Republic of	60	26–27	18	11	39	13	85	37–38	75	19
Malaysia	104	53	26	18	50	28–29	36	8	–	–
Mexico	81	48–49	30	22	69	48	82	36	–	–

Table 16.1 *Cont.*

Country	Power distance		Individualism/ collectivism		Masculinity/femininity		Uncertainty avoidance		Confucian dynamism	
	Index	*Rank*	*Index*	*Rank*	*Index*	*Rank*	*Index*	*Rank*	*Index*	*Rank*
Netherlands	38	14	80	49–50	14	3	53	19	44	14
Norway	31	6–7	69	41	8	2	50	16	–	–
New Zealand	22	4	79	48	58	37	49	14–15	30	8
Pakistan	55	22	14	6–7	50	28–29	70	29–30	0	1
Panama	95	51–52	11	3	44	20	86	39–44	–	–
Peru	64	31–33	16	9	42	16–17	87	45	–	–
Philippines	94	50	32	23	64	42–43	44	10	19	3
Portugal	63	29–30	27	19–21	31	9	104	52	–	–
South Africa	49	18–19	65	38	63	40–41	49	14–15	–	–
Salvador	66	35–36	19	12	40	14	94	48–49	–	–
Singapore	74	41	20	13–15	48	26	8	1	48	15
Spain	57	23	51	34	42	16–17	86	39–44	–	–
Sweden	31	6–7	71	43–44	5	1	29	4–5	33	12
Switzerland	34	9	68	40	70	49–50	58	21	–	–
Taiwan	58	24–25	17	10	45	21–22	69	28	87	21
Thailand	64	31–33	20	13–15	34	10	64	24	56	16
Turkey	66	35–36	37	26	45	21–22	85	37–38	–	–
Uruguay	61	28	36	25	38	12	100	50	–	–
US	40	16	91	53	62	39	46	11	29	7
Venezuela	81	48–49	12	4	73	51	76	32–33	–	–
Yugoslavia	76	42	27	19–21	21	5–6	88	46	–	–
Regions:										
East Africa	64	31–33	27	19–21	41	15	52	18	25	5–6
West Africa	77	43–44	20	13–15	46	23–24	54	20	16	2
Arab Countries	80	47	38	27–28	53	31	68	27	–	–
Bangladesh	–	–	–	–	–	–	–	–	40	13
China	–	–	–	–	–	–	–	–	118	23
Poland	–	–	–	–	–	–	–	–	32	11

From Hofstede, 2001.[2]

Organizational design literature

The appropriate design of an organization depends on many factors, the most salient of which are the strategic intent of the organization[19] and the environment in which the organization operates.[20-23]

The research literature on organizational design[24-28] considers both the structural elements of design and the cultural elements of design.[29,30] Of the structural dimensions, formalization and centralization[24,28,31-33] stand out; of the cultural dimensions, values, learning style and strength[2,34] stand out.

Organizations with high formality are defined as having high division of labor,[35,36] maintaining strict rules[37] and discouraging multiple job skills.[37] High centralization in organizational design exists where communication is controlled by strict vertical, individual command chains,[38] and where communication about and participation in decision making is discouraged.[39] Organizations with high formality and high centralization are often referred to as highly mechanistic in their structure.

Organizations with the obverse structural characteristics are said to be more organic in their structural design. A strong parallel exists on the cultural side of organizational design. Organizations with cultures that encourage participation, two-way communication and decentralize decision making are often characterized as being more organic. They are usually more open about making mistakes, more encouraging of questioning and participation, highly supportive of testing new things, more willing to accept diversity and tolerant of ambiguity.[34] Organizations that fall into the mechanistic category are closed to admitting mistakes, punish mistakes, avoid diversity and are intolerant of ambiguity. Organizational form thus spans the spectrum from organic to mechanistic, with each organization falling somewhere between these two ideal types and having shades of both organic and mechanistic dimensions. The issue is one of relativity: is the organization generally more organic in its structural and cultural dimensions, or is it more mechanistic?

Technology diffusion literature

The research literature on technology diffusion in organizations in the US has shown low correlation between centralization/formalization and the acceptance/adoption/implementation of technology.[40] Meyer and Goes[41] studied the technology diffusion process in 25 hospitals as those organizations were deciding to adopt medical innovations such as computed tomography (CT) scanners, ultrasonic imaging, laser surgery and fiber optic endoscopy. They found only 10% of the variance in adoption success attributable to organization structural variables; they found 40% of the variance, however, attributable to organizational cultural variables such as attitudes, perceptions and especially the climate for innovation created by the organization's leadership.

Organizations most likely to adopt new technical innovations were those with cultures that encouraged their members to try new approaches to meet environmental demands. Van de Ven and Rogers[42] point out that an adoption of technology often falters because the innovation fails to align with the organization's perceived problem, or the expected consequences are perceived by the organization's members as more negative than positive.

Research on computer-related technical innovations in organizations points to the perceived 'uncertainty' created by the innovation as a source of resistance to adoption of the technology.[43] The concept termed 'uncertainty' by these researchers is akin to the dimension of uncertainty avoidance.[2]

Resistance-to-change literature

Just as technology diffusion literature enriches our understanding of the role of organization design in the implementation problem, so too the long-in-history literature on resistance to change and change management adds insight.[44] A primary tenet of this school of thinking is the concept of attitude change. William Bridges[45] purports that attitude change requires a three-phase phenomena:

1 unfreezing (ending)
2 transitioning (neutrality)
3 refreezing (new beginning).

Organizational design frames the capacity for attitude change: most resistance to change in organizations is founded in rational decisions that are based on currently held attitudes of members relative to their position in the organization and the consequences of the change from the point of view of that position.

In his book *Leading Change*, Kotter[46] asserts that technological change needs a visionary leader who is capable of sharing the vision of using the new technology. The leader must also motivate its use and visibly reward those who first begin to adopt and use the new technology. Of greatest importance, according to Kotter,[46] the new technology must become part and parcel of the organization's culture – as integral to the way in which that organization does business.

Organizational learning literature

Many scholars attribute the original work on organizational learning to the work of Cyert and March,[47] Bateson,[48] and Argyris and Schon.[14] Schein[49] points out that there have been so many contributions to the organizational learning literature from so many different fields, such that there now exists considerable confusion with regard to a consensus definition of the term 'organizational learning'. Most scholars do agree, however, that organizational learning speaks to non-transient changes in an organization's behavior as a consequence of its interaction with the environment. There have been many scholars who have explored the concept of style in the study of organizational learning.[14] Despite the many different classifications of organizational style present in the literature, it is Argyris and Schon's (1978) original dichotomy of single-loop versus double-loop learning style that has passed the test of time and is most often researched and alluded to by scholars of organizational learning. This dichotomy has also been reframed: lower-level versus higher-level learning,[50] tactical versus strategic learning[51] and adaptive versus generative learning.[13]

The literature on organizational learning styles does not agree on the 'best style.' Some scholars criticize single-loop learning.[52] Ayas (1996)[53] points out that there is no one best style for an organization to learn. It all depends on the environment in which the organization is embedded. Fiol and Lyles[50] point to the advantages of single-loop learning in stable, more predicable environments. Senge (1990)[15] indicates that in uncertain environments, characterized by discontinuous change, double-loop learning may be the most appropriate organizational learning style.

The concept of organizational learning,[34] at an aggregate level, mirrors the dynamics of the resistance-to-change literature. Organizations with high learning cultures are keen to adopt new things, welcome diversity and embrace change. At the aggregate level, a learning culture stimulates the unfreezing to refreezing phases noted in the resistance-to-change literature. Both organizational learning literature and change management literature, from different vantage points, reach similar conclusions, yet at different levels of aggregation.

DeLong and Fahey[1] argue that culture shapes the assumptions that are relevant to the importance of knowledge, and further state that culture embodies all the unspoken norms or rules about how knowledge is to be distributed between the organization and the individuals in it. Culture dictates what knowledge belongs to the organization and what knowledge remains in the control of individuals and subunits.

Technology acceptance model literature

The Technology Acceptance Model (TAM) was developed by Davis et al.[54] to understand the relationship between attitudes, intentions and behavior of potential IT users. Since its development, over 400 journal citations of the original Davis et al.[54] article have been noted by the Social Science Citation Index. Therefore, the TAM is a well-researched hypothetical construct. Most, but not all, TAM research indicated that if the potential user believes that the IT system will help them accomplish their task, and to a lesser extent will be easy to use, then the potential user will self-report that they will use the IT system.

However, Lucas and Spitler[55] have shown that in real field settings, organizational variables, such as cultural norms and the nature of the job, were far more important in predicting the use of technology than the potential user's perception of likely usefulness or ease of use. Further, Hu et al.[56] report that the TAM did not predict the use of telemedicine by physicians. Hu et al.[56] suggest that cultural and professional/organization variables may be more explanatory of telemedicine use than perceived usefulness or perceived ease of use as measured by TAM.

Barki and Hartwick[57] suggested that the higher the degree of the user's perceived participation in the development of the system, the more likely they would be to use the system. They posited that user involvement entails the execution of a set of activities as well as the psychological state of the user.

The theoretical construct

In our new information technology-rich environment, it is appropriate to raise questions about organizational design in healthcare delivery organizations. In the late 1960s, Perrow,[58] a highly respected sociologist, foreshadowed the issue by suggesting that in US human service organizations, where new technologies are manifest, the organizational structure needs to have:

- less bureaucracy – less programming of tasks
- more moderate rules and regulations
- fewer levels in the hierarchy
- greater coordination by feedback
- greater decentralization in decision making
- a tendency to employ more highly trained professionals.

Perrow's ideas of the late 1960s and early 1970s are, perhaps, even more relevant today in the US.

Most major healthcare delivery organizations in the US have not experienced an organizational design renaissance. Many of today's healthcare delivery organizations were designed to insure quality of care at reasonable costs. Their designs were relevant to the pre-information technology age in which they were conceived in terms of level of centralization and authoritarian organizational culture. With some exceptions, most organization design modifications consist of small changes at the edges of the organization. The central tenet of US organizational design in most healthcare delivery organizations remains: quality results from clear rules, high formalization, high authority and intolerance for ambiguity.

Yet research on implementation of technology in organizations, in general, points to the need to match the characteristics of the technology with the characteristics of the users rather than attempt to change the attitudes, mental models, alliances or culture of the users.[59,60] This is most likely true in healthcare delivery organizations as well.[56] We extend the agrument to the organizations as well as the individuals in the organizations. In the US and Great Britain and elsewhere, we argue, healthcare organizations, which have the utilization of e-health technologies as a strategic intent, need to re-address their organizational designs.

Distinctly, the concern for quality need not be sacrificed in an effort to redesign a more organic system. Anglo-American quality assurance (QA) research and thinking in modern healthcare organization research[61,62] call for greater decentralization so that professionals responsible for care have the power to review and implement necessary changes. This QA research also argues for more participative open and enhanced organizational feedback of results.[63]

The contemporary cultural context in the US and Great Britain is one of low uncertainty avoidance, as shown to be an evolving truth over the past half century, and perhaps longer.[2] In such a cultural environment, new information technologies which may require changes in the normal routine of healthcare delivery are best utilized by organizations which are, we argue, more organic and more often employ double-loop learning. In South Korea and France, cultural environments characterized as high uncertainty avoidance,[2] the organization of choice for implementation of e-health technologies should be a more mechanistic organization, more likely utilizing single-loop learning.

Why is this so? It is so because organizations wanting to learn to utilize the new clinical e-technologies effectively, must adapt to learning styles which are harmonious with their cultures and structures, and with the national culture embedded within the organization's environment.

In national cultures characterized by high uncertainty avoidance, single-loop learning styles often afford speedier organizational learning. This is so as a consequence of high uncertainty avoidance going hand in hand with abhorrence of turbulence, lack of predictability and dislike for experimentation. In such cultural milieu, a single-loop learning style is far less threatening than the more proactive double-loop learning style. Single-loop takes change one predicable step at a time. Double-loop concurrently seeks to anticipate change in the environment and match change in the organization, so as to achieve a desired end-state which is the consequence of the interaction of the two simultaneous change processes. Thus, double-loop learning is far more ambiguous, interactive and complex. High uncertainty avoiding national cultures are more comfortable with more predictable organizational learning of the single-loop style.

Further, organizational structure and culture determine the amount and richness of information provided to its membership.[64] Mechanistic structure and culture restrict the flow of information down the organization. This, in turn, makes double-loop learning more difficult. Double-loop learning requires full and rich information to formulate accurate forecasting models of both environmental future actions and the resultant end-state of the interaction of those environmental future actions with the organization's actions. Therefore, double-loop learning is handicapped by the limited information flow found in mechanistic organizations. However, in organic organizations, information richness is encouraged and as such, double-loop learning proves to be more effective.

Thus, single-loop organizational learning styles are far more comfortable for organizations embedded in high uncertainty avoiding cultures. This does not mean that double-loop learning is precluded in this cultural context. It does occur. However, single-loop learning is the preferred 'modes-operandi'; it is likely to occur more often. When single-loop learning occurs in high uncertainty avoiding cultures, it is more accepted and less resisted by the organization's membership. As a consequence, with other things being equal, single-loop learning, in general, is speedier and more effective than double-loop learning in high uncertainty avoiding cultures. This condition is greatly reinforced when the organization has a culture and structure which are mechanistic rather than organic.

An interesting organizational opportunity arises when three conditions occur:

- a mechanistic organizational culture and structure exists
- a single-loop organizational learning style predominates
- the organization is embedded in a high uncertainty avoiding culture.

That organization is then able to buffer its membership from the anxiety of anticipated, unpredictable change that is potentially concomitant with all learning, and thereby fosters less resistance to speedier and more effective learning.

Figure 16.1 displays the theoretical relationship of the independent variables of national culture, organizational structure, organizational culture and organizational learning style on the resultant speed and effectiveness of e-health utilization, all other variables held constant.

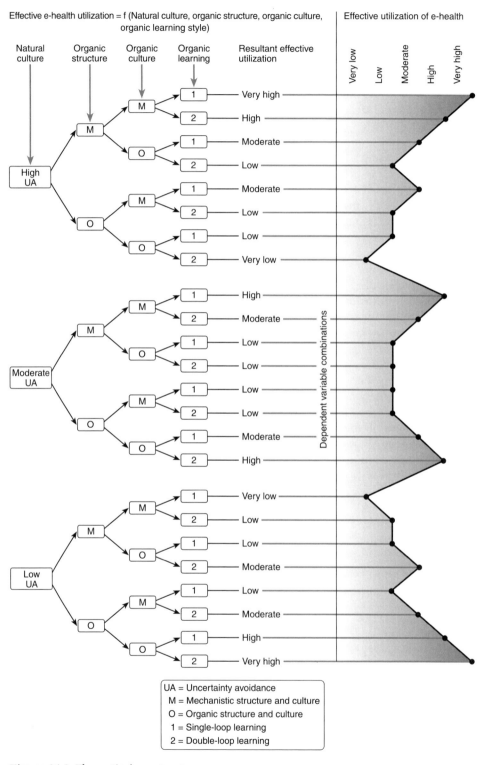

Figure 16.1 Theoretical construct.

Thus, the speediest and most effective e-health utilization in high uncertainty avoiding cultures is seen to arise with mechanistic organizational structures and culture coupled with single-loop organizational learning styles. Similar theoretical constructs are altered for moderate and low uncertainty avoiding national cultural environments.

All that was said for single-loop learning and double-loop learning in organizations embedded in high uncertainty avoiding national cultures is the opposite for organizations embedded in low uncertainty avoiding cultures. Here too, organizations learn with both learning styles: single-loop and double-loop. But, the nature of the cultural values of the membership of such organizations favors double-loop learning. Pro-action and the experimentation associated with pro-action attract such organizational membership towards double-loop learning. The opportunity to concomitantly modify the environment while changing the organization, such that both changes result in a desired end state, is the attractive 'modus operandi' in the low uncertainty avoiding culture.

When coupled with organic organizational cultures and structures, double-loop learning is better received, speedier and more effective than single-loop learning for organizations embedded in low uncertainty avoiding cultures. This still allows for some circumstances in which organizations may choose to employ single-loop learning. It is not an all-or-nothing, on/off situation; it is a continuum along which diverse organizations are positioned. Some predominantly choose single-loop; others choose double-loop learning styles.

We postulate that in high uncertainty avoiding cultures, healthcare delivery organizations that choose mechanistic organization cultures and structures, and predominantly employ single-loop learning, will be more effective at implementing and utilizing clinical e-health technologies. The obverse is hypothesized to be true for healthcare delivery organizations embedded in low uncertainty avoiding national cultures. Figure 16.1 is an attempt to summarize these theoretical constructs pictorially.

Summary of the results of a small pilot study

Our method involved interacting with, interviewing and seeking data on e-health utilization success from healthcare delivery organizations in high uncertainty avoiding national cultures (France, South Korea) and in low uncertainty avoiding national cultures (US, Great Britain), as well as to collect similar information in moderate uncertainty avoiding national cultures (Italy). The results of these case studies are published in detail elsewhere.[65] What follows is a brief narrative summary of our findings.

It was not possible for the authors to test the validity of all the theoretical constructs depicted in Figure 16.1. Rather, it was our choice to conduct a limited number of case studies in healthcare delivery organizations in each of the categories of national culture (low, moderate and high uncertainty avoidance). This was done as a pilot exploration of the reasonableness of the theoretical constructs of Figure 16.1.

In France (high uncertainty avoidance), three healthcare delivery organizations were studied. Full results of this study are available elsewhere.[65] We investigated two organizations in the major metropolitan hub and a third in a provincial capital. The first two organizations used multiple modes of telemedicine (both real-time and store and forward) effectively. We conducted interviews in and observed these organizations. The collected data pointed towards a mechanistic organizational structure and culture in place. Similar findings were obtained for the provincial healthcare delivery organization, through observation; interview data indicated that the telemedicine services, while effective, were not as efficient as those of the metropolitan healthcare delivery organization.

In South Korea (high uncertainty avoidance) we studied one healthcare delivery organization. This was a central urban healthcare delivery organization with a constellation of 12 satellite, affiliate, smaller healthcare delivery organizations. No direct observations were made, but interviews about and demonstrations with a Korean telemedicine system were undertaken. The organization proved to have a highly mechanistic organizational structure and culture; it was seen to be both effective and efficient in its utilization of interactive telemedicine, both for clinical decision making and for patient education.[65]

In Italy (moderate uncertainty avoidance), we observed and conducted interviews in two urban healthcare delivery organizations. One was classified by interview data as slightly mechanistic in structure and culture; the second was slightly organic in structure and culture.[65] Both organizations advertised extensive use of telemedicine. Observation and interviews yielded marginal evidence of the actual utilization of telemedicine. At best, utilization could be rated as moderate to low.

In the US (low uncertainty avoidance), one healthcare delivery organization was observed and interviews conducted. It was in an urban center of Hawaii with multiple telemedicine links throughout the Pacific and Asia, as well as throughout the continental US. Interviews and observational data identified its organizational structure and culture as mechanistic. Review of its telemedicine utilization results yielded very poor scores. Extremely large expenditures on infrastructure and staff resulted in little or almost no telemedicine utilization.[65]

In Great Britain (low uncertainty avoidance), we observed and conducted interviews in two healthcare delivery organizations: one was a large healthcare delivery organization in a major metropolitan hub; the other was a smaller healthcare delivery organization in a rural suburb of a large metropolis. In both organizations we found rather organic structures and cultures. Both were effective in implementing real-time telemedicine. The case for store and forward telemedicine was mixed. While we found high effectiveness of utilization of telemedicine, the frequencies of utilization of all forms of telemedicine at both sites was moderate at best.[65]

Concluding discussion

The data of our qualitative research studies of healthcare delivery organizations in five countries cannot be said to confirm the theoretical constructs of Figure 16.1. However, they do not disprove these constructs and, in fact, our findings can be seen as a pilot study which supports the general theory developed in this chapter.

Our major goal was to offer a theoretical argument for the need for healthcare delivery systems to consider an organizational renaissance. In an environment made turbulent by advances in technology, an organization's dynamics need to match the cultural predilection of its membership if the organization is to be effective and efficient in its implementation and utilization of the new technologies.

Only through a harmonious match of organizational structure and culture to membership national culture predilections can effective and efficient organizational learning emerge. And it is only through organizational learning that new technologies can be effectively utilized.

The cultural context in the US and Great Britain is one of low uncertainty avoidance. In that cultural environment, new information technologies which may require changes in the normal routine of healthcare delivery are best utilized by organizations which are, we argue, most organic. In South Korea and France, cultural environments characterized as high uncertainty avoidance, the organization of choice for implementation of e-health technologies appears to be a more mechanistic organization.

Nonetheless, it must be emphasized that these suggestions are relative. The divide between mechanistic and organic organizational design is not black and white, but rather gray and foggy. Our argument is only to ask executives and researchers in e-health to look at the bureaucratic structure of their organizations; to examine the level of formality and centralization and authoritarian culture and to ask: Is this the appropriate match for the people in our organization whom we depend on to use new e-health technologies?

References

1   DeLong DW and Fahely L (2000) Diagnosing cultural barriers to knowledge management. *The Academy of Management Executive.* **14**(4): 113–27.
2   Hofstede G (2001) *Culture's Consequences* (2e). Sage Publishing, London.
3   Worley CG, Hitchin DE and Ross WL (1996) *Integrated Strategic Change: how OD builds competitive advantage.* Addison-Wesley, New York.
4   Kampas PJ (2003) Shifting cultural gears in technology-driven industries. *MIT Sloan Management Review.* **44**(2): 41–8.
5   Bashshur RL (2002) Telemedicine and healthcare. *Telemedicine Journal and e-health.* **8**(1): 5–12.
6   Ackerman M, Craft R, Ferrante F, Kratz M, Mandil S and Sapci H (2002) Telemedicine technology. *Telemedicine Journal and e-health.* **8**(1): 71–8.
7   Bangert D and Doktor R (2000) Implementing store-and-forward telemedicine: organisational issues. *Telemedicine Journal and e-health.* **6**(3): 355–60.
8   Davis LJ *et al.* (2000) The Pacific Teletumor Board: an innovation in cancer care. *Federal Practitioner.*
9   Pushkin DS *et al.* (1997) Patient and provider acceptance of telemedicine. *New Medicine.* **3**(3): 55–9.
10 Bashshur RL and Gingsby J (1995) Position paper: telemedicine effects: cost, quality and access. *J Medical Systems.* **19**(2): 79–80.
11 Bashshur RL, Sanders JH, Shannon GW (1997) *Telemedicine: theory and practice.* Charles C Thomas, Springfield, IL.
12 Aas IHM (2001) A qualitative study of the organizational consequences of telemedicine. *Journal of Telemedicine and Telecare.* **7**: 18–28.
13 Bangert D and Doktor RH (2000) *Organisational impact of telemedicine.* American Telemedicine Association, Conference Proceedings. Phoenix, AZ.
14 Argyris C and Schon DA (1996) *Organizational Learning II: theory, method and practice.* Addison-Wesley, Reading, MA.

15   Senge P (1990) *The Fifth Discipline: the art and practice of the learning organization.* Doubleday, New York.

16   Hofstede G (1980) *Culture's Consequences.* Sage Publishing, London.

17   Hofstede G (1991) *Cultures and Organizations: software of the mind.* McGraw-Hill, New York.

18   Hofstede G (1994) Management scientists are human. *Management Science.* **40**(1): 4–14.

19   Doz Y and Prahalad CK (1986) Controlled variety: a challenge for human resource management in MNC. *Human Resource Management.* **25**(1): 55–71.

20   Lawrence PR and Lorsch JW (1967) *Organization and Environment: managing differentiation and integration.* Graduate School of Business Administration, Harvard University, Boston, MA.

21   Galbraith JR (1972) *Designing Complex Organizations.* Addison-Wesley, Reading, MA.

22   Porter M (1990) *The Competitive Advantage of Nations.* Macmillan, London.

23   McKelvey B and Aldrich H (1983) Populations, natural selection and applied organizational science. *Administrative Science Quarterly.* **28**: 101–28.

24   Pugh DS, Hickson DT, Hinings CR, MacDonald KM, Turner C and Lupton T (1963) A conceptual scheme for organizational analysis. *Administrative Science Quarterly.* **8**: 289–315.

25   Child J (1973) Strategies of control and organizational behavior. *Administrative Science Quarterly.* **18**: 1–17.

26   Ouchi WG (1987) The relationships between organizational structure and organizational control. *Administrative Science Quarterly.* **22**: 95–113.

27   Weick KE (1977) Organization design: organizations as self-designing systems. *Organizational Dynamics.* **6**: 31–46.

28   Daft RL (1982) Bureaucratic versus non-bureaucratic structure and the process of innovation and change. In: Bacharach SB (ed.) *Research in the Sociology of Organizations,* pp. 129–66. JAI Press, Greenwich, CT.

29   Pfeffer J (1982) *Organizations and Organizational Theory.* Pitman Publishing, Marshfield, MA.

30   Mintzberg H (1983) *Power In and Around Organizations.* Prentice Hall, Englewood Cliffs, NJ.

31   Mackenzie KD (1978) *Organizational Structures.* AHM Publishing, Arlington Heights, IL.

32   Robbins SP (1993) *Organizational Behavior: concepts, controversies, and applications.* Prentice Hall, Englewood Cliffs, NJ.

33   Lin Z and Hui C (1999) Should lean replace mass organization systems? A comparative examination from a management coordination perspective. *Journal of International Business Studies.* **30**(1): 45–80.

34   DiBella AJ and Nevis EC (1998) *How Organizations Learn: an integrated strategy for building learning capacity.* Jossey-Bass, San Francisco, CA.

35   Eisenstadt SN (1986) *Max Weber: on charisma and institution building.* University of Chicago Press, Chicago, IL, p. 46.

36   Rehder RR (1992) Building cars as if people mattered: the Japanese lean system vs. Volvo's Uddevalla system. *Columbia Journal of World Business.* **27**(2): 56–70.

37   Drucker PF (1987) Workers' hands bound by tradition. *The Wall Street Journal.* **August**: 2–18.

38   Womack JP, Jones DT and Roos D (1990) *The Machine That Changed The World: based on the Massachusetts Institute of Technology 5-million dollar 5-year study of the future of the automobile.* Rawson Associates, New York.

39   Zetka JR Jr (1992) Mass-production automation and work-group solidarity in the post-World War II automobile industry. *Work and Occupations.* **19**(3): 255–71.

40   Rogers EM (1995) *Diffusion of Innovations* (4e). Free Press, New York.

41 Meyer AD and Goes JB (1988) Organizational assimilation of innovations: a multi level contextual analysis. *Academy of Management Journal.* **31**(4): 899–923.

42 Van de Ven AH and Rogers GM (1998) Innovations and organizations: critical perspectives. *Communication Research.* **15**(5): 632–51.

43 Gerwin D (1988) A theory of innovation process for computer-aided manufacturing technology. *IEEE Transactions on Engineering Management.* **35**(2): 90–100.

44 Lewin K (1951) *Field Theory in Social Science.* Harper and Row, New York.

45 Bridges W (1991) *Managing Transitions.* Addison-Wesley, Reading, MA.

46 Kotter JP (1996) *Leading Change.* HBS Press, Boston, MA.

47 Cyert RM and March JG (1963) *A Behavioral Theory of the Firm.* Prentice Hall, New Jersey.

48 Bateson G (1972) *Steps to an Ecology of Mind.* Ballentine, New York.

49 Schein EH (1996) Three cultures of management: the key to organisational learning. *Sloan Management Review.* **Fall**: 9–20.

50 Fiol C and Lyles M (1985) Organizational learning. *Academy of Management Review.* **10**: 803–13.

51 Dodgson M (1991) Technology, learning, technology strategy and competitive pressures. *British Journal of Management.* **2/3**: 132–49.

52 Chaston I, Badger B and Sadler-Smith E (2000) Organisational learning style and competences: a comparative investigation of relationship and transactionally orientated small UK manufacturing firms. *European Journal of Marketing.* **34**: 625–41.

53 Ayas K (1996) *Organizational learning and learning organizations for effective innovation management.* Proceedings of the Symposium on Organizational Learning, Department of Management Learning, University of Lancaster, 13–24 September.

54 Davis FD, Bagozzi RP and Warshaw PR (1989) Perceived usefulness, perceived ease of use and user acceptance of information technology. *MIS Quarterly.* **13**(3): 319–40.

55 Lucas HC and Spitler VK (1991) Technology use and performance: a field study of broker workstations. *Decisions Sciences.* **30**(2): 291–311.

56 Hu P, Chau P, Sheng O and Tam K (1999) Examining the technology acceptance model using physician acceptance of telemedicine technology. *Journal of Management Information Systems.* **16**(2): 91–112.

57 Barki H and Hartwick J (1989) Rethinking the concept of user involvement. *MIS Quarterly.* **13**(1): 53–63.

58 Perrow C (1984) *Organizational Analysis: a sociological view.* Wadsworth Publishing, Belmont, CA.

59 Hartwick J and Barki H (1994) Explaining the role of user participation in information systems use. *Management Science.* **40**: 440–65.

60 Venkatesh V and Davis FD (2000) A theoretical extension of the technology acceptance model: four longitudinal field studies. *Management Science.* **46**: 186–204.

61 Williamson JM (1988) Future policy directions for quality assurance: lessons from the health accounting experience. *Inquiry.* **25**: 67–77.

62 Shortell SM, Morrison EM and Friedman B (1990) *Strategic Choices for America's Hospitals: managing change in turbulent times.* Jossey-Bass, San Francisco, CA.

63 Luke R, Krueger J and Modrow R (eds) (1983) *Quality Assurance: professional and organizational issues in healthcare.* Aspen Press, Rockville, MD.

64 Daft RL and Lengel RH (1986) Organizational information requirements, media richness and structural design. *Management Science.* **32**(5): 554–71.

65 Bangert D and Doktor R (2004) Managing implementation of e-health technology. *International Journal of Health & Technology Management.* **6**(1): 121–35.

Index

Page numbers in *italics* refer to figures or tables.